Radioecological Techniques

Radioecological Techniques

Vincent Schultz

Washington State University
Pullman, Washington

and

F. Ward Whicker

Colorado State University
Ft. Collins, Colorado

PLENUM PRESS • NEW YORK AND LONDON

Library of Congress Cataloging in Publication Data

Schultz, Vincent.
  Radioecological techniques.

  Bibliography: p.
  Includes index.
  1. Radioecology — Methodology. I. Whicker, F. Ward. II. Title.
QH543.5.S39   574.5'028   81-22706
ISBN 0-306-40797-3   AACR2

© 1982 Plenum Press, New York
A Division of Plenum Publishing Corporation
233 Spring Street, New York, N.Y. 10013

Printed in the United States of America

Alfred W. Klement, Jr.
Native Texan, Colleague, and Friend

Preface

During the twenty years the authors have been associated with the field of radiation ecology, there has been a diversified and increasing use of radionuclides in applied and basic biological research. Prior to the advent of the atomic age in the 1940s the use of radionuclides as tracers was initiated, and following that period one observed a dramatically increased use in many disciplines. Concurrent with this increase there appeared many books and articles on radionuclide techniques useful to biologists in general. Although only a few ecological applications were evident in these early years, ecologists were quick to see the opportunities available in their field. In the United States, major centers for such activities included Oak Ridge National Laboratory and the U. S. Atomic Energy Commission's Savannah River Plant. At Oak Ridge National Laboratory Dr. Stanley I. Auerbach, director of ecological activities, encouraged with remarkable success the use of tracers by his associates. Dr. Eugene P. Odum had the foresight to see that radionuclide tracers provided the means to solve many problems of interest to ecologists. Consequently, his research included some unique radiotracer applications at the Savannah River Plant. In addition he encouraged others involved in ecological activities at the Savannah River Plant to do likewise. Ecologists such as Dr. Robert C. Pendleton at the U. S. Atomic Energy Commission's Hanford Works applied radionuclides in their research. To these early investigators and to those who followed we owe the oppportunity to write this book.

In 1969 the senior author attempted a compilation of radionuclide usage and published as a report of the U. S. Atomic Energy Commission *Ecological Techniques Utilizing Radionuclides and Ionizing Radiation: A Selected Bibliography,* which was followed by supplements in 1972 and 1979. The limited availability of these publications, the exciting applications listed within them, and our belief that many ecologists are largely unaware of the broad spectrum of feasible applications stimulated us to write this book.

Regretfully we could not describe all the applications but we have attempted to select publications that illustrate their diversity. In addition to the cited references, we have prepared a list of additional references for each chapter. When citing specific research applications we have attempted to paraphrase authors' statements on methods and conclusions without attempting to evaluate the experimental designs or interpretations of data. It has been impossible to do justice to many of the applications we cite; therefore, we recommend that readers consult the cited references for complete details.

We are extremely grateful for the cooperation we received from authors who invested considerable effort in fulfilling our requests for original figures from their publications, even to the extent of preparing new copies. Of the many requests we made, only two were not acknowledged—a tribute to the cooperative attitude of ecologists throughout the world. A. Grauby, Commissariat a l'Energie Atomique (France) and A. Myllymäki, Agricultural Research Centre (Finland) kindly furnished the material we requested but it was received too late to incorporate within the book. Rather than acknowledge the cooperation of each individual here, we refer the reader to citations associated with figures and tables within the book. Others who cooperated but are not acknowledged within the text are James D. Huber, Irene Keller, S. W. O'Rear, Larry Ragsdale, Daryl Skraba, Michael H. Smith and Jay Story.

We appreciate the assistance of Patricia L. Schultz who typed and edited the manuscript and that of April D. Whicker for reading page proofs.

It was a pleasure to work with the capable and efficient editors of Plenum Press: Kirk Jensen, Sponsoring Editor; Larry Goldes, Production Editor; and Richard Millikan, a freelance copyeditor whose remarkable editorial abilities never failed to amaze us.

Last, but not least, we thank individuals, organizations, and publishers who permitted us to use copyrighted material.

Vincent Schultz
F. Ward Whicker

Contents

9. Primary-Productivity Determination

10. Cycling Studies

11. Miscellaneous Techniques and Equipment

Introduction

1.1. General Comments

Although radionuclides were used as tracers prior to the first commercial shipment of radionuclides from Oak Ridge National Laboratory in 1946, it was following this date that extensive contributions were made to the biological and physical sciences that utilize tracer technologies. Today, it would be unusual for an academic institution or a research laboratory not to utilize radionuclides to some degree. One objective of the U.S. Atomic Energy Commission in its early period was promotion of the use of radionuclides and ionizing radiation in research and commercial operations in the United States. The International Atomic Energy Agency (IAEA) assumed this responsibility internationally and is active today in disseminating such knowledge. Undoubtedly, governmental agencies associated with all technologically advanced nations were also engaged in such activities. We are indebted to a wide spectrum of scientists for the enormous literature comprising journal articles, textbooks, symposia proceedings, manuals, and bibliographies on radionuclide and ionizing-radiation applications in the sciences and industry. The history of the production of radionuclides and their use in the United States is presented in *Isotopes and Radiation Technology*, Vol. 4, No. 1, an issue that commemorates the 20th anniversary of the first commercial shipment of radionuclides from Oak Ridge National Laboratory. Worldwide activities are evident in the *IAEA Proceedings Series*. These contributions to the nuclear age contain an overview of perhaps all the significant activities during the early and current years of the nuclear age.

With the advent of textbooks and manuals prepared for courses on the subject of tracer technology, the biological scientist has available a considerable literature on radionuclide techniques. Among these are Arena (1971), G. D. Chase and Rabinowitz (1962), G. D. Chase *et al.* (1964, 1971), Faires and Parks (1973), Hendee (1973a), Tiwari (1974), Wang and Willis (1965), and Wolfe (1964). In addition, a considerable number of literature reviews on the general subject have appeared. Bergner (1966) prepared an extensive review of tracer theory, and Kuzin (1960) reviewed the application of radionuclides in the biological sciences. The enormity of today's literature precludes an entirely comprehensive review of the subject. Today, the researcher seeking information on the application of radionuclides and ionizing radiation in a particular field must gather and integrate widely dispersed material. This appears to be particularly true in the field of ecology, which encompasses many disciplines and for which no single extensive review exists. V. Schultz and Whicker (1972) compiled, for inclusion in a more extensive set of readings on radiation ecology, a set of selected readings on ecological techniques that utilize ionizing radiation.

In this book, we were faced with the enormous task of selecting, from a very large number of papers available, those that would reflect the diversity in ecological techniques that involve radionuclides and ionizing radiation as well as those that illustrate the ingenuity of ecologists and contributions to the understanding of ecosystems. We have directed our efforts to locating pertinent articles, reviews, and bibliographies that should serve to broaden the reader's knowledge of the use of nuclear technologies in ecology.

This book is not a working manual for radiological techniques developed for use in ecology; rather, it was written to familiarize the ecologist and others with the wide assortment of radiological techniques that may lead to unique scientific advances. Since it is impossible to include experimental details for the many references cited, it is obvious that the interested person must consult original publications for such details. Particularly, we have minimized our discussion of sample preparation and radionuclide identification and measurement. It should be emphasized that our brief comments do not do justice to the papers cited. Following the *Literature Cited,* we have appended a list of *Additional Readings*. Such a list is not meant to imply that these publications are of secondary interest, since many could have been used in place of the cited references or included in the text as additional material.

The limitations of this work should be obvious. In addition to those attributed to our subjective selection of references is the common instance of investigators not discussing the positive and negative aspects of their procedures or commenting in detail on sampling, sample preparation, and counting or sampling errors, thus making it impossible to always discuss these essential items. Last but not least, we emphasize methods utilized, rather than overall results of the investigations.

1.2. Relevant Literature

1.2.1. Proceedings and Books

The broad and pervasive nature of ecology made it difficult to decide which references to include within the intended scope of this book. We arbitrarily decided to emphasize work dealing with natural ecosystems and their component parts and to give only minor attention to applications in allied disciplines such as agriculture, archaeology, geology, and hydrology. Considerable literature exists on the application of radionuclide techniques in these allied disciplines. The *IAEA Proceedings Series* includes studies on soil–plant relationships (1962a, 1965, 1972c), weeds (1966b), soil organic matter (1968c), soil physics (1973b, 1974b), entomology (1962b, 1963b), environmental pollution (1971d, 1972a, 1974c, 1975b), hydrology (1963a, 1967, 1970d), and rapid methods for measuring environmental radioactivity (1971c). In addition, a considerable number of other publications in this series are more specific in nature and include techniques discussed in other chapters of this book.

O'Brien and Wolfe (1964b) summarized a selected portion of the literature on radioactivity and radiation as related to insects. A monograph of the American Geophysical Union (Stout, 1967) deals with techniques in the hydrological cycle. Readers interested in techniques utilized in archaeology are referred to Aitken (1974) and Tite (1972) and the bibliography of S. L. Schultz and V. Schultz (1975).

Verkhovskaya (1971) edited the proceedings of a meeting on radioecological methods; Polikarpov and Parchevskiy (1972), those of a meeting on methods of radioactivity determination; and Dohrn (1959), those of a meeting on applications in marine biology.

1.2.2. Manuals

Although some of the textbooks on the subject of radiation biology and radiation techniques contain some laboratory experiments of interest to the ecologist, the best sources of information for persons interested in developing a course on radionuclide techniques or even for those searching for a general review of the subject, including instrumentation as well as techniques, are the training manuals developed by the IAEA and published in its *Technical Reports Series*. Examples are manuals on techniques in soil–plant relationships (IAEA, 1964), entomology (IAEA, 1977), and hydrology (IAEA, 1968d).

Unfortunately, a manual on radiation techniques that encompasses the various disciplines in ecology does not exist. However, two excellent manuals have been developed for the marine radioecologist. One is concerned with methods for marine radioactivity study (IAEA, 1970b), but it is restricted to sampling aspects and analytical procedures for selected radionuclides. The other (IAEA, 1975c) involves design of radiotracer experiments and is highly recommended reading for all aquatic biologists concerned with mineral cycling. In addition to the introduction, this document contains sections on laboratory and field experiments as well as supporting papers concerning tracer experiments with phytoplankton, zooplankton, benthic algae and invertebrates, molluscs, fish, subcellular components, food webs, and compartmental models.

1.2.3. Bibliographies

Various national and international agencies have issued bibliographies on many subjects related to radionuclide and ionizing-radiation techniques and related subjects. The list is too long to include in this book; however, reference sources are available such as the IAEA's periodically released *List of Bibliographies on Nuclear Energy* (publication STI/DOC/11). In addition, a more restricted listing of interest to ecologists can be found on pp. 579–587 in Klement and Schultz (1980).

Entomologists are fortunate in having available four bibliographies compiled by Binggeli (1963, 1965, 1967, 1969) that are in the *IAEA Bibliographical Series*. The literature for the years 1950–1967 was searched, and a total of 6036 references are included. Other bibliographies in this series are referenced in the appropriate chapters in this book.

A bibliography entitled "Nuclear technology in archaeology: Partial bibliography" was published by the U.S. Energy Research and Development Administration (ERDA) (S. L. Schultz and V. Schultz, 1975).

References that deal specifically with the use of radionuclides in studies of wild birds are included in a much broader bibliography on ionizing radiation and wild birds (V. Schultz, 1974).

"Ecological techniques utilizing radionuclides and ionizing radiation: A selected bibliography" is the title of an extensive listing prepared by V. Schultz (1969, 1972, 1975). The subject matter includes terrestrial and aquatic studies and selected references from the aforementioned bibliographies.

1.2.4. Reviews

It was encouraging to find that literature reviews for some disciplines exist, such as those in the fields of entomology, forestry, environmental science, hydrology, aquatic biology, and ornithology. In addition, the literature for more specific subjects within these disciplines and others has been reviewed, e.g., use of radioactive tags for studying animal behavior.

McHenry (1969) discussed tracer techniques in soil-erosion research, Jenkins (1957, 1962a,b, 1963) covered some applications in entomology, and Fraser and Gaertner (1970) reviewed work on radiotracer utilization in forestry research. The broader subject of environmental studies has been considered by Moghissi and Carter (1977) and most significantly by Raaen (1972), who cites 870 references.

Literature reviews of applications in marine and freshwater environments are frequently intertwined. However, Keller (1969) and Amiard (1974a,b) restricted their reviews to the marine environment and V. A. Nelson and Seymour (1972), to oyster research. In a brief review, Rice (1965) discussed radioisotope techniques in fisheries research and referred readers to an "excellent" review by Hooper *et al.* (1961). In addition, Seymour (1964) discussed contributions to understanding aquatic ecosystems and Karzinkin (1962) discussed applications in the fishing industry, Calaprice *et al.* (1971) considered the use of X-ray fluorescence in aquatic biology, and Ichikawa (1973) covered the application of X-rays and radionuclides to ichthyology and fishery science.

Concerning wild birds, Mellinger and Schultz (1975) reviewed the techniques in ornithology as related to behavioral, physiological, and other aspects of the field.

Dating Techniques

2.1. General Comments

Early in this century, it was suggested by Rutherford (Dalrymple and Lanphere, 1969) that the decay of primordial radionuclides could be applied to determine the age of rocks and minerals. The primordial radionuclides such as potassium, rubidium, thorium, and uranium are very long-lived; consequently, their application to geological dating must of necessity be restricted to measurement of long time intervals. W. F. Libby suggested that the cosmogenically produced radionuclide ^{14}C be used to date carbonaceous materials for relatively shorter time intervals. For his work on carbon dating, he received the Nobel Prize. Today, the technique of radiodating geological and biological specimens rests on a foundation of extensive research and has been accepted as a powerful tool by archaeologists, geologists, and biologists. The literature in archaeology is extensive, and the reader is referred to the previously cited bibliography by S. L. Schultz and V. Schultz (1975) and to the books of Tite (1972) and Aitken (1974), as well as to those of Michael and Ralph (1971) and Michels (1973), which deal exclusively with dating methods in archaeology. The methods discussed are those that should be familiar to the archaeologist, namely, radiocarbon dating, potassium–argon dating, fission-track dating, and thermoluminescence dating. Among the references available to the geologist are Hamilton and Farquhar (1968) and York and Farquhar (1972).

Since the radionuclide-dating literature is extensive and our readers may have only a minor interest in the subject, we will describe the concepts briefly.

2.2. Methods and Applications

2.2.1. Carbon-14

Carbon-14 is formed in nature by the cosmic ray bombardment of nitrogen by the reaction

$$^{14}_{7}N + n \rightarrow {}^{14}_{6}C + p$$

Carbon-14, which has a half-life of 5730 years, is present in carbon dioxide of the atmosphere in fixed or equilibrium amounts that depend on the rates of production and depletion. Prior to nuclear-weapons testing and massive burning of fossil fuels, the $^{14}C/^{12}C$ ratio in atmospheric CO_2 was comparatively constant. According to Shilling and Shilling (1964), cosmic ray production is estimated to be 7–10 kg per year, while ^{14}C production from United States nuclear-weapons testing through October 31, 1958, has been 25×10^{27} atoms. They remarked that if ^{14}C is mixed throughout the atmosphere, the tropospheric concentration would be 1.75 times that of the natural equilibrium value and that mixture with oceanic surface waters would reduce this to 1.33 times that of the natural equilibrium value. The burning of fossil fuels, on the other hand, tends to reduce the $^{14}C/^{12}C$ ratio in the atmosphere because the age of most fuels has permitted time for significant decay of ^{14}C.

The importance of carbon in biological entities results from the fact that it occurs in all organic compounds. Consequently, the carbon cycle is of extreme interest. Suggested reading on the carbon cycle is *Carbon and the Biosphere,* the proceedings of a symposium held at Brookhaven National Laboratory in 1972 (Woodwell and Pecan, 1973).

Since ^{14}C occurred in the atmosphere in fixed amounts prior to the Industrial Revolution, and organisms incorporated it within their tissues, it is possible to estimate the date of death of the organism on the basis of the ratio $^{14}C/^{12}C$, which is a function of the initial value and the decay rate of ^{14}C. Since the decay rate of ^{14}C is accurately known and the $^{14}C/^{12}C$ ratio in the sample can be measured, the age can be easily calculated. Aitken (1974) commented that the concentration of ^{14}C in living tissues is about one part of ^{14}C to a million million parts of ^{12}C and that as a result of the decay rate of ^{14}C (half-life 5730 years), the ^{14}C diminishes in nonliving material at about 1% every 83 years. There are various other factors that affect the dating results based on these assumptions. These have been discussed extensively in the literature (e.g., Baxter and Walton, 1971; Olsson, 1968; Suess, 1973).

Carbon-14 has been used to date oceanic water masses, to study water-mass circulation, and also, to a lesser degree, to date remains of marine organisms (Duursma, 1972). The wood rat *(Neotoma)* is noted for the middens it produces.

Wood rat middens at the Nevada Test Site were carbon-dated, and results suggest that the middens studied were deposited between 7800 and 40,000 or more years ago (Jorgensen and Wells, 1964). These middens were located in an area devoid of junipers *(Juniperus osteosperma);* however, it was noted that juniper was one of the major constituents of the middens, indicating a major climatic change in the area since the midden material was deposited. It is interesting that a marmot *(Marmota flaviventris)* skull was collected in a midden dated at 12,700 ± 200 years and that this species is known to occur no closer than 200 km north of the midden site at present.

2.2.2. Potassium–Argon

The stable elements ^{40}Ca and ^{40}Ar are daughters of the natural radionuclide ^{40}K, which has a physical half-life of 1.28×10^9 years. In addition to other dating methods, Aitken (1974) discussed this method quite succinctly. He commented that the method that involves decay of ^{40}K relies on the buildup of ^{40}Ar in volcanic rocks, since argon gas can be detected with a high degree of sensitivity by mass spectrometry. It is not feasible to measure buildup of ^{40}Ca because ^{40}Ca is abundant in most rocks. Contrasted with ^{14}C dating, this method is useful with older material, since ^{40}K has an extremely long half-life, as contrasted with that of ^{14}C. Carbon-14 dating is not generally applicable to dating materials with ages in excess of 50,000 years (Tite, 1972). Duursma (1972) mentioned that the use of the potassium–argon dating method of marine sediments is limited to situations wherein the argon gas is trapped within the material and the ^{40}K is solidly bound to the matrix. Thus, its use in dating marine sediments is restricted to glass shards of volcanic origin. Details concerning the method are presented by Dalrymple and Lanphere (1969).

2.2.3. Uranium Series

The uranium series offers other unique opportunities to date igneous rocks and sediments. Tite (1972) and Aitken (1974) discussed the procedure of dating by using members of the series. These radionuclides are in equilibrium in older rocks, and the amounts at equilibrium are proportional to their half-lives. The isotopes of interest to us are ^{230}Th, ^{226}Ra, and ^{231}Pa. Dating of ocean sediments by means of the ^{230}Th (ionium) method depends on the fact that ^{230}Th is precipitated from seawater, while the uranium parent remains in solution. Consequently, the concentration of ^{230}Th in the sediment is no longer supplemented, and it decays at a half-life of 8×10^4 years. This implies that if the sediment has been deposited uniformly, the concentration of ^{230}Th will decrease with increasing sediment depth and that the age of deposition can be estimated, provided certain assumptions are valid (Duursma, 1972). More reliable results can be obtained from the $^{231}Pa/^{230}Th$ ratio (Aitken, 1974). In addition to dating marine sediments, the uranium-series method has been used in dating bone, shell, and stalagmite deposits. Duursma (1972) compiled an extensive table on the use of primordial radionuclides in ocean studies that includes dating.

2.2.4. Other Dating Techniques

Thermoluminescent and fission-track dating are two other methods that should be included in the family of nuclear dating techniques. The thermoluminescent method has been used for dating pottery, terra-cotta, hearths, ovens, and burnt stone. It is based on the emission of measurable light when ground-up pottery samples are twice heated rapidly. The extra light in the first heating is called "thermoluminescence" and has as its source constituents in the pottery. It is the result of exposure of these minerals to a weak flux of ionizing radiation from the radionuclides present in the parent pottery material and the surrounding burial soil (Aitken, 1974). The amount of light emitted is proportional to the total radiation exposure, and thus to the age of the specimen.

Uranium fission in minerals and glass causes damage in the lattice by recoiling fragments. The fission-track density can be measured and used as a basis for dating, since it is a function of uranium content and time.

Neutron Activation

3.1. General Comments

Activation analysis has become an important technique for the environmental biologist as well as for others. By means of bombardment with neutrons, high-energy photons, or charged particles, stable elements can be transformed to radionuclides. These radionuclides can be measured relatively easily, and the results can be interpreted in terms of the type and quantity of stable elements present in the sample of interest. Although several types of bombardment may be used to transform stable elements to radionuclides, slow neutrons are usually employed. Details concerning the procedure are described in many sources (e.g., Schulze, 1969; Hendee, 1973b). In addition, publications of direct interest to the environmental scientist are fairly numerous (Leddicotte, 1969; Byrne *et al.*, 1971; Pillay and Thomas, 1971; Filby and Shah, 1974).

Schulze (1969) lists advantages and limitations of activation analysis as follows:

Advantages

(a) The ultimate sensitivity is excellent for nearly every element and is, for many elements, better than can be obtained by any other technique.

(b) Non-destructive analysis is possible.

(c) It is generally possible to determine several elements in a single sample, even when non-destructive methods are used.

(d) Provided that no pre-irradiation chemical manipulation is attempted, the technique is free from blank errors caused by the use of contaminated reagents.

(e) Post-irradiation chemical treatment is greatly facilitated by freedom to use carrier techniques, thus eliminating the necessity for rigorous microchemical procedures in the determination of trace constituents.

(f) In principle, activation analysis allows the opportunity of distinguishing between different isotopes of an element. This facility has been usefully exploited in a number of clinical and physiological investigations.

Limitations

(a) Since the technique is based on characteristics of atomic nuclei, it does not give any information about the chemical form in which a particular element is present.

(b) Near the limit of detection, the main source of error in activation analysis lies in the fluctuations associated with the statistical character of nuclear disintegrations. This statistical error is still present even when the element in question occurs in amounts well above the limit of detection. . . . It is, however, fair to add that activation analysis is only used for macro-determination when speed and convenience, rather than sensitivity, are decisive. So far, the main uses of the technique have been in microdetermination of elements close to—or beyond—the limits of sensitivity offered by other methods. Though several elements can often be determined in a single sample, it is generally not possible to obtain a complete survey of all trace constituents, as can for example be expected from spectrographic analysis.

(c) Though the chemical and instrumental methods used in activation analysis are relatively simple and inexpensive, the irradiation stage of the technique requires access to a nuclear reactor or some other source of sub-atomic particles or radiations. A considerable volume of work is necessary to justify the cost involved in the provision of such resources—though the marginal cost of providing irradiation facilities with an already established reactor or accelerator is quite small.

At least three excellent bibliographies on activation analysis are available. One edited by Lutz (1970a) is restricted to oceanography, another covers only pollution analysis (Lutz, 1970b), and the other, more general in nature, was edited by Lutz *et al.* (1972). In addition, the previously cited bibliography of S. L. Schultz and V. Schultz (1975) lists uses of the technique in archaeology.

Activation analysis has been readily accepted by the scientific community, as is clearly evident from Figure 1. Let us now inspect some unique applications in terrestrial and aquatic ecology.

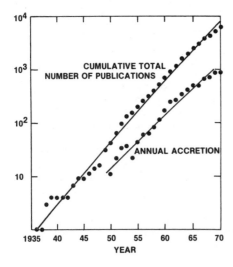

Figure 1. Growth rate of literature on activation analysis. From Lutz *et al.* (1972).

3.2. Applications

3.2.1. Terrestrial

Hair samples from antelope *(Antilocarpa americana)*, elk *(Cervus cana-densis)*, horse *(Equus caballus)*, moose *(Alces alces)* and mule deer *(Odocoileus hemionus)*, as well as an intact and cast skin of a rattlesnake *(Crotalus viridis)*, were exposed to a neutron flux in the Materials Testing Reactor at the Idaho National Engineering Laboratory, Idaho Falls, Idaho (Kennington and Ching, 1966). Other than the hair of one of three horses and the rattlesnake skin, which were collected in the vicinity of Idaho Falls, the other specimens came from animals collected in Wyoming. Figure 2 presents the gamma-ray spectra for the five mammals and three horses, which illustrate a dissimilarity among the species of nuclides present and the proportionate amount of each. The investigators concluded: "It would appear that although differences in habitat, range, and physiological condition may produce certain differences in the amount and com-osition of trace elements found in the hair, these differences are superimposed on a general species or perhaps generic pattern." A comparison of hair samples from three different horses revealed quite similar patterns (Figure 2a). Contin-uation of this study to evaluate variability within species and relate the obser-vations to habitat and life histories of the five species should prove of interest to a big-game biologist.

In an attempt to locate natal areas of North American waterfowl, Devine and Peterle (1968) utilized rectrices and wing bones of birds collected from various localities. The bones were ashed and the rectrices cleaned and pulverized prior to exposure to a neutron flux. The gamma-ray spectra were then compared. The radioisotopes of Na, Ca, Al, Mn, and Cl were used in the study. Canada geese *(Branta canadensis)* collected in Oregon could be differentiated from those collected in Colorado and Wisconsin. Differentiation was on the basis of the amount of Mn in rectrices. In each of the 6 samples from Oregon, the levels of Mn were higher than in all the 12 samples from Colorado and Wisconsin com-bined. No consistent differences were observed among waterfowl species or regions of collection.

Interesting innovations of a tagging procedure were to study the tracing of several foods of granivores in the field (Smigel *et al.*, 1974) and also to study the survival rate of a beetle in the field (Bate *et al.*, 1974). In both studies, items were marked with a stable element, and during the course of the study, samples of interest were collected in the field, neutron-activated, and identified as to whether or not the sample had been previously marked with the stable tracer element.

The granivores studied by Smigel *et al.* (1974) were the Merriam kangaroo rat *(Dipodomys merriami)* and the desert pocket mouse *(Perognathus penicil-latus)*. Seeds were solution-tagged with stable isotopes of rare elements, and the

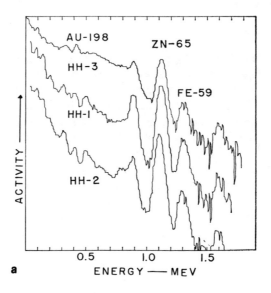

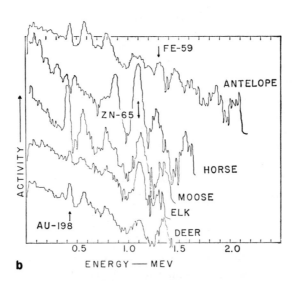

Figure 2. Results of activation analysis of ungulate hair. (a) Gamma-ray spectra of three samples of horse hair. (b) Gamma-ray spectra of hair from five mammals. The authors note that the scales of the spectra are the same, but the actual position on the y-axis has been ignored to allow the comparison. From Kennington and Ching (1966). Copyright 1966 by the American Association for Science.

seeds were then distributed in the environment. Feces of granivores from the study area were collected and exposed to a neutron flux, and determination of the presence or absence of the rare-element tag from the seed was made and quantified if observed. Considerable procedural material is presented in the paper, including pilot studies that involved laboratory experiments utilizing the two previously mentioned species and the eastern chipmunk *(Tamias striatus)* and deer mouse *(Peromyscus maniculatus)*. The stable tracers studied were In, Sm, Dy, Mn, Ba, and Zn. The selection criteria were based on the need for an element with a high isotopic abundance, a relatively short half-life of its isotope, and availability in water-soluble form. Since Ba and Zn have long irradiation times and Mn was present in significant amounts in control fecal material, these elements were eliminated as viable tracers.

Bate *et al.* (1974) immersed live elm bark beetles *(Scolytus multistriatus)* in a solution of 0.01% gold, placed them on elm *(Ulmus)* twigs, and collected live beetles at a later date. All beetles were subjected to a neutron flux, the tagged beetles were identified, and the survival rate was estimated.

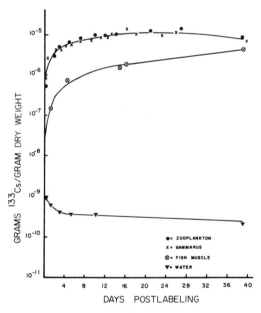

Figure 3. Concentration of tracer ^{133}Cs in some of the components of East Twin Lake as a function of time postlabeling (biotic samples in terms of g ^{133}Cs/g dry wt.; water samples in terms of g ^{133}Cs/ml) From Hakonson *et al.* (1973).

3.2.2. Aquatic

The kinetic behavior of cesium was studied in a montane zone lake in the northern Colorado Front Range by introducing stable ^{133}Cs uniformly into a 5-hectare lake, followed at a later date by neutron activation of various types of samples and measurement of the resulting radionuclide ^{134}Cs (Hakonson *et al.*, 1973). Since the lake was used by fishermen, it was not desirable to introduce a radioactive tracer into the lake; thus, this procedure appeared satisfactory even though it required use of an irradiation facility in Denver, Colorado. Some of the results of this study are presented in Figure 3. The authors commented that this approach might be useful in studies of ecosystems in populated areas where use of a radiotracer would not be desirable.

Thatcher and Johnson (1973) discussed the use of neutron activation of trace elements in water and aquatic biota. Numerous papers on the application to specific aquatic systems exist. Among these are the work of Lucas *et al.* (1970), who studied trace elements in Great Lakes fishes, and Piper and Goles (1969), who determined trace elements in seawater.

In the field of radiation ecology, we are interested not only in the cycling of a radioactive element within an ecosystem but also in its stable form, as well as that of elements of the same chemical family. The use of activation analysis in this context for the determination of stable elements has been discussed by Fourcy *et al.* (1967) with an application to two experimental systems.

Autoradiography

4.1. General Comments

When a radioactive substance is placed on a surface containing a photographic emulsion, the ionizing radiations affect the silver halide in the emulsion and a blackening is observed when the emulsion is developed. The result is a self-portrait, or what is known as an autoradiograph. Today, the silver halide is usually silver bromide in a gelatin matrix (Hendee, 1973a). According to Rogers (1973), the first autoradiograph was produced by Niepce de St. Victor in 1867 when he observed blackening on emulsions of silver chloride and iodide when the emulsions were exposed to uranium nitrate and tartrate. Henri Becquerel, using uranyl sulfate exposed to sunlight, observed blackening on a photographic plate. Rogers (1973) remarked that autoradiography did not become a scientific technique until 1924, when Lacassagne and associates used the process to study the distribution of polonium in biological specimens. Today, it is a widely accepted technique used to observe the location of radioactivity within physical or biological specimens.

It meets our purpose to say that intensity of blackening at a point is a function of exposure time and the concentration of activity in the sample at the point. In addition, the specific ionization of the radiations is an important consideration, since those with low specific ionization will produce hardly any blackening, while hard beta radiation produces diffuse autoradiographs. Soft beta radiation with a high specific ionization is effective for producing high-contrast autoradiographs, e.g., ^{3}H, ^{14}C, ^{35}S, and ^{45}Ca. Alpha-emitting radionuclides produce very high-resolution autoradiographs. Proper emulsion selection must be balanced with a fine grain to increase resolution and with the need for high sensitivity to reduce exposure time.

Although autoradiography has been used to some extent in environmental sciences, it is in other biological disciplines that it has found its greatest use.

There are books available to the scientific community that deal solely with this subject (e.g., Gude, 1968; Baserga and Malamud, 1969; Rogers, 1973). In addition, the subject of autoradiography appears to be an integral part of books on the general subject of radionuclide techniques (e.g., Hendee, 1973a, Chapt. 16; Faires and Parks, 1973, Chapt. 20).

4.2. Applications

4.2.1. Terrestrial

Environmental radioactivity resulting from atmospheric nuclear-weapons testing is detectable in all components of the ecosystem. Autoradiography as a method of detection was utilized by Hawthorn and Duckworth (1958) in studying the presence of radioactive strontium in deer antlers. A 2-mm transverse section of the antler was placed on X-ray film and exposed for 82 days. The autoradiograph disclosed a concentration of activity in the peripheral zone of the antler (Figure 4).

The introduction of tracer amounts of radionuclides into an organism followed by application of the autoradiographic technique to study the distribution of the tracer after a period of time is common practice. In a study of the calcium distribution in leaves of dogwood trees *(Cornus florida),* Thomas (1968) injected ^{45}Ca into the stems of living trees. He compared his autoradiographic results with those from a chemical analysis and, on the basis of his results and the literature, concluded:

> Radiocalcium distribution in leaves, as shown by autoradiograms, is affected by calcium availability, age of tissues within the leaf, leaf age, and leaf vigor. In addition, distribution of a radioisotope as revealed by autoradiograms can be altered (from no apparent radioactivity to uniform distribution throughout) by varying film exposure time and developing procedures. Although autoradiograms are useful in many phases of plant nutrition research, this technique alone may not indicate where the stable element is concentrated on a total-leaf basis.

A very interesting study involving autoradiography was conducted by Plummer and Kethley (1964). These investigators were interested in the foliar absorption of various nutrients by the pitcher plant *(Sarracenia flava).* One portion of the study involved the movement of certain nutrients from food to carpenter ants *(Camponotus* sp.) and then via their exoskeleton to the liquor within the sarcophageal region of the plant and finally within the plant. Ants were starved for 2 months, permitted to feed on a lump of sugar saturated with ^{32}P or ^{35}S solution, removed from the feeding chamber, and confined until defecation occurred. The ants were then permitted to feed on nonradioactive sugar until the unincorporated radionuclide was flushed from the alimentary canal, after which they were washed to remove possible external deposits of the radionuclide. Finally, the ants were placed in the insect-free sarcophaguses of the pitcher plants. Then, 30 days later, autoradiographs of the insects and pitcher-plant leaves were made. It was established that nutrients do follow the path from food to ant to liquor to plant leaf.

Utilizing autoradiography and plant residues labeled with ^{14}C, Grossbard (1973a) studied the decomposition of these residues. Also using ^{14}C, Waid *et al.* (1973) used an autoradiographic technique to detect active microbial cells in nature.

The application of radiotracers to pesticide research has also resulted in the application of autoradiography in the study of concentration of a pesticide within an organism as well as within the ecosystem. Nishimura *et al.* (1971) injected ^{203}Hg(NO$_3$)$_2$ into the cervical vein of laying coturnix quail *(Coturnix coturnix japonica)*. At various times after injection, the quail were killed, carcasses sheared of feathers, frozen, and sagittal sections about 30 μm thick prepared. Autoradiographs were prepared by exposing the film to a section for 1 week (Figure 5). It was observed that

> . . . high radioactivity was distributed in the blood, liver, kidney, ovary, ova, bone, lung, pancreas, and intestinal wall of the sample obtained at 1 hour; in the liver, kidney, ovary, ova, and the wall and contents of the intestine at 24 hours; and in the liver, kidney, and ova at 48 hours. At 96 hours, the activity of ^{203}Hg remained only in the kidney and ova.

In a study of the utilization of carbon from herbicides by microorganisms, Grossbard (1973b) sprayed soil with ^{14}C-labeled atrazine, incubated it for 2 months, then autoradiographed a soil sample. The autoradiograph revealed that there was a greater accumulation of ^{14}C associated with plant fragments than with the mineral portion of the soil. In a study of the uptake and possible incorporation of the radiocarbon, the microscope slides containing a gelatin–soil mixture used to prepare the autoradiograph described above were incubated for 2 months after the original coverslips were replaced with sterile ones. During the incubation, it was observed that microorganisms grew over the coverslips. After further processing, autoradiographs were prepared and revealed that

> . . . uptake and possible incorporation of ^{14}C, derived from a herbicide, by microorganisms is feasible. However, far more work and greater replication is needed in order to determine whether this observation is of frequent occurrence, and thus of major ecological importance.

In another study of a pesticide, high-resolution autoradiography was used to study the location of ^{3}H-labeled DDT and its metabolites in two insects, the

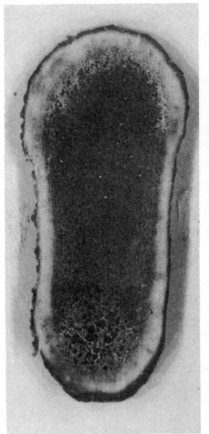
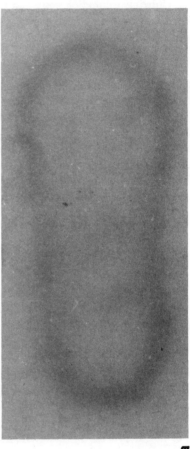

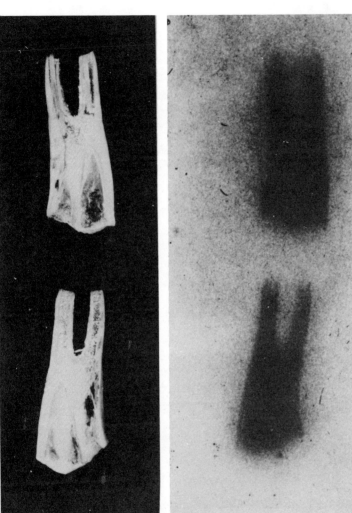

Figure 4. Autoradiograph of a portion of a deer's antlers and halves of a sheep's premolar. (a) Cross section of a deer's antler (i) and the autoradiograph produced from it (ii). (b) Two halves of a sheep's premolar from Ben Lawers, Perthsire (i), and the corresponding autoradiograph (ii). From Hawthorn and Duckworth (1958).

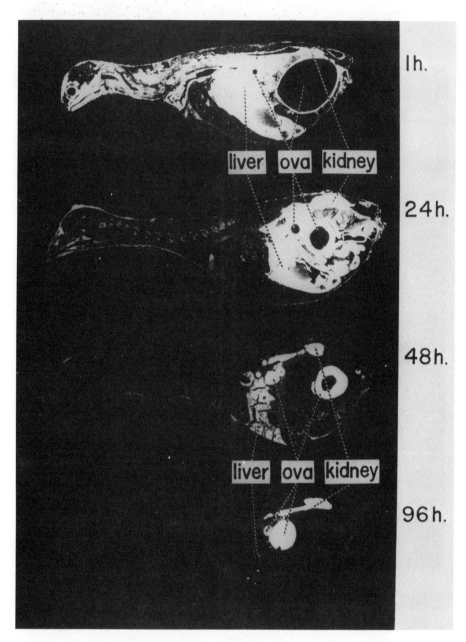

Figure 5. Autoradiographs of laying quail injected intravenously with ^{203}Hg(NO$_3$)$_2$, taken 1, 24, 48, and 96 hr after injection. From Nishimura *et al.* (1971).

American cockroach *(Periplaneta americana)* and the tobacco budworm *(Heliothis verescens)* (Coons and Guthrie, 1972). The tagged pesticide was injected into adult female cockroaches and into the 6th instar of the tobacco budworm; after 5–6 hr, the insects were dissected and autoradiographs of the nervous system were made.

4.2.2. Aquatic

Autoradiography has been utilized in marine and freshwater biological studies. Such studies include the use of fallout radionuclides in natural systems as well as the use of radionuclides in controlled laboratory and field studies.

Growth rate of the giant clam *(Tridacna gigas)* at Bikini Atoll was studied by Bonham (1965), who observed the deposition of ^{90}Sr from the 1956 and 1958 nuclear tests in the growing shell as determined by autoradiography. The fallout ^{90}Sr produced definite lines on the autoradiographs, which corresponded to specific time periods (Figure 6). Using a similar procedure, Knutson *et al.* (1972) studied the growth rates of corals *(Fayia speciosa, Goniastrea parvistella, G. retiforms, Porites lutea, Psammocora togianensis)* collected in 1971 at Eniwetok Atoll, which was the site of various nuclear tests from 1948 to 1958. Vertical sections less than 2 cm thick were placed for 40 days on X-ray film. The darkened bands on the autoradiograph were due to ^{90}Sr and were related to specific series of tests (Figure 7). This information was used in conjunction with X-ray observations to compare ages determined by the two methods:

> The agreement between ages based on radioactivity inclusions and those determined by density band counting encourages us to measure growth rates on the basis of density bands in those corals which do not contain radioactivity.

Cross *et al.* (1968) studied the distribution of ^{65}Zn in two marine crustaceans, a benthic amphipod *(Anonyx* sp.) and a euphausiid *(Euphausia pacifica)*. The organisms were collected off the Oregon coast, placed in containers of seawater and ^{65}Zn, removed after 8 days, sectioned, and autoradiographed. The investigators observed that the ^{65}Zn was localized predominantly in the exoskeleton and myofibril interstitial spaces. They discussed this observation in relation to ^{65}Zn cycling in the marine ecosystem.

Using ^{33}P in conjunction with autoradiography, Fuhs and Canelli (1970) studied phosphate uptake in individual freshwater algae. Rose and Cushing (1970) were interested in the major sorption site of ^{65}Zn on mats of Columbia River periphyton. They cultured periphyton communities on paraffin blocks that were placed for 24 hr in a container of filtered river water containing ^{65}Zn. The paraffin blocks and periphyton were embedded under vacuum and sectioned, and

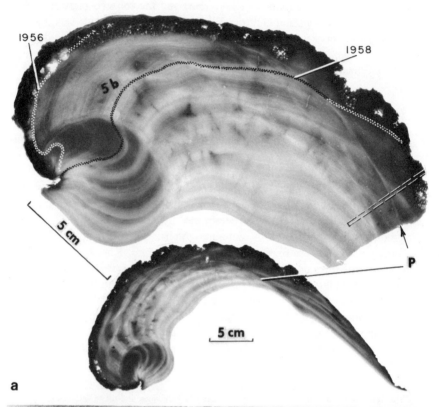

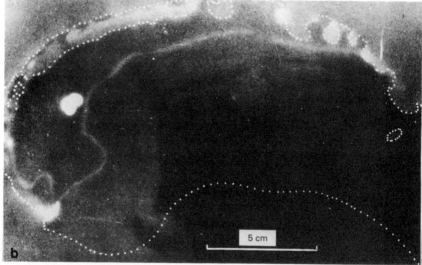

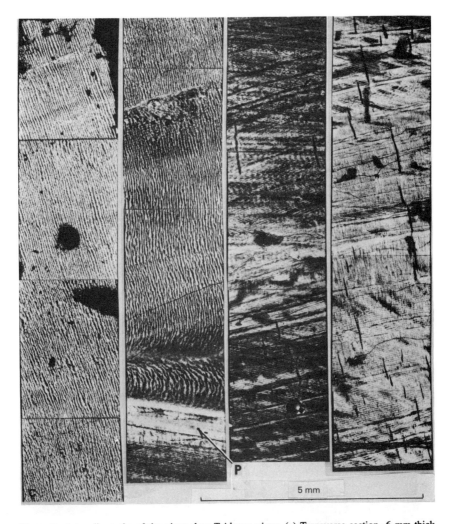

Figure 6. Autoradiographs of the giant clam *Tridacna gigas*. (a) Transverse section, 6 mm thick, of a *Tridacna gigas* shell near the umbo. *Top:* Basal portion to a scale 2.5 times the bottom figure, showing by stippled lines the positions of the layers of radioactivity traced from the autoradiograph (P) Pallial mark. *Bottom:* Entire section. (b) Autoradiograph of the basal portion of the section of a *Tridacna gigas* shell shown in (a). Retouching was limited to the dotted lines indicating the outlines of the shell and eroded areas. The two light undulating lines that originate near the umbo resulted from the beta activity of ^{90}Sr presumed to have been deposited in 1956 and 1958. Radioactivity is also evident in the umbonal cleft and elsewhere on the outer surface as well as in the eroded spaces. The white spot at left of center resulted from ^{45}Ca mixed with the ink used to label the section *5b* [see (a)]. (c) Composite photomicrograph of a thin transverse section ground to a thickness of 15–20 μm. The section was removed from the position indicated by dashes at the right side of (a) *(top)*. Length and width of section: 41 by 2 mm. The continuous strip is divided for convenience into four columns starting with the outside of the shell at the upper left. (P) Pallial mark. From Bonham (1965). Copyright 1965 by the American Association for the Advancement of Science.

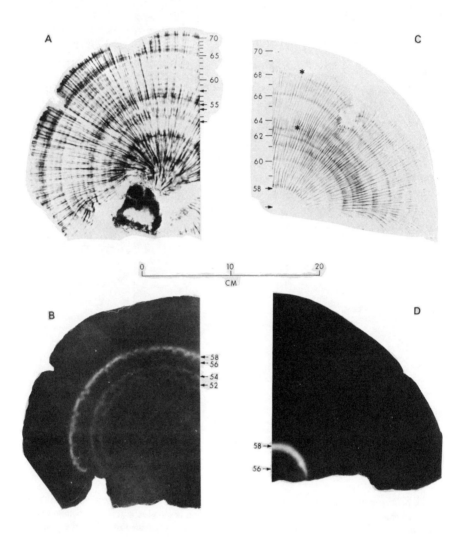

Figure 7. (A) X-radiograph of a cross-sectional slice of sample 1; annual bands are indicated by index lines and dates; arrows show the locations of (B) dated radioactivity bands. (B) Autoradiograph of sample 1, with dates of test series associated with observed bands. (C) X-radiograph of sample 2; the circles indicate the locations of intraseasonal bands less intense or less continuous, or both, than the annual bands. (D) Autoradiograph of sample 2. The pictures are positives printed from X-ray negatives, so that dark areas correspond to the denser portions of the coral. To index bands near the center of the coral, half of each radiograph is shown. From Knutson *et al.* (1972). Copyright 1972 by the American Association for the Advancement of Science.

the sections were used to prepare autoradiographs. The authors observed that ^{65}Zn was sorbed mainly on the upper surface of the community (Figure 8).

A common procedure for the measurement of primary productivity in aquatic ecosystems is the ^{14}C method proposed by Steeman Nielsen (e.g. 1963). The method does not permt the determination of individual contributions of the various phytoplankton species present in a specific ecosystem. A method that involves autoradiography of ^{14}C-labeled algal cells was developed by Maguire and Neill (1971) to investigate this matter. Briefly, the method involves labeling the algal cells by means of the Steeman Nielsen procedure, exposing the labeled cells to a radiosensitive emulsion, and determining the proportion of "silver grains" produced by each species. The authors discuss the procedures in considerable detail, and their paper is recommended reading for persons interested in primary productivity.

Radionuclide-labeled organisms, particularly insects and small mammals, have been used in dispersal studies. Berlin and Rylander (1963) used radionuclide-tagged bacteria and autoradiography in the study of the spread of bacteria in water. *Escherichia coli* were grown in a carrier-free medium containing ^{35}S. The number of labeled bacteria in water samples was estimated by the viable-count method and autoradiography. The authors conducted a field study by introducing radiolabeled bacteria into the effluent from a household septic tank and studying the dispersion of these bacteria in a Baltic Sea inlet.

Studies of cell division using autoradiography and ^{3}H are common; however, applications of the technique to organisms other than laboratory animals are less so. One example is the study of Polikarpov and Tokareva (1970), in which the technique was used to study the cell cycle in marine dinoflagellates.

Although laboratory studies have value for specific purposes, it is in the natural ecosystem that we must determine the behavior of a pesticide and its possible effect. Studies of the cycling of radionuclide-labeled pesticides in natural ecosystems are limited, since introduction of radionuclides into the environment involves public-health and public-relations issues as well as possibly difficult technical considerations. However, an ecosystem study was conducted by spraying a 4-acre marsh in western Sandusky Bay, Ohio, with ^{36}Cl-labeled DDT. One aspect of the study involved the incorporation of the pesticide in some invertebrates of this aquatic ecosystem as determined by autoradiography (Webster, 1967). An amount of the pesticide suitable for mosquito control was applied to the study area by helicopter. Samples of leeches *(Erpobdella punctata)*, amphipods *(Hyallela* sp.), and copepods *(Cyclops bicuspidatus, Diaptomus organensis)* were collected, fixed, sectioned, and autoradiographed. It was observed that leeches contained the pesticide or a ^{36}Cl-compound, but none was detected in amphipods or copepods.

Using a model ecosystem, Metcalf (1972) studied pesticide biodegradability and ecological magnification by means of autoradiography and thin-layer chrom-

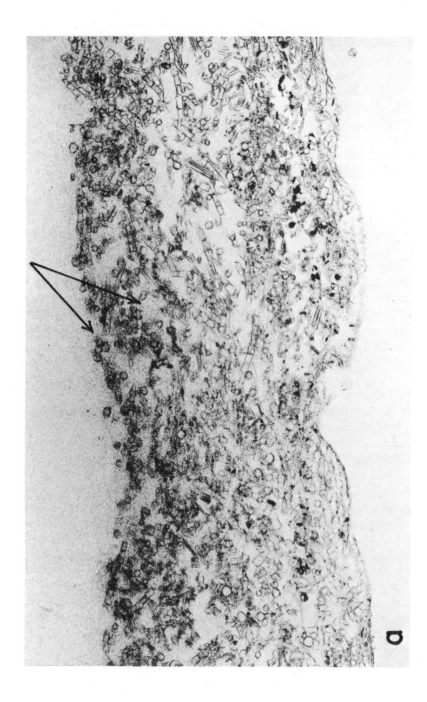

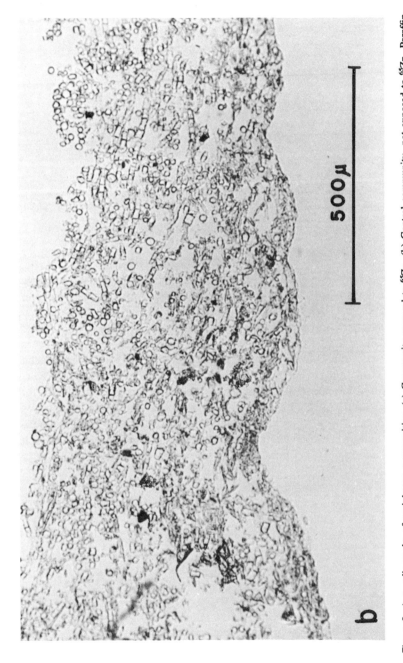

500μ

b

Figure 8. Autoradiographs of periphyton communities. (a) Community exposed to ^{65}Zn. (b) Control community, not exposed to ^{65}Zn. Paraffin substrates were at the bottom edge of both communities. Arrows indicate the darkened band of ^{65}Zn deposition. From Rose and Cushing (1970). Copyright 1970 by the American Association for the Advancement of Science.

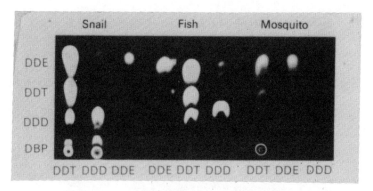

Figure 9. Autoradiograph of thin-layer plate with extract of fish, snail, and mosquito larvae from model ecosystems containing ^{14}C-labeled DDT, 2,2-bis-(p-chlorophenyl)-1,1-dichlorethane (DDD), and 2,2-bis-(p-chlorophenyl)-1,1-dichloroethylene (DDE). From Metcalf (1972).

otography. The model ecosystem consisted of an aquarium comprising an aquatic and a terrestrial portion. The terrestrial portion contained the plant *Sorghum halepense* and the aquatic portion, the blue-green alga *Oedogonium cardiacum,* plankton, water fleas *(Daphnia magna),* and snails *(Physa* sp.). The leaves of the terrestrial plant were treated with the labeled pesticide, and the 4th instar of the salt marsh caterpillar *(Estigmene acrea)* was permitted to feed on the leaves of the plant until the leaves were consumed. Labeled insect feces contaminated the aquatic ecosystem. After 26 days, mosquito larvae *(Culex quinquefasciatus)* were introduced into the system, and after 30 days, the top minnow *(Gambusia affinis)* was added. After 33 days, the experiment was terminated, samples of water and organisms were collected, and organic extracts and water were examined by thin-layer chromotography. Autoradiography and serial scintillation counting of the radioactive areas were used to study the degradation products (Figure 9).

Radiation Sources and Dosimeters

5.1. General Comments

Radiation sources and dosimetric methods were developed by radiation ecologists interested in the effects of ionizing radiation on species, communities and ecosystems. Radiation may be considered as a form of stress that can be applied with safety and precision to natural ecosystems. Community responses to radiation stress reveal many basic aspects of ecosystem structure and function, and for this reason, radiation may be considered as a technique to develop fundamental ecological knowledge. The general subject of radiation sources and dosimeters has been discussed in symposia and in journals (e.g., International Atomic Energy Agency, 1960, 1973c; Attix, 1967; Spurny and Sulcova, 1973). Sparrow (1960) discussed the uses of large sources in botanical research and cited many references on sources utilized by investigators.

In general, ecologists and biologists investigating the effects of ionizing radiation on individual organisms have used as radiation sources practically every means available from dental X-ray equipment to the sophisticated gamma-ray sources available at a national laboratory. Similarly, many types of dosimeters have been used. A very interesting historical paper on radiation sources, dosimetry, and some concepts associated with the study of effects of ionizing radiation on organisms, communities, and ecosystems is that of Platt (1963). Ideas proposed by Platt in this paper, which was presented to the First National Symposium on Radioecology, September 1961, bore fruit in later years.

5.2. Radiation Sources

The wide diversity of radiation sources utilized in irradiation of single organisms restricts our comments concerning such sources to referring the reader to irradiation procedures described in the many papers on the subject of biological effects of ionizing radiation on the single organism. To do otherwise would present an impossible task and detract from other matters of more relevance to our anticipated audience. We would prefer to discuss those radiation sources that were specifically developed for ecological studies.

Early observations on effects of ionizing radiation on wild plants occurred in the vicinity of sources utilized for specific botanical studies with domestic plants, e.g., at Brookhaven National Laboratory (Sparrow and Woodwell, 1963). In addition, Dr. Robert B. Platt, Plant Ecologist at Emory University, observed what appeared to be ionizing-radiation effects in natural ecosystems at the site of an unshielded nuclear reactor (Figure 10). As a result of these observations, Platt and his associates initiated the first study of the effects of ionizing radiation on an ecosystem. A description of the study plan was published (Platt and Mohrbacher, 1959), and some observations were presented at the First National Symposium on Radioecology in 1961. The radiation source was a 10-MW reactor that was operated for the U.S. Air Force by Lockheed Nuclear Products. It was an air-shielded, pressurized, light-water-moderated and cooled reactor, producing a high neutron and gamma flux. Selby *et al.* (1961) discussed in some detail the characteristics of this reactor, its operation, and its effects on the environs. Since the ecologist could not control the level and time distribution of radiation to the ecosystem, the next step was to conduct controlled experiments that required radiation sources developed exclusively for ecological studies.

A 2500-Ci ^{137}Cs gamma facility was established at Emory University for ecological research (Platt *et al.*, 1964) to be used to interpret further some of the observations made at the air-shielded reactor (Figure 11). The organisms or communities of interest were brought to this facility for irradiation.

At the Savannah River Ecology Laboratory, a mobile radiation source was developed that could be used within the permanent study area adjacent to the laboratory or trucked into the field to specific sites of interest (Golley and McCormick, 1966; McCormick and Golley, 1966). It consisted of 9200 Ci ^{137}Cs encased in a stainless steel capsule that was placed in a lead container (Figure 12). This versatile source played an important role in the recognition of the Savannah River Ecology Laboratory as a center for ecological research in the United States. When the source was placed in the permanent study area (Figure 13), plant study plots or cages of animals could be irradiated at known levels corresponding to given distances from the source. Plant communities not available within the permanent field could be studied by moving the source to the sites of these communities.

Both large and relatively small radiation sources placed in fixed positions were utilized by ecologists in various vegetation types: in the United States, in an oak–pine forest (Woodwell, 1963), a shortgrass prairie (Fraley and Whicker, 1973a,b), a desert-shrub community (French, 1964), and an aspen forest (Ru-

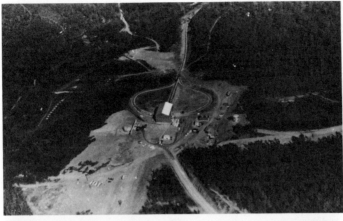

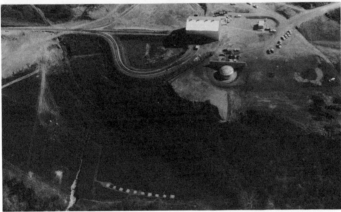

Figure 10. Aerial views of the Lockheed Reactor Site. *Bottom view:* The reactor is in the rectangular aluminum building at the intersection of the three railroad spurs, the control rooms are underground and to the right, and the 500-foot entrance tunnel extends to the right. A row of experimental plots extends leftward from bottom center. Most of the plots are along radii rather than arcs. Courtesy of R. B. Platt.

dolph, 1974); in Puerto Rico, in a tropical rain forest (H. T. Odum and Drewry, 1970); and in France, in oak-dominated communities (Fabries *et al.*, 1972).

The shortgrass-vegetation radiation field consisted of 1.2 hectares in north-central Colorado and included a 8750-Ci ^{137}Cs source that was suspended 1 m above the ground surface. The radiation field was divided into six sectors: a control sector shielded from radiation, two chronically irradiated sectors, and

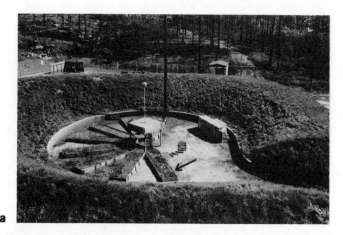

Figure 11. Emory University gamma-radiation field. (a) An experimental community on a simulated granite outcrop (←) is at the right of the radiation field. A wall of high-density concrete blocks placed between the community and the radiation source under the sky shield is used to control the duration and total dose of irradiation received by the experimental community. The simulated outcrop used as a control in this study is located behind the earthen bunker within the fenced area. (b) Profile view of ^{137}Cs-source operating mechanism. (1) Source capsule; (2) electromagnet; (3) raising and lowering limit switches; (4) electromagnet supply cable assembly; (5) motor drive assembly for mechanically raising and lowering electromagnet; (6) weather shield; (7) source position indicator lights; (8) lead and steel sky and transient shields; (9) concrete structural base and source-down radiation shield; (10) circuit control center with the fused switches for major electrical components of operating mechanism; (11) vent pipe for hydraulic brake for oil bath; (12) source-down position seat in 30-inch oil bath 5 feet below ground level; (13) pipe containing positive-readout detector for monitoring source-down position. (a) From McCormick and Platt (1962). (b) From Platt *et al.* (1964).

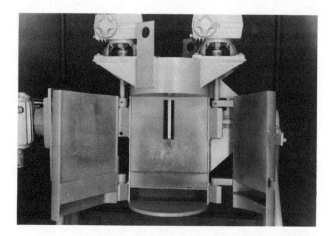

Figure 12. Savannah River Ecology Laboratory ^{137}Cs source. Front view of cask, showing location of gears (E, F) to open doors (B, C) to expose cesium capsule (A). From Golley and McCormick (1966).

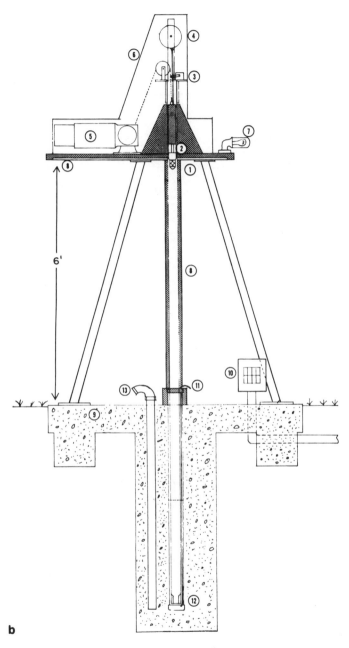

b

Figure 11. *(continued)*

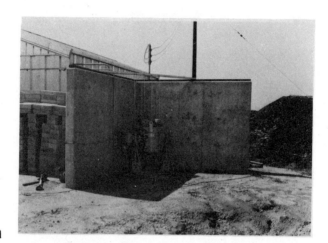

a

b

Figure 13. Savannah River Ecology Laboratory gamma-radiation field. (a) View of cask in place in gamma field before renovation of shielding. The cables that control the doors extend through the concrete wall into the control house. (b) View of ^{137}Cs-source shielding, including concrete shield and earthen bunkers (1), and also showing location of control house (3), farm gate (4), mirror to view source (5), barbed wire and hog fence surrounding the bunker (2), and the source (6). From Golley and McCormick (1966).

three sectors that were seasonally irradiated (Figure 14). A source of this magnitude produces very high exposure rates near the irradiator.

Another study that involved high levels of ionizing radiation was one located in an oak–pine forest in central Long Island, New York. This study, conducted at Brookhaven National Laboratory, involved a 10,000-Ci ^{137}Cs source that was stored below ground when not in operation (Figure 15). The study plans included establishment of 16 radii marked at 20-m intervals to aid in locating study plots. Details of the source and study design are presented by Woodwell (1963) and Woodwell and Hammond (1962).

Research in a tropical rain forest in Puerto Rico utilized a semiportable 10,000-Ci ^{137}Cs source to deliver chronic irradiation to the ecosystem and its components (H. T. Odum and Drewry, 1970) (Figure 16). When in operation, the source was suspended 6 ft above a ground platform. As with the other radiation sources described, safety features were an important consideration in the operation of this source. On completion of the studies in Puerto Rico, this gamma-radiation source was reencapsulated with 10,000 Ci ^{137}Cs and installed at Rhinelander, Wisconsin, in the Enterprise Radiation Forest (Rudolph, 1974). When in operation in this aspen forest, the source was approximately 5 ft above ground.

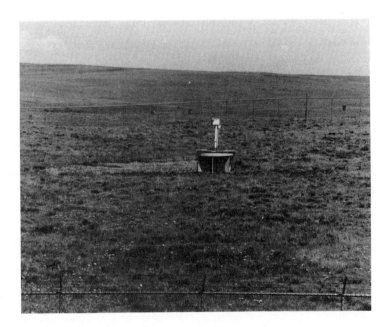

Figure 14. Shortgrass-prairie gamma-radiation field. Courtesy of F. W. Whicker.

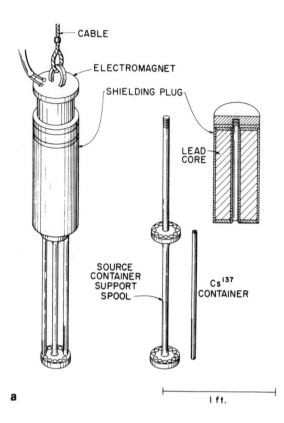

CABLE

ELECTROMAGNET

SHIELDING PLUG

LEAD CORE

SOURCE CONTAINER SUPPORT SPOOL

Cs^{137} CONTAINER

a

I ft.

In southeast France at the Cadarache Nuclear Research Center, a Mediterranean-type phytocenose was subjected to chronic gamma radiation from a ^{137}Cs source of 1200 Ci. The mechanical aspects of the source consisted of a vertical tube 3 m in height in which the radioactive component moved from a lead chamber in the ground to the top of the tube, which contained a lead shield to prevent the escape of radiation from the study area. (Fabries, Grauby and Trochain, 1972).

To our knowledge, only one study utilizing a radiation source in the field was conducted to evaluate the effects of exclusively low levels of ionizing radiation on an ecosystem. This interesting study was developed by Dr. Norman R. French at the U.S. Atomic Energy Commission's Nevada Test Site. A 20-acre circular area, enclosed with a rodent-proof fence, was irradiated by a 33,000-Ci ^{137}Cs source located in the center of the circular area (French, 1964). A shield of varying thickness was used in an attempt to develop a reasonably uniform radiation level over the circular area. The shield was fixed permanently at the

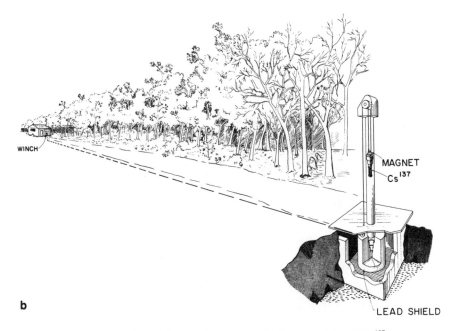

Figure 15. Brookhaven National Laboratory ^{137}Cs source. (a) Source container. The ^{137}Cs as cesium chloride crystals is in six stainless steel tubes supported in the cylindrical bracket. (b) Handling mechanism. The cable to the source passes through a 4-inch pipe buried 30–40 cm beneath the soil surface. From Woodwell (1963).

top of a tower, and the source was moved up the 50-ft tower to a position above the shield during periods of irradiation (Figures 17 and 18).

5.3. Dosimeters and Dosimetry

Dosimetry is the procedure of estimating the quantity of ionizing radiation delivered to an object or area, or the energy absorbed from this amount of radiation, or both. The instruments used to determine this are called "dosimeters." Selection of an appropriate dosimeter depends on the types of ionizing radiation of interest as well as on the conditions under which they are measured. The ecologist is faced with problems that are unique, as contrasted with those faced by the health physicist interested in human exposure. Of course, the ecologist dealing with individual animals in cages or plants in pots deals with a much simpler problem than the ecologist irradiating an ecosystem and its various

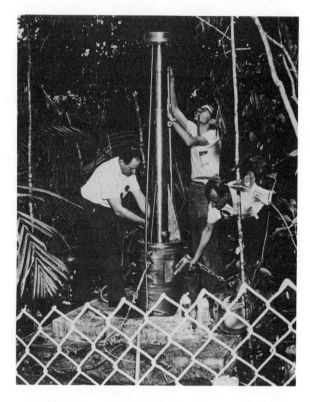

Figure 16. Puerto Rico tropical rain forest ^{137}Cs source. Source almost ready for irradiation, December 1966. The small fence was removed prior to irradiation. From H. T. Odum and Drewry (1970).

components. Animals in a field situation may spend much of their time underground and thus be shielded from radiation emitted from a radiation source above ground, and terrain shielding may result in differential exposures to plants and animals at the same distance from the source. If the radiation source is waste material on the ground surface, the animal's ventral area will probably receive a higher dose than its dorsal area.

Radiation ecologists have attached various types of dosimeters to small animals in an attempt to estimate the radiation dose. Kaye (1965) studied the use of silver-activated metaphosphate-glass dosimeters, which measure dose by radiophotoluminescence, in ecological research at Oak Ridge National Laboratory. These solid-state dosimeters, measuring 1 × 6 mm, were injected subcutaneously into cotton rats *(Sigmodon hispidus)* (Figure 19a). The rats were then released on radioactive sediment of White Oak Lake, a waste-disposal impoundment that had been drained. Readings from dosimeters placed on the ventral and dorsal aspects of animals disclosed that average ventral readings were larger than average dorsal readings (Figure 19b). Kaye also studied the exposure rate as a function of distance above the lake bed by suspending dosimeters at 1-ft intervals above the surface (Figure 19c). In addition to making field observations, he compared characteristics of various commercially available dosimeters, such as response as a function of photon energy and net fluorometer readings as a function of absorbed dose. Blaylock and Witherspoon (1965), also working at Oak Ridge National Laboratory, studied the influence of temperature and sunlight on fluorescence of Toshiba low-Z rods, which were also used by Kaye in his investigations. The laboratory study of the influence of temperature disclosed an increase for ^{137}Cs gamma rays and no change for ^{137}Cs beta radiation (Figure 20a). These investigators observed that predosed dosimeters faded exponentially when exposed to sunlight for 30 hr and that this fading was related to the initial dose (Figure 20b). As a result of these observations, several kinds

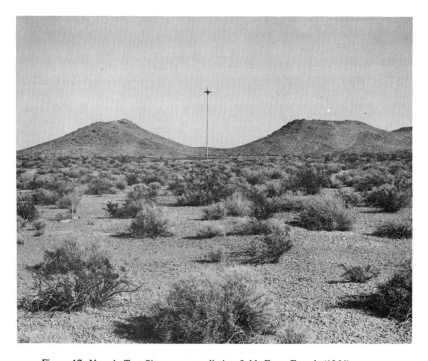

Figure 17. Nevada Test Site gamma-radiation field. From French (1964).

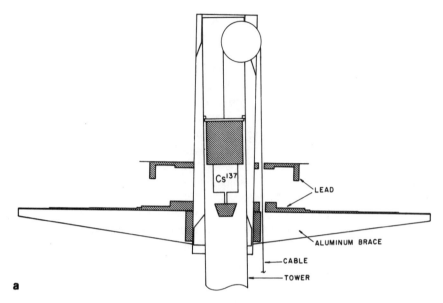

Figure 18. Nevada Test Site ^{137}Cs source. (a) Diagram of source and shield. (b) Diagram of structure that supports the source and shield. From French (1964).

of shields were used, and the shielded dosimeters were tested over the White Oak Lake bed (Table 1). Chapuis *et al.* (1973) discussed the use of glass dosimeters at the ecosystem irradiation site in France.

The radiation flux throughout the 20-acre circular enclosure at the Nevada Test Site was determined by placing thermoluminescent dosimeters in holes drilled in the tops of stakes placed at various sites within the enclosure. The dosimeter consisted of a glass-capillary tube (0.8×6.0 mm) that was filled with $CaF_2 \cdot$ Mn or LiF. When utilized with the pocket mouse *(Perognathus formosus)*, it was placed in a polyethylene tube (Figure 21a), which, in turn, was attached externally to the rodent by a single suture to the neck skin (Figure 21b). Using the hypodermic syringe method of Kaye, investigators placed the dosimeter beneath the skin of the side-blotched uta lizard *(Uta stansburiana)*. The distribution of the ratio, animal/surface exposure, for the pocket mouse and side-blotched uta in the enclosure (Figure 21c,d) was presented by Lucas and French (1967) in addition to the information on attachment of the dosimeters. Turner and Lannom (1968) discussed the procedure of measuring radiation doses to the side-blotched uta as well as to the whip-tail lizard *(Cnemidophorus tigris)* and the leopard lizard *(Crotaphytus wislizenii)* on this study area. French (1964) commented that external attachment of dosimeters provided for ease of detach-

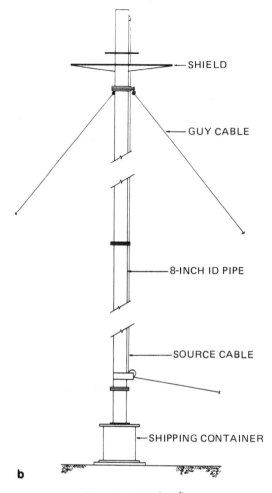

b

Figure 18. (continued)

ment, and such attachments were not etched by body fluids as were subcutaneous implants. Etching would interfere with light transmission from the rod. He further commented that the thermoluminescent dosimeter rods have advantages over phosphate glass rods, since the former lack energy dependence and have a greater sensitivity.

Thermoluminescent dosimeters have been used in aquatic environments. Guthrie and Scott (1969) used lithium fluoride dosimetry in a freshwater pond to measure the radiation dose to chironomid larvae. Cesium-137 was added to the pond and allowed to disperse through the water. Following pilot studies in

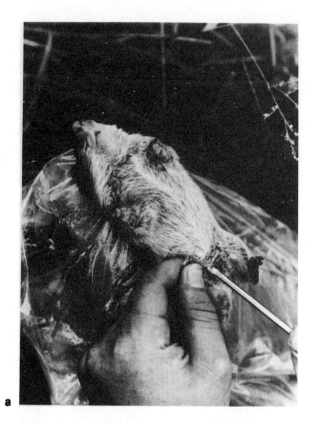

a

Figure 19. Glass-rod dosimeter insertion in cotton rats *(Sigmodon hispidus)* and results. (a) Subcutaneous insertion of glass-rod dosimeter in the field. The glass rod is in a nylon capsule held in the orifice of the implantation needle. (b) Average absorbed dose rate for 38 cotton rats on the radioactive White Oak Lake bed. (c) Exposure rate above the radioactive White Oak Lake bed. Toshiba low-Z rods were tied at 1-ft intervals to a nylon cord affixed normal to the soil surface. Each rod was contained in a small nylon capsule (wall thickness 0.047-inch). From Kaye (1965). Copyright 1965 by The Ecological Society of America.

an aquarium, the authors selected a cylindrical dosimeter coated with silicon rubber to prevent leaking (Figure 22a). The dosimeters were placed at 1-m intervals on a weighted cord that rested on the bottom of the pond and were arranged to be at the intersections of 1-m^2 grids. A plot of the resulting isodose lines is presented in Figure 22b. In another study at White Oak Lake, Blaylock (1966) used metaphosphate glass-rod dosimeters to estimate the dose from radioactive sediments to *Chironomus* larvae in which he was studying chromosomal aberrations. Lithium fluoride powder was placed in a 2.4-mm-diameter heat-

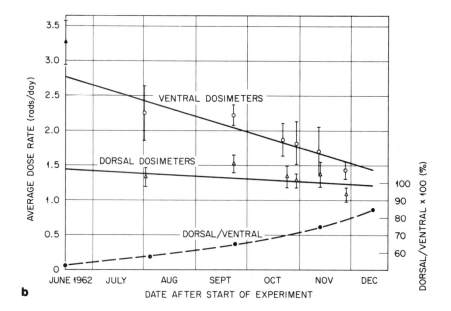

b

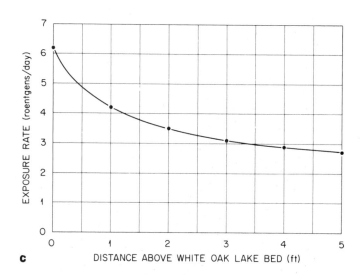

c

Figure 19. (*continued*)

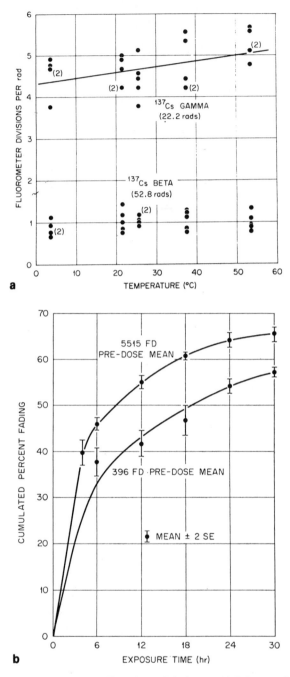

Figure 20. Environmental factors that affect glass-rod dosimetry. (a) Influence of temperature on Toshiba II glass response to ^{137}Cs. (b) Fading in unshielded Toshiba II glass exposed to sunlight. From Blaylock and Witherspoon (1965). Reproduced from *Health Physics* **11**:549–552 (1965) by permission of the Health Physics Society.

Table 1. Fading Characteristics of Shielded Glass Rods[a]

Type of shielding	4-Hour exposure to sunlight			24-Day exposure on White Oak Lake bed		
	Number	Predose (FD)[b,c]	Fading (%)[b]	Number	Cumulated fluorescence (FD)[b,c]	Loss (relative to black nylon) (%)
Unshielded	5	5365 ± 154	39.8 ± 2.7	5	110 ± 2.7	61.7
White nylon capsule (translucent, 2 mm thick)	5	5240 ± 144	19.2 ± 0.2	5	132 ± 2.9	54.1
Black nylon capsule (opaque, 2 mm thick)	5	5317 ± 192	1.2 ± 0.5	5	287 ± 6.3	0
Clear lucite capsule (transparent, 2.25 mm thick)	5	5355 ± 162	13.7 ± 2.8	—	—	—

[a] From Blaylock and Witherspoon (1965). Reproduced from *Health Physics* **11**:549–552 (1965) by permission of the Health Physics Society.
[b] Means ± 2 S.E.
[c] Fluorometer division.

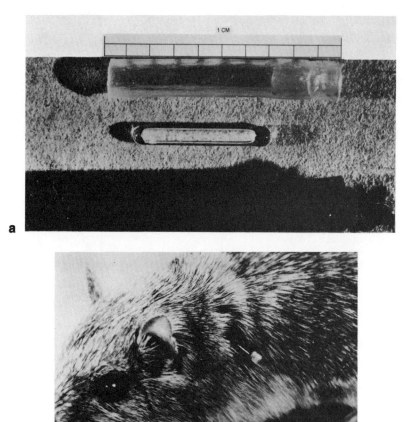

Figure 21. Glass-rod dosimetry and results at the Nevada Test Site gamma-radiation field. (a) Dosimeter container. (b) Dosimeter assembly fastened by a single stitch to the neck of the rodent. Dosimeters could be removed periodically for reading and replaced with unexposed units. (c) Distribution of gamma-ray exposures of *Perognathus formosus* during the winter of 1964–1965. The

shrinking, light-impervious tubing and used by Watson and Templeton (1973) to study the radiation dose to aquatic organisms in the Columbia River downstream from effluent release from Hanford reactors. Dosimeters were suspended in a 1-m length of pipe that was, in turn, attached to the underside of a float. The function of the pipe was to reduce exposure of the dosimeter to light, which

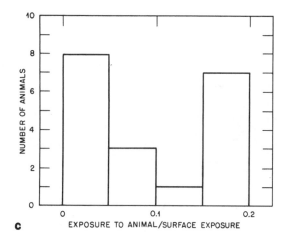

c

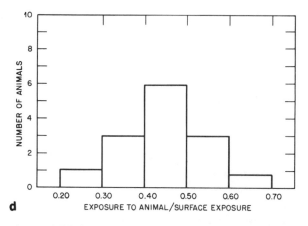

d

readings of the rodent-carried dosimeters have been divided by the exposure that would have resulted
if the animal had remained on the ground surface. (d) Distribution of gamma-ray exposures of *Uta*
lizards during April 1965. Same normalization of abscissa as in (c). From Lucas and French (1967).

consequently reduced algal growth on the dosimeter. Doses to benthic organisms
were estimated from dosimeters tied to the top and bottom surfaces of rocks.
Initially, studies related to fish involved attaching dosimeters below the dorsal
fin or implanting them into the abdominal cavity and maintaining the fish in a
fenced enclosure in the river. As a result of fluctuating water levels, this ex-

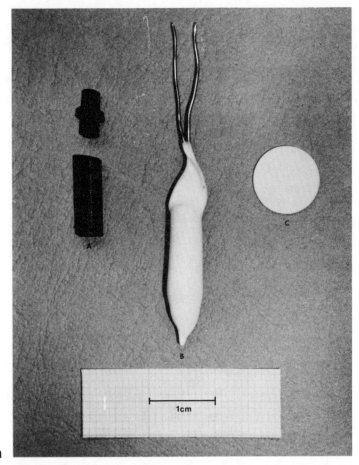

Figure 22. Lithium fluoride dosimetry and results from a pond habitat. (a) Equipment. (A) Cylindrical dosimeter with sealing plug; (B) cylindrical dosimeter filled with 47 mg LiF powder and coated with a silicone–rubber waterproofing compound; (C) Teflon disk dosimeter. (b) Isodose plot of radiation-dose distribution in pond as of October 1967. From Guthrie and Scott (1969).

periment was terminated and dose estimates made of killed fish, frozen after capture, on or in which the dosimeters had been placed. Lappenbusch *et al.* (1971) also used the dosimeter in estimating dose to periphyton in the Columbia River. Thermoluminescent dosimeters were used in a Baltic Sea bay to study the diffusion of low-level radioactive wastes from Studsvik (Gyllander, 1966).

It is obvious that radiation-dose distribution in a study area exposed to chronic high levels of ionizing radiation must be established if the effects of

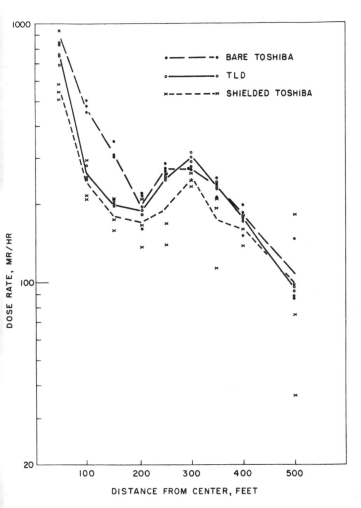

. Dose rate at ground level along a radius at the Nevada Test Site gamma-radiation field.
s were measured in August and September 1964. (TLD) Thermoluminescent dosimeter.
nch (1964).

eral techniques are available for measurement of exposure. Ionization chambers were
most accurate dosimeters available for most purposes, but measurements are expensive
ime and the chambers are impractical for use in large quantities. Film badges are
ap, convenient to handle in large numbers and have a wide range of sensitivity.
sphate glass dosimeters are less accurate than either badge or ionization chambers at
ranges, but can be used with a precision of about 5–10 per cent for total exposures
from approximately 10 r through several hundred r. Their small size makes them

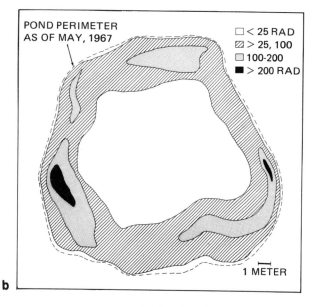

b

Figure 22. (*continued*)

ionizing radiation on the ecosystem are to be determined and related to dose
level. Usually, the air dose was determined throughout the study area, and as
noted above, the dose to specific organisms was determined. The dose distributions on the previously discussed study areas involving a fixed or transient
radiation source in an ecosystem have been determined by use of the dosimeters
described as well as with film badges and ion chambers. The results are specific
to the specific ecosystem and to the radiation source. Details concerning the
radiation-dose distribution for specific sites can be found in the papers cited
above; for the tropical rain forest, in papers by Hall (1970) and McCormick
(1970); and for the aspen forest, in the paper by Salmonson *et al.* (1974).
Difficulties vary from the extreme of those in the uncontrolled study utilizing
the air-shielded Lockheed Reactor (Cowan and Platt, 1963), which involved
considerable heterogeneity of dose as a result of terrain and tree shielding (Figure
23), to the relatively less complicated situations in the oak–pine forest (Figure
24) and the desert-shrub study area at the Nevada Test Site (Figure 25). It is
obvious that even in the latter two, the dose distribution is less uniform than
desired.

Woodwell (1963) adequately summarizes the subject of dosimeters and
dosimetry as follows:

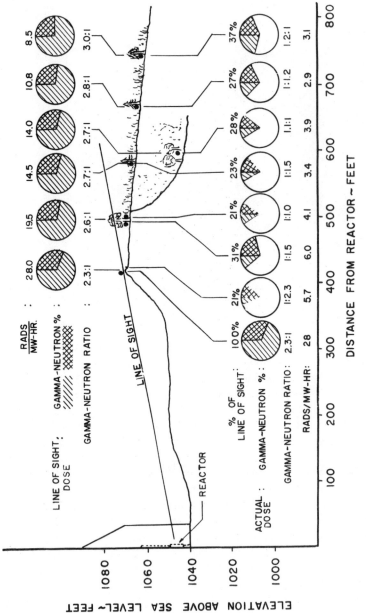

Figure 23. Effects of terrain and vegetation shielding at Stations 46–53 on the east–southeast beam line. The detection stations are located in a mature oak–hickory forest stand. The upper circles show the expected line-of-sight dosages and the gamma/neutron ratios, and the lower circles show these quantities under actual conditions. The station at 595 feet is located in a wooded ravine about 20 feet below the adjacent stations. From Cowan and Platt (1963).

Figure 24. Radiation exposure rates and frequency distribution at the Brookhaven National Laboratory gamma-radiation field. (a) Exposure rates at various distances. Curve is the mean of about 600 measurements of exposure made among six distances. (b) Frequency distribution of dose along an arc at each of two distances. The skewness and spread of these curves are attributable to shielding. From Woodwell (1963).

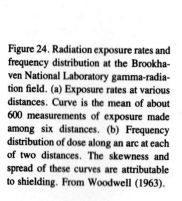

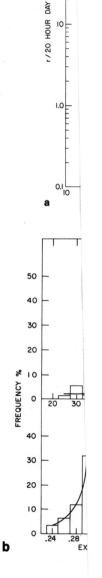

particularly well adapted to animal studies. Perhaps the most promising technque for ecological studies involves the thermo-luminescence crystals. With proper equipment lithium fluoride crystals can be used with total exposures as low as 1 mr ± 0.25 mr and as high as 80,000 r and would seem to be ideally suited for use in ecology. In addition to this wide range of sensitivity they have very low energy and dose-rate dependence making them suitable for many field applications.

6

Behavioral Studies

6.1. General Comments

Population ecologists are concerned with the analysis of natural populations. It is a fact that sooner or later the number of individuals in any population will change and that observations on laboratory populations may not explain the reasons behind changes in free-ranging populations. Consequently, the importance of field studies should not be underrated. The subject of population dynamics entails the numerical estimate of various population attributes such as total numbers, birth and death rates, immigration, and emigration, as well as the effect of various environmental parameters on these attributes. With the current interest in ecological modeling, it is essential that accurate estimates of population parameters be obtained. Development of radionuclide-tracer technology provided the opportunity for ecologists to apply new techniques to ecological investigations related to population dynamics, such as in conjunction with tag–recapture procedures for population estimation, determination of home range, and other behavioral aspects of populations.

Prior to the introduction of radiotracer technology, identification of animals involved mutilation, such as toe-clipping and ear-notching, and other methods such as banding and marking with streamers or paint. Limitations to these standard methods include difficulties in making observations, e.g., when the animals are in burrows; difficulties associated with initial capture and recapture of large numbers of animals; behavioral modification due to handling; and the possibility of increased vulnerability to predation. The use of a radionuclide tag overcomes some of these disadvantages but has limitations that are unique, such as the need for somewhat sophisticated equipment; legal aspects associated with introducing a radionuclide into the environment; possible effects of ionizing radiation on the organism; and the impossibility of distinguishing among individuals tagged with the same radionuclide, which may be overcome with numbered metal bands.

The radiotracer method of tagging involves using radioactive paint, bands, rings, wires introduced internally or used externally, physiological tagging, or, as discussed in Chapter 3, neutron activation of a stable element introduced as a tag. Certain methods are applicable to group marking and others to individual marking. When selecting a radionuclide as a behavioral tag, one must consider such characteristics as toxicity, physical half-life, biological half-life if used as a physiological tag, energy emissions, and detection equipment available. Last but not least, the objectives of the study and the characteristics of the organism to be studied must be taken into consideration.

Although there is a need for a general manual on the subject of tracer methodology for ecologists interested in population dynamics, none exists. There are review papers concerned with specific groups of animals, and these will be cited in the appropriate sections to follow. There exist two outdated review papers of a general nature, Pendleton (1956) and Tester (1963), the latter being restricted to vertebrates.

6.2. Invertebrates

Applications of radionuclides in behavioral studies of insects are numerous, while applications to studies of other invertebrates are very limited. The primary sources of references to behavioral applications in entomology are the excellent bibliographies of Bingelli (1963, 1965, 1967, 1969) and limited comments available in O'Brien and Wolfe (1964a). Radioactive and nonradioactive marking methods are summarized for insects by Dobson (1962) and Southwood (1966). Gangwere *et al.* (1964) discuss both marking methods for insects, with emphasis on Orthoptera. Table 2, which was prepared by them, summarizes the methods of administration of radionuclides to insects. We will now consider some applications to organisms of various classes of the phylum Arthropoda.

The isopod, *Armadillidium vulgare,* was studied by Paris (1965) in a California grassland habitat. The primary objective of the research was to document the movements of this species. Studies of movements prior to this investigation were unsuccessful, since the animal was very difficult to relocate. Paris tagged the individuals collected from his study area by first denying them food for at least 48 hr and then making available rodent pellet food that had been soaked in a solution of ^{32}P. A total of 1000 tagged individuals were released in each of the four studies conducted. Initially, the investigator was concerned that the beta emitter would not be detected as a result of shielding by materials above the organism. However, experimental conditions involving light litter and soil minimized this concern. The relatively short half-life of ^{32}P was sufficient for the study objectives, for repeating the study on the same area, and also from the standpoint of ease of decontamination. Released animals were relocated with a

Table 2. Use of Radioactive Materials in Marking and Studying Insects[a,b]

Means of administering isotope	Comments
External application	
1. Organisms reared in or exposed to natural or artificial media containing isotope. (9, 10, 23, 28, 29, 35, 38, 66, 68, 74)	1. Not suitable for Orthoptera, which are terrestrial in habit.
2. Organisms placed in contact with isotope residue on glass plate.** (49*)	2. For most insects, probably less efficient and less permanent than No. 1; not very suitable for Orthoptera; dosage fluctuates; contamination of environment results.
3. Organisms dipped individually in isotope solution.** (67*)	3. Same comments as for No. 2; isotope readily washes off.
4. Organisms sprayed with aqueous solution of isotope in closed chamber.	4. Comparatively inefficient method, often dangerous to technician; contamination as with No. 2 above.
5. Pieces of radioactive wire or metal foil attached to cuticle by adhesive agent. (6, 24, 72, 75)	5. Partly satisfactory for adult Orthoptera, but not for nymphs, which lose tag with each molt; dosage controlled; administration difficult with small species.
Internal application	
6. Organisms given nonliving food or drinking water containing isotope.** (1*, 5*, 12, 31, 38, 47, 48, 65, 81)	6. Suitable for most Orthoptera, particularly omnivorous species, though perhaps not efficient; dosage fluctuates; careful selection of isotope necessary to ensure retention.
7. Organisms given food-plant grown in, dipped in, or otherwise treated with isotope solution. (8, 25*, 29, 33*, 40, 41*, 53, 64*, 65)	7. Entirely suitable for phytophagous Orthoptera, but not for carnivores; dosage fluctuates; careful selection of isotope necessary, as in No. 6, and dependent on uptake and localization by plant.
8. Predators or parasites given radioactive host animal. (29, 80)	8. Entirely suitable for predators or parasites, but not for herbivores; dosage fluctuates; selection of isotope necessary, as in No. 6, and dependent on host uptake and localization.
9. Isotope solution placed between mouthparts with pipette. (49*)	9. Satisfactory for some species; probably inefficient; dosage difficult, particularly in the case of small species.
10. Isotope injected into spiracles or body cavity with microsyringe.** (1*, 49*)	10. Excellent method, but difficult with small species; dosage controlled, with limitation based on the isotope used, some being readily excreted; injection into body cavity much superior to that in spiracles.
11. Pieces of radioactive wire or metal foil inserted into body cavity. (3)	11. Excellent method, but difficult with small species; dosage controlled; later removal of source of radioactivity may be difficult.

[a] From Gangwere et al. (1964).
[b] Numbers in parentheses are those of papers cited in the source reference; a single asterisk indicates a paper dealing, at least in part, with Orthoptera. Methods tested on 5 or more individuals of an orthopteran (the house cricket, *Acheta domesticus*) are marked with double asterisks.

Geiger–Müller (GM) tube mounted at the end of a 6-ft handle and used in conjunction with a survey instrument equipped with earphones.

Mark–recapture estimates of population size were made by E. P. Odum and Pontin (1961) of the yellow ant *(Lasius flavus)* near Oxford, England, by utilizing ^{32}P tagging and by Erickson (1972) of the California harvester ant *(Pogonomyrmex californicus)* in San Diego County, California. Although the methods of labeling differed in details, both studies utilized a method of "soaking" the ants in a solution of ^{32}P. Although E. P. Odum and Pontin (1961) observed secondary tagging of nontagged ants, presumably from ingestion of feces or fluid from tagged ants, they had no difficulty in separating the two on the basis of the degree of tagging. The number of tagged ants released at the collection site varied from about 400 to 1000. At a later date, ants were collected and fastened with cellophane tape to ruled paper, which was then attached to a moving belt and passed through a scanning instrument. Radioactive ants were automatically recorded, and this information was utilized in determining the number of tagged individuals in the sample. Erickson (1972) did not describe the instrumentation used in his study to detect tagged individuals. Both publications include a comparison of mortality of tagged and untagged ants, with no effect of radiation apparent in the studies.

In a study of dispersion of the leaf bug *(Orthotylus virescens)*, Lewis and Waloff (1964) marked samples with either ^{32}P or ^{35}S. Insects containing either of the two radionuclides were identified by autoradiography. Labeled insects were released in two sections of the study area, and by subsequent recaptures, within and outside the study area, a "considerable edge effect" on the movement of the insects was observed. The investigators devised a procedure for labeling a group of individuals that one might call "soaking" (Figure 26). Polystyrene plastic dishes, 9.5 cm, were used, and holes 2.5 cm in diameter were made in each base and lid with a hot metal tube. A stopper was used in the upper hole, and a nylon net covered the lower opening. A radioactive solution was used to soak a piece of lens tissue that adhered by surface tension to the underside of the lid; the lid and base were then held together with a rubber band. Through the hole in the lid, 100 insects were introduced, the stopper was replaced, and the dishes were stacked. After a period of time to permit labeling, the petri dishes were taken to the field, where the insects were released. The investigators

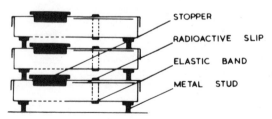

STOPPER

RADIOACTIVE SLIP

ELASTIC BAND

METAL STUD

Figure 26. Stacked polystyrene dishes modified for the presentation of radioactive solutions to batches of *Orthotylus virescens*. From Lewis and Waloff (1964).

compared this method of labeling with that of permitting insects to feed on labeled plant seedlings and cuttings and concluded that the procedure using the lens tissue was the more satisfactory method. The autoradiographic detection of marked individuals involved placing all insects on strips of adhesive "cellotape," sealed between two strips of very thin polythene, and placing this between two X-ray films for film exposure for a 4-week period. Since the beta radiation of the ^{32}P penetrated the polythene and cellotape easily, images were produced on both films, while the differential shielding of the two resulted in an image on only one of the films when an insect containing the ^{35}S, a relatively weak beta emitter, was involved.

In a study of the dispersal of adult blackflies (Diptera: Simuliidae), ^{32}P was placed in a tub containing aerated water and rocks along with the fly larvae and pupae. Two hr later, the rocks were returned to the stream from which they had been collected. By means of traps, a total of about 261,600 adult flies were collected from various sites. The investigators, Baldwin et al. (1966), attempted to identify radiolabeled flies using a low-background scaler, but, as a result of the effort involved, decided to use an autoradiographic procedure. The latter method could detect individuals giving less than 10 cpm above background.

Utilizing radionuclide tagging of ticks (order Acarina), Sonenshine and his associates have contributed to knowledge of the ecology of this important organism through both laboratory studies (Sonenshine, 1968; Sonenshine and Yunker, 1968) and field studies (Sonenshine and Clark, 1968). Sonenshine (1968) reported on the mass rearing and long-term survival of tagged ticks. He used six radionuclides (Table 3), which were inoculated into engorged female

Table 3. Radioactivity in Progeny (Eggs and Larvae) of *Dermacentor variabilis* Females Inoculated with Seven Different Radiochemicals[a]

Radiochemical	Number of inoculations	Mean activity/ inoculation (μCi)	Mean radioactivity (all ticks) in cpm over background	
			All eggs	All larvae[b]
[^{14}C]Glycine	33	38.5	91.4	45.0
[^{14}C]Glucose	7	17.5	122.0	93.1
Cerium-144	1	0.04	2.5	ND
Cesium-137[c]	3	0.09	8.5	ND
Strontium-90[d]	4	0.05	18.5	9.5
Phosphorus-32	6	5.8	211.6[e]	26.0
[^{3}H]Glycine	4	25.0	6.0	ND

[a] From Sonenshine (1968).
[b] (ND) Not determined.
[c] Activity was determined with a gas-flow counter. Activity was also determined with a solid scintillation detector, and with very similar results.
[d] Including 1 *Amblyomma americanum*.
[e] Egg-laying ceased shortly after day 1; the parent ticks died.

ticks according to the procedure described by Sonenshine and Yunker (1968); one such procedure is shown in Figure 27. Sonenshine observed that most treated adults produced young and that the degree of labeling was related to the inoculated dose. Differences in degree of tagging of young ticks was related to day of oviposition and to the radiochemical used. An effect of the level of radioactivity in the inoculant was observed, with no hatching of eggs when the label exceeded 637 cpm above background. Field trials (Sonenshine and Clark, 1968) were conducted in Virginia and Montana using larvae of *Dermacentor variabilis* and *D. andersoni*. The labeled larvae were obtained by inoculating the adult female with [^{14}C]glucose or [^{14}C]glycine. *Dermacentor variabilis* larvae, totaling 42,400, were released on the Virginia study area, and *D. andersoni* larvae, totaling 22,500, on the area in Montana. Numerous tagged individuals were gathered from small mammals collected in both areas the first year of study (1966) and from small mammals collected in Virginia the following spring.

6.3. Vertebrates

6.3.1. Fish

Fish-marking is one of the common tools the fisheries biologist uses to study growth, survival, and movement. In addition to marking by mutilation, the biologist uses various types of metal and plastic tags and radio transmitters and has at his disposal various dyes and chemicals suitable for marking, including radionuclides. Arnold (1966) reviewed the literature on use of dyes and chemicals in fish-marking and included critical comments and suggestions for future research. His section on the use of radionuclides was brief because very few applications had been published other than the Russian articles that he cited. Although he did not cite specific literature on use of radionuclides as a fish tag, Seymour (1958) presented an excellent discussion of four questions he raised: "Is the use of radioisotopes practical? What are the hazards in handling radioisotopes? What isotope and what form of the isotope should be used? What are the procedures for obtaining isotopes?" Seymour concluded that tagging by standard methods was more practical and that use of radionuclides at the time he prepared his paper was restricted by law to nonfood fishes. Further, he concluded that hazard to the worker would be negligible provided reasonable care was taken and that the amount of a radionuclide needed would require the researcher to be licensed.

Radionuclides that occur as waste products of nuclear testing, that is, fallout, and those from reactor operations at Hanford have been used as "natural radionuclide tags." Utilizing the fallout radionuclides ^{55}Fe and ^{54}Mn, Forster (1968) studied the migration patterns of salmon in the northwest Pacific. He concluded:

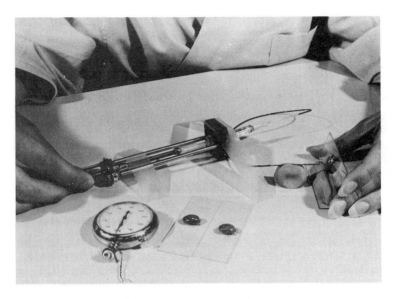

Figure 27. Apparatus for inoculating engorged female ticks. The micrometer drive serves to control the volume and speed of delivery of the inoculum. The tick is secured with double-stick tape; the micropipette is held and oriented with plasticine. From Sonenshine and Yunker (1968).

The chinook and coho salmon, which feed more on smaller fishes than sockeye and migrate more north and south, show this pattern by an inverse relation of Mn^{54} and Fe^{55} specific activities to distance from source. The sockeye salmon show relatively high specific activities for Mn^{54} and Fe^{55} due to a combination of feeding on a lower trophic level and more east–west migration patterns. Those salmon with migration patterns close to the fresh water plume of the Columbia River, a well-known source of Zn^{65}, also reflect these differences in their Zn^{65} and Mn^{54} gamma spectra.

The ^{65}Zn in the Columbia River plume, which is assimilated by coho salmon *(Oncorhynchus kisutch)*, was used as a tag by Loeffel and Forster (1970) in a study of the movement of stocks of this species. Individuals swimming in the coastal waters of Cook Inlet, Alaska, to Oregon accumulate ^{65}Zn to levels at least several times background. The researchers postulated that further study of the change in ^{65}Zn levels should be able to differentiate different stocks of coho salmon and that " . . . most coho salmon originating in northeastern Pacific streams can be separated from Bering Sea fish using levels of ^{65}Zn activity as the identifying mechanism even when captured on the high seas." Their research, however, failed to conclusively establish migratory patterns.

Scott (1961) studied the feasibility of using ^{59}Fe to mark brook trout *(Salvelinus fontinalis)*. A solution of ^{59}Fe was injected through the ventral body wall

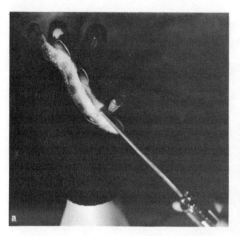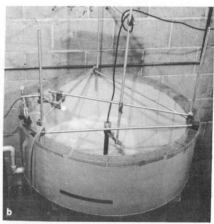

Figure 28. Equipment utilized in a study of the feasibility of using ^{59}Fe to mark brook trout (*Salvelinus fontinalis*). (a) Radioassay of Group I trout, using needle scintillation probe. (b) Constant-geometry tank for radioassay of Group II trout. (c) Relationship between $\log_{10}$ (count rate) and time for Group I trout, from radioassay by the needle scintillation probe over the heart–liver region. Values plotted are geometric means for all fish assayed on each day. From Scott (1961).

of the fish using a 1-ml tuberculin syringe. A needle scintillation probe and a tank with a specialized GM tube placed at the center were used for radioassay (Figure 28a,b). The investigator observed that the biological half-life of ^{59}Fe was probably at least 2 years (Figure 28c), which would be similar to that of ^{55}Fe. ^{59}Fe and ^{55}Fe have physical half-lives of 45.1 days and 2.6 years, respectively, but the latter has the disadvantage of a very weak emission. Scott concluded that ^{55}Fe should provide a suitable lifetime mark for most species of fish and that the method of injection used is useful only for larger fish. Although ^{55}Fe is present in fallout, he believed that this would not be of any serious consequence. For short-term experiments, the investigator preferred the use of ^{59}Fe, since the gamma emissions of this radionuclide make it relatively easy to detect with portable gamma spectrometers. Because most of the iron in a fish is in the blood and thus would be removed when the fish is cleaned and because iron is absorbed from food in relatively small amounts rarely exceeding 10%, there should be no health hazard to man.

Postlarval flounder (*Paralichthys* spp.) were marked either by introduction of stable cobalt followed by neutron activation or by marking with ^{60}Co or ^{144}Ce that was made available in the food or introduced into water occupied by the small fish (Hoss, 1967). The direct use of tracers resulted in satisfactory marking, but the radionuclide obtained from the water was retained longer by the fish than that obtained from the food. Some of Hoss's data on the biological turnover of

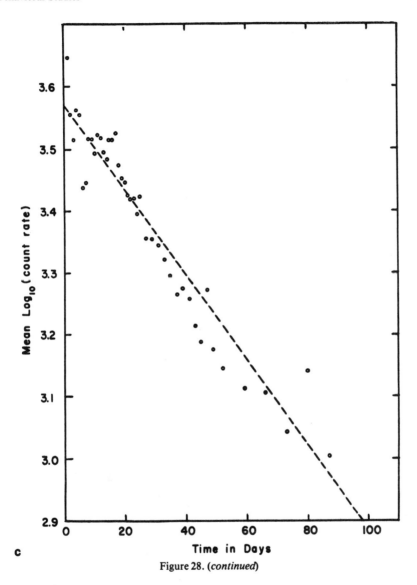

c

Figure 28. (*continued*)

^{60}Co in fish marked by feeding or retention in seawater containing the nuclide are presented in Figure 29 and Table 4. Data from fish marked by retention of ^{144}Ce in seawater are presented in Figure 29a. The studies involving neutron activation of stable cobalt disclosed that no difference existed in cobalt levels of fish containing natural levels from those placed in water containing 0.244 μg cobalt/ml., while a difference was apparent when the level was raised to 15.62 μg cobalt/ml. (Figure 29b,c).

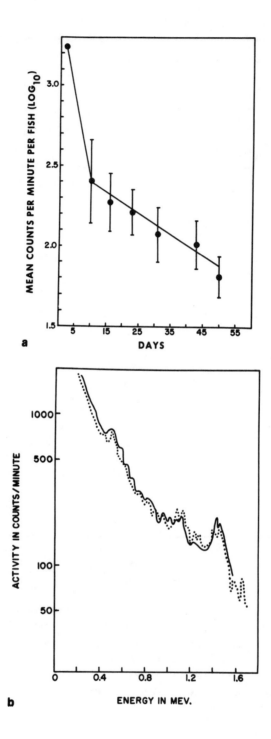

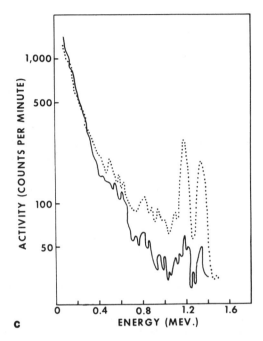

Figure 29. Some results of an investigation of marking paralichthid flounders with radionuclides. (a) Cerium-144 remaining in flounder held in flowing seawater, after they had been marked in seawater containing 1.0 μCi ^{144}Ce/ml. Vertical brackets indicate 1 S.D. (b) Comparison of gamma spectra of flounder containing a "natural" level (—) and an increased level (. . . . .) of cobalt. The level of cobalt in flounder was increased by uptake from water containing 0.244 μg cobalt/ml. (c) Comparison of gamma spectra of flounder containing a "natural" level (—) and an increased level (. . . . .) of cobalt. The level of cobalt in flounder was increased by uptake from water containing 15.62 μg cobalt/ml. From Hoss (1967).

Table 4.   Summary of ^{60}Co Experiments[a]

Expt. No.	Number of fish marked	Average weight (mg)	Method of marking	Concentration of isotope in water (μCi/ml)	Marking time (hr)	Days in flowing sea water	Mean cpm/fish at end of experiment
5	10	54	Water	0.01	48	26	16
6	10	41	Water	1.00	24	62	1086
7	10	79	Food	0.01	48	3	32
8	10	93	Food	1.00	24	55	531

[a] From Hoss (1967).

6.3.2. Amphibians and Reptiles

In recent years, considerable interest has developed in the ecology of amphibians and reptiles, with one aspect of investigation concerning movements above and below ground. Since nearly all these animals spend a considerable amount of time underground, it has been difficult to study movements. In the spring and summer of 1955, Karlstrom (1957) utilized a ^{60}Co tag on the Yosemite toad, *Bufo canorus,* in an attempt to locate toads below the surface of the ground. The tag was made by hollowing a split-shot fishing sinker, filling the cavity with a solution of ^{60}Co, heating the sinker to cause evaporation of the solution and leave ^{60}CoCl$_2$ residue, and crimping it into a flattened form. The exterior of the flattened sinker was filed smooth and covered with four or five coats of plastic to prevent lead and radionuclide poisoning. In the field, the tag was inserted subcutaneously in a 1-cm dorsal incision in the toad. Since ^{60}Co has a relatively long half-life (5.26 years) and relatively high gamma energy, it appeared suitable for the study. Based on a literature review of radiation effects on the frog, *Rana pipiens,* and on other considerations, Karlstrom utilized in the field tags containing 20–30 μCi. Actual experiments concerning radiation sensitivity of this species were not conducted; however, limited observations were made on three California toads *(B. boreas halophilus).* Field detection of the tagged toads was by means of a GM detector* and a scintillometer, with earphones being used in conjunction with the counting system. An experimental 200-μCi tag had a practical surface detection range of approximately 4 ft and from 12 to 15 inches below the surface with a scintillometer. The investigator commented that an 800-μCi experimental tag was detectable at a distance of 17 ft on the surface and 2 ft below the surface. The GM detector was useful if the tag exceeded 40 μCi.

In an investigation on the ecology of the Manitoba toad, *Bufo hemiophrys,* Breckenridge and Tester (1961) conducted movement studies above and below the surface utilizing a wire tag of ^{182}Ta. Radioactive tantalum was selected as an appropriate tag because it has high gamma-ray energy and a relatively short half-life (115 days) and was available in wire form. Using an adapted syringe and needle in which a 1-mm-diameter × 5-mm-long piece of wire (100 μCi ± 50%) was inserted, the investigators tagged the toads with a subcutaneous dorsal implant. Effects of implantaton on 12 toads disclosed no effect on growth. In a few cases, a detrimental physical effect was observed. Using a scintillation counting system, they could detect a tagged animal on the surface at a distance of about 20 ft; an animal with a 4-month-old tag was detected in 22 inches of silty clay loam soil; and a newly tagged individual, in 16 inches of water 4–5 ft away. The tag proved to be highly successful as an aid in locating animals

---

* The terms "detector" and "counter" are commonly interchanged in the literature. Correctly "detector" refers to that portion of the counting system sensing the radiation event while "counter" refers to that portion recording the event.

on the surface. This study of movement during hibernation is unique and, to the best of our knowledge, the first to use a radionuclide tag on an amphibian to study hibernation. When a toad was observed to begin hibernation, thermocouples spaced at 4-inch intervals were placed into the ground 12 inches laterally from the toad, and temperature readings were taken throughout the hibernation period. At another site, a 3-inch-diameter hole 6 ft deep was dug with a soil auger, also 12 inches laterally from the toad. By lowering a probe into the hole to locate maximum radiation readings, the investigators determined the position of the toad during the hibernation period. Figure 30 illustrates some of the results. It is interesting to note that the toad moved vertically during the hibernation period.

Shoop and his associates applied radioactive tags to salamanders to study movement. An 18-gauge wire (3–5 mm long) of ^{182}Ta (20–48 μCi) was inserted into the abdomen of the salamander, *Plethodon jordani,* in a field study in North Carolina (Madison and Shoop, 1970). In the field, these tagged individuals could be located at a distance of about 2 m with a scintillometer. In another study (Shoop and Doty, 1972), a 10-μCi ^{182}Ta tag was inserted into the dorsal tail musculature of the marbled salamander *(Ambystoma opacum)*, and the animals were released in a Rhode Island study area. Placing newly hatched ambystomatid salamander larvae in a solution of pondwater and ^{24}NaCl (half-life 15 hr) for 4 hr, Shoop (1971) successfully tagged the larvae. The detection of these larvae under field conditions was extremely successful, although the tag was not detectable after 3 days. In a comparison with nontagged controls, the investigator observed no significant differences in mortality.

Dispersal of three species of snakes from a hibernaculum in Utah was observed by Hirth *et al.* (1969), who used a 400-μCi ^{182}Ta tag. The wire tag was inserted beneath the skin in the ventral basal tail segment, using the procedure of Breckenridge and Tester (1961). A total of 196 snakes were tagged after emergence. Tagged snakes could be detected at a distance of 9 m on the surface and 30 cm below the surface at a distance of 3 m. Radiation-produced necrosis was observed on some of the snakes.

6.3.3. Birds

The use of radionuclide tagging in investigations of bird behavior has been relatively limited when contrasted with studies involving mammals. Griffin (1952) attached small capsules containing ^{65}Zn to leg bands on semipalmated plovers *(Charadrius semipalmatus)* to study nest attentiveness. Tester (1963) reported on a study by the Canadian Wildlife Service to investigate nest attentiveness of mallards *(Anas platyrhynchos)* by using ^{90}Sr and a GM tube positioned on opposite sides of nests. Further, Tester reported that blue grouse *(Dendragapus obscurus)* were labeled with 500 μCi ^{86}Rb attached to a standard patagial wing

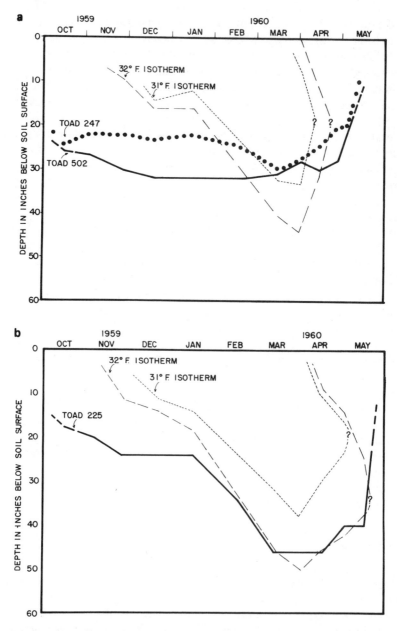

Figure 30. Hibernation movements of the Manitoba toad *(Bufo hemiophrys)* determined with a [182]Ta tag. (a) Relationships between depths of wintering toads 247 and 502 (sites were 8 ft apart) and positions of 31 and 32°F isotherms in the soil. (b) Relationships between depth of wintering toad 225 and positions of 31 and 32°F isotherms in the soil. (c) Relationships between depth of wintering

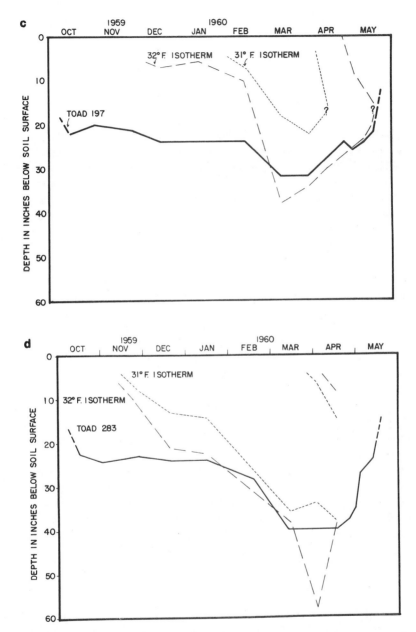

toad 197 and positions of 31 and 32°F isotherms in the soil. (d) Relationships between depth of wintering toad 283 and positions of 31 and 32°F isotherms in the soil. From Breckenridge and Tester (1961).

band by researchers at the University of British Columbia in an unsuccessful attempt to track the birds. In addition, Wilkinson (1950) developed a device utilizing polonium to measure the length of time a bird was in flight. The device incorporated a steel ball that, when the bird's wings were folded, mechanically shielded a photographic film from alpha rays from the polonium source; when the wings were in motion, the steel ball moved and the film was exposed. The time of flight was then correlated with the degree of exposure. Ward (1967, 1968) used ^{182}Ta sheathed in platinum attached to aluminum bird bands that were fastened to the carmine bee eater *(Merops nubicoides)* and the white-flanked flycatcher *(Batis molitor)*; frequency of nest visits was recorded by a radiation detector attached to a portable rate meter and recorder. Storteir and Palmgren (1971) studied the daily activity pattern of the black guillemot *(Cepphus grylle)* during the breeding season by placing a radioactive tag on the adult bird, which permitted recording the incubating rhythm and feeding frequency. When the reactors were operating at Hanford, waterfowl on the Columbia River within and below the reservation accumulated radionuclides released into the river from reactor effluent. By means of this onsite "natural" tagging with ^{65}Zn and ^{32}P, Hanson and Case (1963) studied waterfowl dispersion from the vicinity of Hanford. Basically, the procedure included collection of duck heads offsite and onsite followed by a scan for ^{65}Zn and an analysis for ^{32}P. During the 1960–1961 hunting season, ^{32}P was detected in 41% of 601 waterfowl collected offsite within a radius of 50 miles from Hanford (Figure 31). In addition, seasonal fluctuation of tagging incidence indicated the arrival of unmarked migrants. Extending the findings of Hanson and Case, investigators in Colorado (Glover *et al.* 1967) scanned 6594 mallard wings for ^{65}Zn that would have been obtained at Hanford, in order to study the movement of the mallard duck between the Pacific and Central Waterfowl Flyways. Only ducks shot in Oregon and Washington contained significant amounts of ^{65}Zn. McCabe and LePage (1958) indirectly labeled young birds by implanting calcium phosphate pellets containing ^{45}Ca in the breast muscle of the ring-necked pheasant *(Phasianus colchicus)* hen prior to nesting. Some radioactive calcium passed to the eggs and consequently was detectable in the leg bones of juvenile pheasants that hatched from these eggs. The leg bones of birds killed by hunters were collected and analyzed for ^{45}Ca to determine the contribution of labeled hens to the fall population.

6.3.4. Mammals

Of all behavioral studies of vertebrates, those of small mammals have shown the widest use of radionuclide tagging. Perhaps this is the result of the relatively small home range of these mammals as well as the interest of population ecologists in interpreting the population dynamics of this group. Gerrard (1969) reported 36 studies that utilized external or subcutaneous radionuclide marking

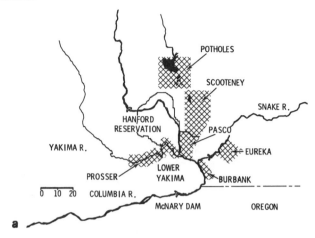

ALL WATERFOWL - ALL LOCATIONS

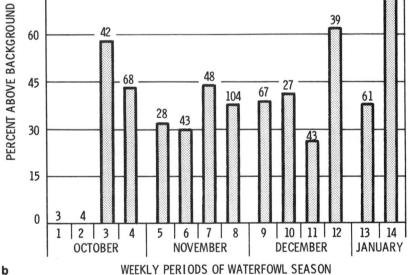

Figure 31. Dispersion of waterfowl naturally tagged with ^{32}P and ^{65}Zn. (a) Major areas of sport hunting from which samples were obtained, Hanford environs, State of Washington. (b) Percentage of waterfowl heads collected at weekly intervals during the 1960–1961 waterfowl hunting season in the Hanford environs that contained measurable amounts of ^{32}P and ^{65}Zn. The number of heads examined is at the top of each bar. From Hanson and Case (1963).

Table 5. Summary of Characteristics of Some Radioactive Isotopes Used or Suggested for Use in Tracing Mammals[a]

Isotope	Half-life	Main γ energies (MeV)	Specific γ-ray constant (R/mCi/hr at 1 cm)	Dose rate at 1 m from 1 Ci (rads/hr in tissue)	β Rays[b]	Other radiations[c]	Toxicity (IAEA classification)[d]	Used or suggested by[d]	Remarks
Antimony-124	60 days	0.6, 1.69	9.8	0.94	+ + + +	−	Medium upper	Punt and van Nieuwenhoven (1957)	Used in capsules on rings.
Bromine-82	35.4 hr	0.55, 0.78	14.6	1.40	+ + + +	−	Medium lower	Griffin (1952)	Suggested only.
Calcium-45	165 days	None	—	—	+ + + + (0.245 MeV)	−	Medium upper	Twigg and Miller (1963), Rongstad (1965), Meslow and Keith (1968)	Implanted in absorbable form by Rongstad and by Meslow and Keith. Fed in bait by Twigg and Miller.
Carbon-14	5760 yr	None	—	—	+ + + + (0.159 MeV)	−	Medium lower	Soldatkin (1961)	Fed to animals
Chromium-51	27.8 days	0.323	0.16	0.015	−	+	Medium lower	Michielsen (personal communication), Myllymäki et al. (1971)	Leg ring. Fed in bait.
Cobalt-60	5.25 yr	1.17, 1.33	13.2	1.27	+ + + +	−	Medium upper	Godfrey (1953 et seq.), Linn and Shillito (1960), Barbour (1963), Hamar et al. (1964)	Barbour implanted Co alloy wire, gave no comment on biological activity. Otherwise used in capsules on rings, or implanted.
Gold-198	2.7 days	0.412	2.3	0.22	+ + + +	+	Medium lower	Kaye (1960), Cope et al. (1961)	Implanted by Kaye, biologically inert. Used on rings by Cope et al.
Iodine-131	8.04 days	0.36	2.2	0.21	+ + + +	+	Medium upper	Gifford and Griffin (1960), Johanningsmeier and Goodnight (1962), Gentry (1971), Myllymäki et al.	Injected in two inert forms by Bailey et al.; some biological activity, not toxic. Radioactive paint tried by Bailey et al. not successful. Otherwise used in capsules on rings, or implanted.

Radionuclide	Half-life	γ energies (MeV)	γ-ray constant		β rays	Toxicity	Persistence	References	Use
Iron-59	45 days	1.1, 1.29	6.4	0.61	++++	−	Medium lower	Griffin (1952), Gentry (1971)	Fed in bait.
Lanthanum-140	40.2 hr	0.49, 1.6	11.3	1.1	++++	−	Medium lower	Griffin (1952)	Suggested only.
Phosphorus-32	14.3 days	None	—	—	++++ (1.71 MeV)	−	Medium lower	Jenkins (1954), Miller (1957), Hamar et al. (1963), Rudenchik (1963), Shura-Bura et al. (1960), Stoddart (1970), and many others	Injected or fed to animals; biologically active, nontoxic.
Selenium-75	121 days	0.14, 0.27, 0.28	2.0	0.19	–	+	Medium lower	Frigerio and Eisler (1968)	Incorporated into epoxy resin for tag or implant.
Silver-110m	253 days	0.66, 0.89	14.3	1.37	++++	+	Medium upper	Michielsen (in Linn and Shillito, 1960)	Whole leg ring made radioactive.
Sodium-22	2.6 yr	0.51, 1.28	12.0	1.15	++++ (0.54 MeV)	+	Medium upper	Frigerio and Eisler (1968)	Suggested only, for incorporation into epoxy resin for tag or implant.
Strontium-89	51 days	0.91 (very few)	—	—	++++ (1.46 MeV)	−	Medium upper	Shura-Bura and Kharlamov (1961)	Injected or fed to animals; no information about toxicity.
Strontium-90	28 yr	None	—	—	++++ (0.54 MeV)	−	High	Soviet workers (see Kulik, 1967)	Used for ectoparasite work.
Sulphur-35	87.2 days	None	—	—	++++ (0.167 MeV)	−	Medium lower	Rudenchik et al. (1967), Korneyev (1967a,b)	Fed or injected.
Tantalum-182	115 days	0.068, 1.12, 1.22	6.8	0.64	++++	+	Medium upper	Graham and Ambrose (1967)	Implanted, biologically inert.
Zinc-65	245 days	1.11	2.7	0.26	+	+	Medium lower	Griffin (1952), Gentry (1971), Nellis et al. (1967)	Used in capsules on rings on birds, fed in bait. Used as feces tag, fed, or injected.

[a] From G. N. A. Bailey et al. (1973). Physical data of radionuclides are from *The Radiochemical Manual*, 2nd ed., 1966 The Radiochemical Center, Amersham, England. The half-life gives an indication of persistence; γ energies and γ-ray constant give data that are related to strength of γ emission and therefore to ease of detection; dose rate, presence of β rays, presence of other radiations, and toxicity are all important when considering the possibility of tissue damage.

[b] Each + indicates that β rays are emitted by up to 25% of disintegrations (i.e., + + + + = 75–100% of disintegrations emit β rays).

[c] Other emissions (e.g., X-rays) were not quantified; only their presence (+) or absence (−) was recorded.

[d] See source for references.

of small vertebrates and invertebrates. Although the literature citation for small mammals was adequate, only three references were cited for invertebrates. Small-mammal ecologists interested in the application of radionuclide marking are fortunate in having available the excellent review of G. N. A. Bailey *et al.* (1973). Their review was concerned with the development of the technique and use of ^{131}I as a tag for small mammals. The review included 80 citations and an excellent table (Table 5) summarizing the characteristics of some radionuclides, citations on their use, and comments on how the animal was marked. The salient techniques covered in the literature review were inert implants, external tags, physiological tagging, and special techniques. The authors also suggested injection of ^{131}I in an inert form and external attachment of Ag^{131}Iodide either as paint placed on dorsal neck fur or enclosed in a thin-walled tube attached to a leg band. In a discussion of the use of ^{131}I, the authors concluded that the leg-band procedure was satisfactory and that other procedures were less satisfactory for various reasons.

It is impossible for us to improve on this review; however, to maintain continuity in our presentation, we have selected some references to illustrate the diverse nature of small-mammal tagging applications. It is obvious that selection of the appropriate radionuclide for a specific study is determined by characteristics already discussed in this chapter, e.g., physical and biological half-life, high-energy gamma emissions and low beta emissions, characteristics of the animal being studied, and the detection equipment available.

Let us first consider the most commonly used tagging method, use of an external tag. Godfrey (1953) developed a technique for locating nests of *Microtus agrestis* in which he live-trapped pregnant females, attached leg bands containing ^{60}Co, released the vole into the study area, and located them in the nest with GM equipment. In a study of shrews, Linn and Shillito (1960) modified Godfrey's tag of 100 μCi ^{60}Co to 50 μCi. Rather than embed the radionuclide in plaster of Paris in a brass tube that had been soldered to the leg band, they used a 1-mm stable cobalt rod inserted into a nickel tube that was activated to produce ^{60}Co. They stated that the nickel tube and solder used to attach it to the leg band shielded the animal from beta radiation, but did not serve as a barrier for the gamma radiation. Michielsen's use of a silver band irradiated to produce ^{110m}Ag was discussed by them. Selenium-75, which has a half-life of 120.4 days, has the desirable property of being a gamma emitter that decays by electron capture rather than emitting charged particles, thus minimizing dose to the skin; use of ^{75}Se has been discussed by Frigerio and Eisler (1968), who developed an automatic monitor of nest and burrow activity. They suggested the use of ^{22}Na (half-life 2.602 years) as an alternative to ^{75}Se when larger animals or longer observation periods are desirable. Both radionuclides can be attached to bands with epoxy resin.

In addition to use of radioactive bands, the technique of insertion of radioactive wire subcutaneously in a small mammal has been developed. Gold-198 wire inserted subcutaneously in the lower abdominal region with the hypodermic procedure previously discussed was used as a tag in a study of movements of the eastern harvest mouse *(Reithrodontomys humulis humulis)* by Kaye (1960, 1961). This radionuclide was selected because it has a relatively short half-life (2.693 days) and a gamma energy adequate for the study. The tag activity varied from 0.7 to 4.5 μCi, with the former being detectable at a maximum distance of 9 ft with a GM counter and remaining detectable for 1 week. The 4.5-μCi tag could be detected at 20 ft, but the high activity prevented accurate location of the animal, since it exceeded the capacity of the monitoring equipment. Figure 32 illustrates the monitoring equipment and its use in the field; Figure 33 illustrates the large number of observations attainable in a relatively short period of time, an impossible task if live traps were used, which would, in addition, disturb the animals. Johanningsmeier and Goodnight (1962), in a study of the meadow vole, *Microtus pennsylvanicus,* used [131]I (0.5 μCi; half-life 8.070 days) as the tag introduced by the subcutaneous hypodermic procedure; however, rather than inserting the radioactive material directly under the skin, they first placed it in a polyethylene capsule. Utilizing a GM counter arrangement similar to Kaye's, they were able to track a tagged animal for as long as 2 weeks.

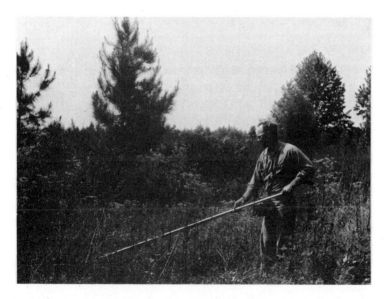

Figure 32. S. V. Kaye demonstrating the use of detection equipment in a study of movements of harvest mice *(Reithrodontomys humulis humulis)* tagged with [198]Au. Courtesy of S. V. Kaye.

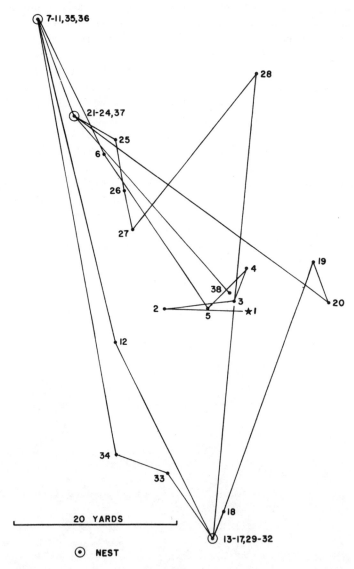

Figure 33. Movements of harvest mouse *(Reithrodontomys humulis humulis)* No. 1, tagged with [198]Au, between August 27 and September 1, 1958.(★) Point of initial release. From Kaye (1961).

Various types of radioactive tagging procedures have been developed for studying bats. Punt and van Nieuwenhoven (1957), in an attempt to locate bats in caves in The Netherlands, utilized a numbered aluminum band with one end lengthened and folded over a rod of ^{124}Sb (half-life 60.3 days); C. E. Gifford and Griffin (1960) evaporated a solution of ^{131}I in the fold of a metal band used to locate bats in caves; Cope et al. (1961) evaporated a solution of ^{198}Au placed on the inner surface of U.S. Fish and Wildlife Service numbered aluminum bands and used these bands to locate bats in rafters and brick walls; Davis et al. (1968) used a ^{60}Co wire injected beneath the skin of the forearms of bats in their study of colonial behavior.

In Section 6.3.2, we discussed the procedure of Breckenridge and Tester (1961) in studying the movement of toads beneath the ground surface by lowering a probe periodically into a vertical hole and noting the depth at which the maximum reading was attained. Kenagy and Smith (1970, 1973) developed an interesting procedure involving a radioactive tag and applied the principle of gamma-ray attenuation in soil to study the depth of heteromyid rodents in their burrows. They investigated the gamma-ray attenuation by burying ^{60}Co, ^{24}Na, ^{64}Cu, and ^{198}Au to depths ranging to 1 m in various soils, concluding that accurate determination of the depth of the source was possible. They presented a model of gamma-ray attenuation for different soils and radionuclides. Of particular interest to an ecologist is their use of the technique with ^{198}Au in a study of kangaroo rats (Dipodomys microps and D. merriami) and a pocket mouse (Perognathus longimembris) in burrows as related to burrow temperature. Some of the characteristics of ^{198}Au detection pertinent to the study are illustrated in Figure 34.

An automatic monitoring procedure more elaborate than that proposed by Frigerio and Eisler (1968) was described by Graham and Ambrose (1967) for continuous monitoring of the meadow vole in a field enclosure that contained a scintillation probe mounted on a rotating boom with a recording ratemeter (Figure 35a,b). Tantalum-182 wire (50–75 μCi) was placed subcutaneously in a vole, the vole was released into the enclosure, and the monitoring device was activated. An example of the records obtained is presented in Figure 35c. The investigators concluded that they could locate a resting animal within 1 ft; however, if the animal moved when the boom passed over it, a skewed peak resulted and there was loss of accuracy in locating the animal.

Investigators utilizing radioactive tags should be concerned with possible biological damage to the organism, and they often comment in their papers on this matter, e.g., on the desirability of shielding the animal. Two papers of interest on this subject are those by Barbour and Harvey (1968) and Cosgrove et al. (1969). The former conducted a comparative laboratory study of the behavior of tagged and nontagged small rodents (Microtus ochrogaster and Baiomys taylori). Animals containing a subcutaneously implanted tag of ^{60}Co

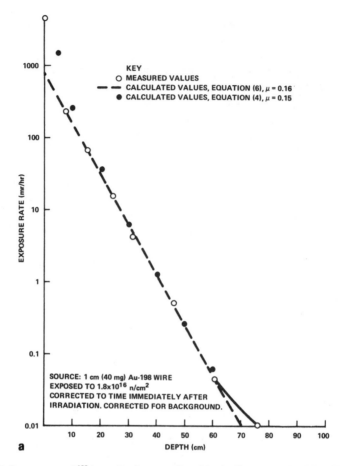

Figure 34. Some aspects of ^{198}Au application to studies of depth of burrows and activity of heteromyid rodents. (a) Sensitivity of ^{198}Au detection in soil. (b) Resolution of ^{198}Au detection in soil. (c) Model for measurement of a line source in soil. (ℓ) Length of line source; (d) depth of source; (h) horizontal distance of point (p) from a point on surface directly above source. From Kenagy and Smith (1970).

wire (55 μCi) did not have a behavior pattern significantly different from that of those not tagged. Cosgrove *et al.* (1969) observed malignant tumors associated with dorsal, interscapular subcutaneously implanted ^{60}Co wire tags in three long-tailed deer mice *(Peromyscus maniculatus)*. These wires were encapsulated in nylon to shield the animal from beta radiation. At 10 months after implant, a tumor developed at the site of the implant in one mouse (Figure 36). Another mouse died 15 months after implant without a tumor present, but there was a whitening of the fur over the wire site. The remaining mouse developed a tumor

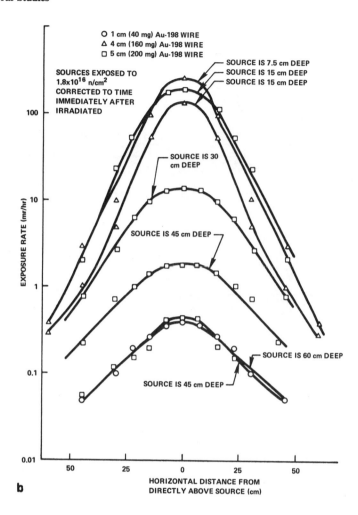

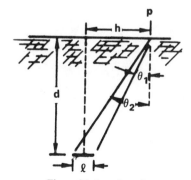

Figure 34. (*continued*)

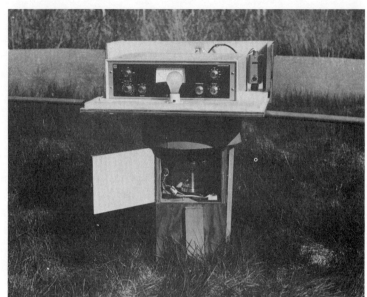

a

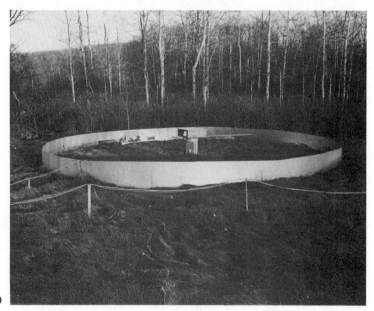

b

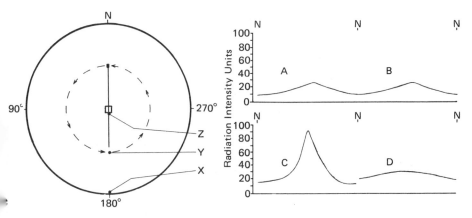

Figure 35. Facilities utilized in a study of activity patterns of the meadow vole *(Microtus pennsylvanicus)* marked with a ^{182}Ta wire. (a) Enclosure with detection unit. The probe is on the end of the boom, which rotates once each 6 min. (b) A log/linear ratemeter housed in an insulated box (cover removed for photograph). The stationary base contains the motor, the "commutator," and a cam-operated microswitch. (c) Position and motion of the boom in the enclosure (a); the three positions used to calibrate each radioactive vole are X, Y, and Z. The records that result from a vole's being present in these three positions are shown at the right: (A, B) from position X; (C) from position Y; (D) from position Z. (a–c) From Graham and Ambrose (1967). (a, b) Photographs courtesy of F. C. Evans.

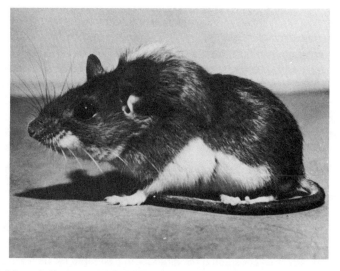

Figure 36. Mouse 1. *Peromyscus maniculatus* showing dorsal tumor. Note the white fur overlying the ^{60}Co wire. From Cosgrove *et al.* (1969).

at the initial wire site 20 months after implant. The tag had moved to the left side of the animal during this period. A necropsy of each tumor was conducted, described, and photomicrographed. The authors concluded:

> In our mouse 1, the tumor and the radioactive wire coincided anatomically, but a cause and effect relation is not provable. In our mouse 3, the wire was immediately adjacent to the tumor. We have held a few untagged *P. maniculatus* in our colony for periods of from 1 to 4 years and have observed no tumors in these to date. However, we do not know the expected incidence and types of tumors in aged *P. maniculatus*. Nevertheless, in view of the hematologic effects and tumors present in the tagged animals, we suggest that caution be exercised in interpreting data from animals containing radioactive tags for long periods of time.

Dose data were not available from the mouse lacking a tumor; however, dosimetry of wires removed from the mice containing tumors revealed an exposure contact of approximately 2 R/day for mouse 1 and approximately 15.7 R/day for the other mouse.

Physiological labeling can be accomplished either by direct injection of a radionuclide into the body of an animal or by utilizing, in the laboratory or field, bait labeled with a radionuclide. The direct method relies on the ability of the investigator to capture an animal, and there is the uncertainty that the animal is representative of the population of interest. The bait procedure does not require initial capture, but here again the question is whether or not the animal is representative of the population under study. Both methods require another capture of the animal if a mark–recapture estimate of the population is desired, including the various assumptions inherent in the method of estimation. If the objectives of a study involve movement of a mammal, one might collect feces to see whether they contain the tag, rather than capture the live animal.

In a grassland habitat in southern Finland, Myllymäki *et al.* (1971) utilized apples labeled with ^{32}P, ^{51}Cr, and ^{131}I as bait in an attempt to mark the small mammal *Microtus agrestis*. The experimental design included establishment of trapping grids on which trapping was conducted for 8 days. The central trapping grid was surrounded by belts in which the different tagged baits were placed. These belts were separated by a bait-free zone that was 5 m wide. Prebaiting, not conducted on the central grid prior to trapping this grid, was commenced 1 day after baiting with labeled apples. The primary objective of the study was to investigate the behavioral characteristics of various components of the population and to utilize these data to improve the population estimate. The available detection equipment and the radionuclide cost restricted the choice of radionuclide labels. Individuals marked with ^{32}P were detectable when whole-body counts were made, but the marked feces were, in general, almost undetectable; thus, the investigators considered the radionuclide suitable for their purpose. The detection of ^{32}P was done in the field, after which, in the laboratory, the investigators inspected the spleen—which is rich in red blood cells containing protein-bound chromium—for ^{51}Cr and the thyroid—which concentrates iodine—for ^{131}I. The rate of removal of the unmarked and marked animals classed as juveniles and subadults and of those in the additional classifications of reproductive status, was studied. Referring to these data, the investigators, in addition to other comments, stated:

> 1). The rate of removal of unmarked "sedentary" insiders is most rapid for the reproductive males, then for the reproductive females, the non-reproductive subadults and juveniles, being the slowest. 2). The contribution of invaders, e.g., isotope-labelled individuals, is much greater in reproductive males than in reproductive females. . . . the percentage of invading subadults (all males) is slightly higher than that of reproductive males. The rate of invasion of juveniles is clearly lower than that of other groups. . . . 3). The great agility of reproductive males and subadults (males), compared with females and juveniles, is illustrated by the higher proportion of long-distance (I-131 and Cr-51 marked) invaders in the former groups than in the latter.

The results showed a "remarkable edge effect" on the total catch, and this was due mainly to invasion by individuals outside the trapping grid.

In another study wherein the major objective was the investigation of movement of small mammals as related to removal trapping, Gentry et al. (1971) established a trapping grid in a lowland hardwood forest in South Carolina on which prebaiting with radioactive peanut butter was conducted for 5 days prior to trapping. The peanut butter was labeled with either ^{59}Fe, ^{65}Zn, or ^{131}I, with the baits assigned to an inner square grid, concentric middle band, and concentric outer band, respectively (Figure 37a). After 5 days of prebaiting, investigators removed the bait and commenced trapping, utilizing untagged peanut butter as bait on the inner square, which had been baited previously with the ^{59}Fe- and ^{65}Zn-labeled peanut butter. Trapping continued for 36 consecutive days on this area, while trapping commenced on day 18 on the remaining areas, which had been prebaited with ^{131}I-labeled peanut butter. All animals captured were scanned for the three isotopes in a multichannel pulse-height analyzer (Table 6). As a result of the satisfactory biological half-lives of the selected radionuclides, the tagged animals could be detected for a reasonable period. For example, the short-tailed shrew (Blarina brevicauda) labeled with either ^{65}Zn or ^{131}I was detected on days 21, 25, 30, 36. The investigators commented that the tags could be detected for longer periods than those reported for tags of basic fuchsin dye or colored wool, which are eliminated from the digestive tract more rapidly; e.g., the dye may be present for 8 days and the colored wool for 6 days. Of the animals captured on the inner grid, which had been prebaited with ^{59}Fe- and ^{65}Zn-labeled peanut butter, 36% contained two isotopes and 9% none. Of the animals captured in the outer concentric band, which had been baited with ^{131}I-labeled peanut butter, 63% contained one isotope (mostly ^{131}I) and 32%, none.

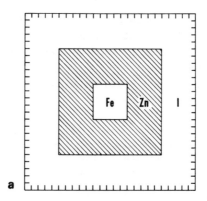

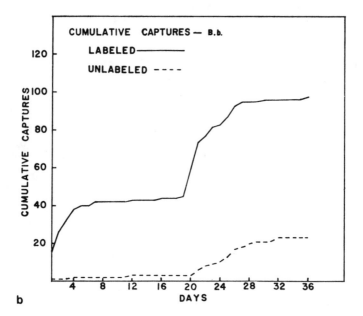

The use of different radionuclides permitted observation of different segments of the population at the same time. The experimental design differed from that of the previous investigators, since Gentry and his associates prebaited the primary trapping grid and also placed labeled bait in this grid; there was no buffer zone between study zones; and labeled baiting was discontinued prior to trapping. Some of the results are illustrated in Figure 37b,c.

Both projects discussed above involved the capture of tagged and nontagged animals in the population to see whether the animals had been marked as a result of consuming the bait. Other studies of movement of small animals involve the

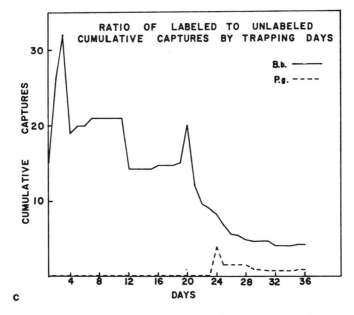

Figure 37. Experimental grid and a portion of the results of a study of radionuclide-tagged small-mammal populations. (a) Diagram of the experimental 26 × 26 [14.1 hectare (ha)] grid. The areas prebaited with a given isotope are listed. (^{59}Fe) 36-station grid (0.6 ha); (^{65}Zn) 220-station concentric band (4.5 ha); (^{131}I) 420-station concentric outer band (9.0 ha). (b) Cumulative captures of labeled and unlabeled *Blarina brevicauda* (B.b.) over the total 36 days of trapping. The outer concentric band of the 26 × 26 grid was trapped only during the last 18 days (days 19–36). The isotopes used for labeling were ^{59}Fe, ^{65}Zn, and ^{131}I. (c) Ratio of labeled to unlabeled cumulative captures of *Blarina brevicauda* (B.b.) and *Peromyscus gossypinus* (P.g.) by trapping days. The middle 16 × 16 grid was trapped for the entire 36 days, while the surrounding concentric band was trapped for the last 18 days (days 19–36). The isotopes used for labeling were ^{59}Fe, ^{65}Zn, and ^{131}I. From Gentry *et al.* (1971).

Table 6. Number of Isotopes Detected in the Bodies of Small Mammals Removed from the Middle 16 × 16 Grid and the Outer Band[a]

Area	Species	Number of isotopes			
		0	1	2	3
Middle	*Blarina brevicauda*	3	27	19	1
16 × 16 grid	*Peromyscus gossypinus*	0	1	0	0
	Microtus pinetorum	2	2	0	0
	Ochrotomys nuttalli	0	0	1	0
Outer	*Blarina brevicauda*	20	46	3	0
band	*Peromyscus gossypinus*	8	5	0	0
	Microtus pinetorum	1	4	1	0
	Ochrotomys nuttalli	1	3	0	0

[a] From Gentry *et al.* (1971).

radionuclide tagging of an animal and determination of whether or not feces collected in the study area contained the radionuclide. Miller (1957) injected the meadow vole *(Microtus pennsylvanicus)* with ^{32}P and detected animal movement by the presence of the radionuclide in feces collected throughout the study area. Since the study area was adjacent to a residential area and because ^{32}P was relatively safe, this radionuclide was chosen as an appropriate tag. Further, subcutaneous injection of 200 μCi ^{32}P was used in preference to feeding labeled bait to the animal, since the injected material had a longer biological half-life. At 2 weeks after injection of the mouse, ^{32}P could still be detected in a sample of five fresh droppings at a distance of 5 cm with a GM survey meter. The short detection distance makes it impractical to survey feces over a large area; consequently, defecation sheets of aluminum (4 × 4 inches) were placed in a grid pattern. One rodent was selected from a sample of eight caught in the center of the 1-acre study area, tagged, and released where captured. A field-survey meter was used to establish the background radiation associated with the defecation squares and was followed by periodic checking of the squares for counts above background that could be due to tagged feces or urine or both. Difficulties with the detection procedure are discussed in detail by the investigator.

In a feces-tagging study of larger mammals, Nellis *et al.* (1967) fed or injected animals with 2 μCi ^{65}Zn (half-life 243.6 days) per kg body wt. The animals studied were "rabbit," "bobcat," "fox," and "opossum." The time in days that the ^{65}Zn was detectable in the feces was about 1 year if the radionuclide was injected into the animal; for animals that were fed an aqueous solution of 10 μCi, this period was, in general, on the order of 1 month (Table 7).

A very interesting study of the home-range length of the water vole *(Arvicola*

Table 7. Detectability Time of ^{65}Zn by Two Methods of Administration[a]

Animal	Method of administration[b]	Amount (μCi)	Time detectable in feces (days)
Rabbit 1	Injected (i.m.)	6	300+
Rabbit 2	Injected (i.m.)	6	300+
Bobcat 1	Fed	80	400+
Bobcat 2	Fed	10	35
Bobcat 4	Injected (i.p.)	10	400+
Fox 1	Fed	10	30
Fox 2	Injected (i.p.)	10	300
Opossum 1	Fed	36	180
Opossum 2	Fed	10	35
Opossum 3	Fed	10	140+
Opossum 4	Injected (i.p.)	10	300

[a] From Nellis *et al.* (1967).
[b] (i.m.) Intramuscularly; (i.p.) intraperitoneally.

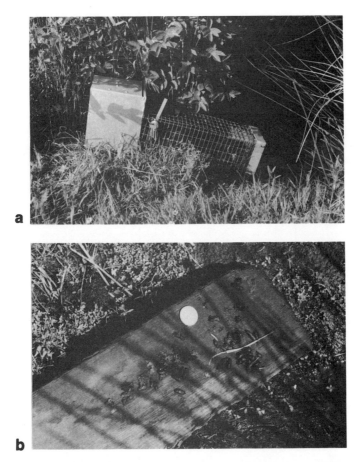

Figure 38. Movement of water voles *(Arvicola terrestris)* as determined with a ^{32}P tag. (a) Water vole trap. (b) A water vole latrine at station II, July 1968. The sixpenny piece (diameter 19.5 mm) gives an idea of scale. From Stoddart (1970). Courtesy of the British Ecological Society.

terrestris) was conducted by Stoddart (1970) in Scotland in which he compared the home-range length obtained by conventional capture–recapture procedures with that obtained by using a radionuclide feces tag. The mammal was trapped and tagged by subcutaneous injection of 20 μCi ^{32}P, and the tagged feces on defecation boards were located by use of a GM survey meter (Figure 38). The rate of ^{32}P excretion and a comparison of the length of home range estimated by the tagged feces and capture–recapture techniques are given in Figure 39. Stoddart observed that range lengths estimated by the capture–recapture procedure are shorter than those estimated by the tagged-feces method. Figure 39 shows how quickly the length can be estimated by the tagged-feces method,

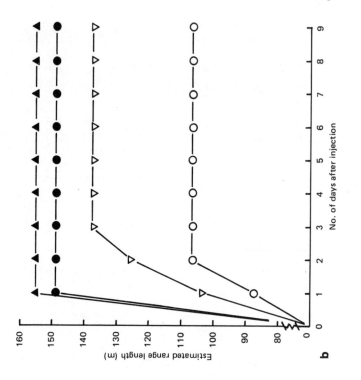

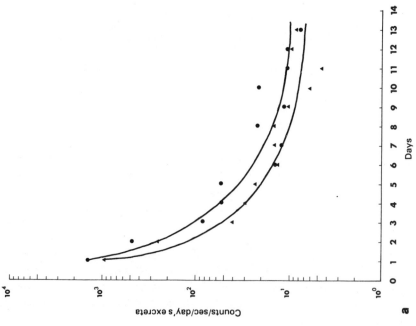

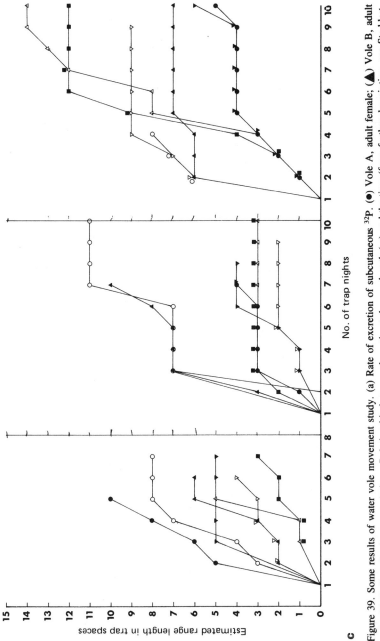

Figure 39. Some results of water vole movement study. (a) Rate of excretion of subcutaneous ^{32}P. (●) Vole A, adult male; (▲) Vole B, adult male. (b) Radioactive-isotope technique: Relationship between the estimated range length (m) and the time (for a further description, see Stoddart, 1970). (○) H24; (▽) O63; (▲) 144; (●) O76. (c) Capture–recapture technique: Relationship between the estimated range length (in trap spaces) and time (trap nights). (a) Linear-threes trapping system; (b) clumped threes; (c) clumped fives (for a further description, see Stoddart, 1970). (●) 144; (○) 073; (▲) 076; (▼) 098; (▽) 063; (■) 139. From Stoddart (1970). Courtesy of the British Ecological Society.

about 3 days. Concerning the use of the ^{32}P-labeled-feces method in determining home-range length, he commented that a disadvantage was that only one animal could be observed at a time and that 14 days would have to elapse after injection before another could be tagged and studied. He did not observe any deleterious effect due to the injection of ^{32}P in his animals. It was suggested that the most serious error could be due to the use of defecation boards not placed to reflect the true range boundaries.

Let us now consider a method of physiological tagging that involves introduction of a radionuclide into an adult female with transmission of the radionuclide to her young during pregnancy. Such tagging of young permits assignment of individuals to marked females. This technique, used by McCabe and LePage (1958) to label young pheasants, was described in Section 6.3.3. The usefulness of a radionuclide in this technique depends on the biological and physical half-lives of the radionuclide, its energy level, and the site of incorporation within the organism. Since calcium is an essential element and a "bone-seeker," it appeared that an isotope of this element would be suitable; thus, ^{45}Ca, a soft beta emitter with a physical half-life of 165 days, was utilized.

One study using this radionuclide was made by Twigg and Miller (1963), who fed crushed wheat containing 3.92 μCi ^{45}Ca to adult male and female brown rats *(Rattus norvegicus)*. Periodically, adults and young were sacrificed and skeletal parts were ashed and counted. All tested parts of the skeleton of tagged individuals contained counts at least 4 times background 113 days after ingestion of the labeled bait. Offspring of females tagged during the last week of pregnancy were identifiable for 10 weeks. The investigators concluded that the method was effective in marking adult females and their offspring.

Rongstad (1965) successfully labeled with ^{45}Ca the young of cottontail rabbits *(Sylvilagus floridanus)*, snowshoe hares *(Lepus americanus)*, and thirteen-lined ground squirrels *(Citellus tridecemlineatus)*. He used a technique similar to that of McCabe and LePage (1958) for marking adult females. Calcium-45-labeled calcium oxalate was mixed with vegetable shortening to delay release of the radionuclide, and this mixture was placed in gelatin capsules. In all three species, the capsule was inserted beneath the skin in the middle of the animal's back. Detection of the radionuclide in bone was accomplished by cleaning, ashing the bone, and then counting. At times, impacted capsules were observed (Figure 40); at other times, none was detected. Rongstad discusses in considerable detail his methods and observations including distribution of ^{45}Ca in the skeleton and turnover rates (Figure 41). A very interesting result of his efforts was that following an initial implant, more than one litter of cottontail rabbits would be labeled and the degree was a function of capsule strength and of the specific bone counted (Table 8). He also observed that there was a small carryover of ^{45}Ca in marked adults and that the first litters were detectable until 2 weeks past weaning. It is desirable in some population studies not to sacrifice the captured

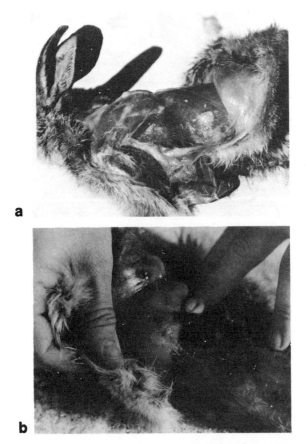

Figure 40. Calcium-45 labeling of cottontail rabbits *(Sylvilagus floridanus.)* (a) Remains of capsule 42 days after implant. (b) Remains of capsule 208 days after implant. From Rongstad (1965). Reproduced from *Health Physics* **11**:1543–1556 (1965) by permission of the Health Physics Society.

animals; therefore, Rongstad removed one toe from each foot of the smaller mammals, which provided sufficient material for ashing and counting. Concerning suitable doses, Rongstad stated:

> Thirty microcuries of ^{45}Ca implanted in a female thirteen-lined ground squirrel labeled her offspring for a year or more after birth. Sixty microcuries of ^{45}Ca labeled all four litters of snowshoe hares and could be detected until the September following birth. Sixty microcuries of ^{45}Ca were in most cases sufficient to label all cottontail litters, but 175 μCi insured labeling fifth and sixth litters and prolonged the time of detection.

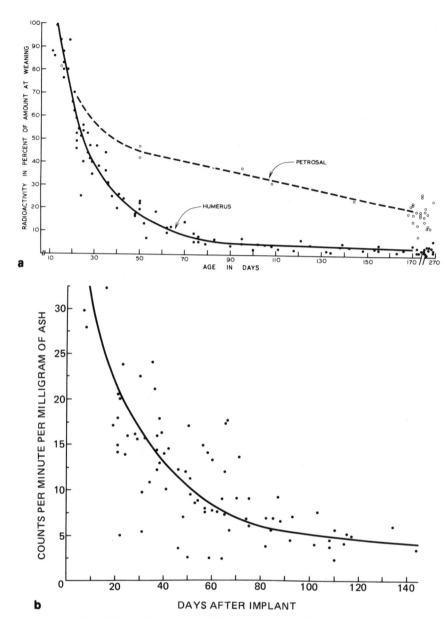

Figure 41. Specific activity of ^{45}Ca in bone ash of labeled cottontail rabbits *(Sylvilagus floridanus)*. (a) Decline with age of the specific activity of ^{45}Ca in bone ash of cottontail rabbits. Calcium-45 was received through the milk while the animal was suckling. Since all values were corrected for decay, the actual radioactivity at 164 days would be 50% of that shown. The lines were visually fitted to the dots. (b) Decline in specific activities of ^{45}Ca in bone ash of suckling cottontail rabbits with time after females were implanted. Each dot represents the specific activity of a different litter. Days after implant: Number of days after implant that the litters were born. The line was visually fitted to the dots. From Rongstad (1965). Reproduced from *Health Physics* **11**:1543–1556 (1965) by permission of the Health Physics Society.

Table 8. Calculated Time (Days) after Implantation That Offspring of Implanted Female Cottontails Remained Detectably Radioactive[a]

	Humerus			Petrosal		
	Capsule strength			Capsule strength		
Litter	50 μCi	100 μCi	200 μCi	50 μCi	100 μCi	200 μCi
1st	380	544	708	761	925	1089
2nd	284	448	612	665	829	993
3rd	177	341	505	558	722	886
4th	127	291	455	508	672	836
5th	103	267	431	484	648	812
6th	18	182	346	399	563	727

[a] From Rongstad (1965). Reproduced from *Health Physics* **11**:1543–1556 (1965) by permission of the Health Physics Society.

Meslow and Keith (1968) applied the technique developed by Rongstad in a study of demographic parameters of a Canadian showshoe hare population. Since toe-clipping patterns of juveniles were used to identify individuals during the summer, the investigators analyzed the removed toe for the presence or absence of ^{45}Ca. Utilizing a simple Lincoln index with these data, they estimated the total number of adult females in the spring population according to the equation proposed by Rongstad (1965):

$$\frac{\text{Radioactive young in the sample}}{\text{Total young in the sample}} = \frac{\text{Number of females implanted}}{\text{Total number of females present}}$$

Iodine-125 was injected intraperitoneally into lactating eastern chipmunks *(Tamias striatus)* to identify their young (Roberts and Snyder, 1973). Since the transmission of iodine through milk is well documented, a radioisotope of iodine was used in this study. Iodine-125 was selected, since it had a weaker gamma emission and thus was of less hazard to the investigators than ^{131}I. It also has a longer physical half-life (60 days) than the latter (8.070 days). The effective half-life of ^{125}I in the eastern chipmunk is about 11.5 days and that of ^{131}I is about 5 days. Each lactating female was injected periodically during lactation with 20–50 μCi ^{125}I. The investigators did not observe any effects attributable to radionuclide tagging; in fact, survival of tagged individuals was higher than that of controls. They suggested that in future studies adjacent lactating females be injected with different isotopes, to distinguish among their litters, and also that initiation of injection be delayed until the first juveniles appeared in the population, to reduce the total dose required.

Hydrological Studies

7.1. General Comments

The science of hydrology concerns the properties and distribution of water and snow, including such facets as tracing groundwater, sediment, and surface-water movement. Hydrological techniques utilizing radionuclides are rather well established. Two excellent bibliographies on the subject have been published [International Atomic Energy Agency (IAEA), 1968e, 1973e]. In addition, the IAEA (1966c) has published a guide to safe use of radionuclides in hydrology. This publication contains a description of techniques used in various countries (Table 9). Readers interested in applications to sediment transport and water movement in the sea are urged to read the excellent paper by Duursma (1972).

7.2. Sediment Movement

The use of radionuclides in the study of sediment transport has been a topic for discussion in the symposia on isotopes in hydrology sponsored by the IAEA (1963a, 1967, 1970d) as well as by a special panel of the IAEA (1973a). Methods for labeling sediments are summarized in Table 10, and a comprehensive list of investigations of sediment transport in saltwater environments is presented in Table 11. In addition to preparing these tables, Duursma (1972) summarized his opinion by stating that radionuclides are used in sediment studies more than are luminophor tracer techniques and that on shipboard, *in situ* detection of radionuclides is easier than for luminophors and the latter must, in general, be collected and analyzed at a later date. He mentions that the exception is the detection of luminophores on beaches at night with use of ultraviolet light. The fact that radionuclides physically decay permits studies on the same area at future times,

Table 9. List of Techniques and Quantities of Radioisotopes Used[a]

Country	Date	Nature of experiment	Isotope used Nature	Isotope used Amount
France	—	Riverbed silt and pebble	^{182}Ta–^{51}Cr–^{192}Ir	10–500 μCi/pebble
	June 62	Flow-rate measurement	^{82}Br	
	July 62	Groundwater tracing		
		a. Harbor zone	^{82}Br	10 mCi
			^{82}Br	20 mCi
		b. Rhone valley	^{82}Br	5.4 mCi
			^{82}Br	100 mCi
			^{82}Br	18 mCi
			^{82}Br	18.5 mCi
Germany Netherlands U.A.R.	May 62	Filtration rate	^{131}I ^{82}Br	10–30 μCi 10–30 μCi
Greece	Mar. 61	Tracing groundwater	^{3}H	1000 Ci
	Feb. 62	Tracing groundwater	^{3}H	400 Ci
Japan	1960	River engineering and flow rate	^{131}I	1.5 Ci
	1961	River engineering and flow rate	^{131}I	600 mCi
			^{24}Na	750 mCi
			^{131}I	60 mCi
		Littoral drift	Glass ^{65}Zn ^{60}Co ^{46}Sc	160 mCi
		Riverbed variation	Sealed ^{60}Co or ^{137}Cs source	2 mCi 25 mCi
	Aug–Nov. 56 June 57	Water infiltration	^{131}I	100 mCi 60 mCi 200 mCi
			^{32}P	50 mCi 200 mCi
			^{86}Rb	200 mCi
			^{3}H	1 Ci
	1962	River dilution and flow	^{24}Na +	13.5 mCi
			NH$_4$Br, nonradioactive	100 kg

Table 9. *(Continued)*

Country	Date	Nature of experiment	Isotope used	
			Nature	Amount
Sweden	1960–1962	Water flow, water tracing, etc.	^{3}H (HTO) ^{51}Cr EDTA	100 mCi–2.5 Ci 200 mCi–250 mCi
United Kingdom		Flow rate of river	^{24}Na ^{82}Br ^{3}H	2.1 mCi–90 mCi 9 mCi–30 mCi 470 mCi–4.2Ci
		Investigation of underground pool	^{131}I	50 mCi
		Sand transport	Glass ^{46}Sc ^{191}Ir ^{65}Zn	— — —
United States	1961	Open-channel flow	^{198}Au	166 mCi–2048 mCi
Yugoslavia		Groundwater tracing	^{3}H	200 mCi
Kenya	1964	Lake-water tracing	^{3}H	1500 Ci
Canada	1958–1963	Groundwater-flow measurements	^{3}H ^{35}S ^{85}Sr ^{90}Sr ^{106}Ru	— — — — —
India	1965	Silt movement in sea bed between India and Ceylon (Sethusamudram Tracer Experiment)	^{46}Sc	60 Ci
Israel	1957–1965	Aquifer characteristics Groundwater velocity, groundwater mixing and storage	^{60}Co as $K_3Co(CN)_6$	Up to 1 Ci in single study

^{a} From IAEA (1966c). The list is far from exhaustive; it is intended merely to give the reader a rough idea of the scope.

Table 10. Methods for Labeling Sediments with Radionuclides[a]

Method	Radionuclide	Type of sediment to which applicable	Advantages and shortcomings	References[b]
Surface labeling				
Precipitation from solution by reduction with formaldehyde or SnCl₂; also by exchange with predeposited Ag for ¹⁹⁸Au	^{198}Au ^{110}Ag	Sand, silt	Simple, efficient method. No loss of radionuclide.	Antier et al. (1965), Bougault et al. (1967), Campbell (1964), cf. Courtois (1967), Jeanneau (1967), Petersen (1963)
By wetting with aqueous radionuclide solution and subsequent heating to 500°C, or by wetting with alcoholic solution, drying, and heating	^{192}Ir, ^{46}Sc, ^{110}Ag, ^{140}Ba, ^{140}Ba-La, ^{198}Au, ^{60}Co	Sand, pebbles	Simple method, highly efficient for Ag and Au. Ba–140 (separated from daughter) has weak radiation. After release, radiation increases as ¹⁴⁰La is built up.	Becker and Götte (1965), Dolezal et al. (1965), Smith and Eakins (1958)
By precipitation through boiling radionuclide solution with cleaned sand, or precipitation by changing pH	^{51}Cr	Sand, silt	Simple method, but fixation not too efficient and loss possible.	Bougault et al. (1967), Peterson (1960)
By thermal decomposition of (NH₄)₂Cr₂O₇ at 200–260°C	^{51}Cr	Sand, silt	Efficient method for large quantities of sand. No loss from abrasion. Safety measures necessary.	Campbell and Seatonberry (1967)
By ion exchange on waterglass-treated sand	^{51}Cr	Sand	Needs special equipment for preparations. Loss is possible.	Meyn (1965)
By fixing with glue (caseinet), or albumen, adding additional layers of glue for protection; drying at 90°C	^{65}Zn, ^{32}P, ^{110}Ag, ^{95}Zr	Sand	Applicable only on small scale.	Gibert and Cordeiro (1962), Lodhi and Ali (1967)

Method	Tracer	Sediment	Remarks	References[b]
By adsorption from neutral solution	^{59}Fe, ^{32}P	Silt	For sewage solids. Loss to be expected.	Putman et al. (1956), Scalf et al. (1968)
By adsorption of stable element onto silt, release in environment, subsequent sampling, and neutron activation of these samples	Co, Ta	Silt, clays	No radioactivity in environment.	Groot et al. (1970)
Incorporation				
Incorporation of stable elements in glass, subsequent grinding, followed by neutron activation	Ta, Sc, Cr, Ir, Tm, Au, Sc	Sand, silt	Needs nuclear reactor and space in reactor. Possible baking together of glass particles during activation. No loss by abrasion.	Cf. Courtois (1967), Petersen (1965)
Incorporation of radionuclide in melt of glass with subsequent grinding	^{46}Sc	Sand, silt	Preparation too hazardous.	Cf. Courtois (1967)
Incorporation of preheated-to-750°C ion-exchanger Ionic-C50 (green sand)	^{46}Sc	Sand, silt	Easy to prepare aboard ship. Some loss at heavy grinding. No problems of grain size.	Arlman et al. (1960), Pilon (1965)
General				
Discussions on methods, safety, theory, and detection techniques				Anonymous (1965a,b), Courtois (1967, 1968), IAEA (1971), Case et al. (1970a,b), Hartley (1965), Courtois and Sauzay (1970), Sauzay (1968), Romanovsky (1968)
Detection equipment and computer analysis				
Theories of sediment distribution				
Economic aspects				

[a] From Duursma (1972).
[b] See source for references.

Table 11. Investigations Using Radionuclide Markers to Study Sediment Transport[a]

Radionuclide	Total activity (Ci)	Type of sediment	Weight added (kg)	Place, year	References[b]
Argentina					
^{110}Ag ads.	—	Natural	>300	Channel construction from La Plata River to Panama de la Palmas and Puerto Nuevo Rivers	Gomez-Ruiz et al. (1970)
^{110}Ag ads.	0.200	Sand	100	Port of Mar del Plata, 1963	Lachica and Baro (1963)
Australia					
^{51}Cr ads.	200	Sand	300	Botany Bay, 1965	Campbell and Seatonberry (1967)
	60	Sand	90	Newcastle, 1966	Ellis and Miles (1968)
Belgium					
^{95}Zr/Nb } fallout $^{103/106}$Ru }	—	Silt, clay	—	Coastal engineering, Belgian coast, 1963	Bastin (1965)
Brazil					
^{198}Au ads.	—	Sand, silt	—	Dredging navigation channel, Port of Rio de Janeiro	Maestrini et al. (1970)
Cambodia					
^{192}In }	1.5	Ground glass	0.3	Mekong, Stung-Sen, 1963	Anguenot et al. (1965)
^{182}Ta } inc. glass	0.2	Ground glass	0.04	Mekong, Stung-Sen, 1963	
^{170}Tm }	2.0	Ground glass	00.4	Mekong, Stung-Sen, 1963	
Denmark					
^{51}Cr ads.	4	Sand	2.5	Estuary of Thyrobon, Baltic Sea, Coast of Jutland, 1960	Cf. Courtois (1967)
France					
^{51}Cr inc. glass	0.68	Ground glass	25	Beach at Cannes, 1955	Cf. Courtois (1967)
^{182}Ta holes in pebbles	0.4	Pebbles	800 pebbles	Mouth of Var, 1956	Cf. Courtois, (1967)
^{46}Sc inc. glass	3.75	Ground glass	0.6	Mouth of Adour, 1956–1957	Cf. Courtois, (1967)
^{182}Ta inc. glass } ^{192} Ir inc. glass } n. activated	Some Ci	Ground glass } Ground glass	Some kg	Rhone estuary, 1961–1965	Cf. Courtois (1967) Cf. Courtois (1967)

Tracer	Material	Activity	Quantity	Location	Reference
^{192}Ir inc. glass n. activated	Ground glass	Some Ci	Some kg	Coast south of Roussillon, 1964, 1965, 1966	Cf. Courtois (1967)
^{198}Au ads. ^{192}Ir inc. glass	Natural sand Ground glass	Some Ci 0.08	Some kg 0.5	Seine estuary	Giresse and Courtois (1966)
^{198}Au ads.	Sand	3	0.800		
Natural activity	Natural sediment		—	Mouth of Frayere (Gulf of La Napoule)	Pautot (1968)
Germany ^{51}Cr ads.	SiO$_2$, sand	Some 100 mCi to some Ci	Some kg to some 100 kg	Estuary of Jade, 1959 Estuary of Eider Estuary of Weser, 1960 Estuary of Elbe	Fahse (1965) Schulz (1965)
^{46}Sc inc. glass ^{51}Cr ads.	Ground glass SiO$_2$, sand	— Some 100 mCi to some Ci	— Some kg to some 100 kg	Bay of Lübeck, 1961 Oste and Elbe, 1959 Estuary of Jade, 1962 Beach of Stakendorf, Baltic Sea, 1962 Fehmarn Belt, Baltic Sea, 1963 Island Sylt, Westerland, 1963–1964	Klein (1965) Schulz (1965) Petersen (1965)
^{46}Sc inc. glass ^{192}Ir ads. + fixed	Ground glass Gravel	2–3 —	100 —	Beach at Schleswig-Holstein	Petersen (1965), Dolezal et al. (1965), Runge (1969)
India ^{46}Sc inc. glass	Ground glass	16	1.78	Channel of Port of Bombay	Cf. Courtois (1967)
Japan ^{46}Sc ^{60}Co inc. glass ^{65}Zn	Ground glass	Some mCi to some Ci	10 kg/injection	Port of Tomakowai, 1954–1962 Keike, 1957–1960 Fukue, 1959–1961 Isohama, 1960–1961 Coast of Kashimanada, 1962	Cf. Courtois (1967)
Netherlands ^{46}Sc ads. inc.	Ionac-C50, ion exchanger	Some Ci	Some 100 kg	Rhine delta, Europort construction, 1957–1965	Pilon (1965)

(Continued)

Table 11. (Continued)

Radionuclide	Total activity (Ci)	Type of sediment	Weight added (kg)	Place, year	References[b]
Pakistan					
^{198}Au ads.	—	Sand	—	Hydraulic channels	Lodhi and Ali (1967)
^{110}Ag ads.	—	Sand	—	Hydraulic channels	
Portugal					
^{110}Ag ads.	0.8	Sand	4000	Estuary de Mandeco and mouth of the Tage, 1957	Cf. Courtois (1967)
^{32}P adh.	4	Sand	100	Port of Povoa de Varzim, 1959–1960	
Romania					
^{192}Ir	—	Sand	—	Gulf of Eforia	Gaspar et al. (1968)
South Africa					
^{198}Au	0.08	Sand	1.6	Gordonsbay	Bain et al. (1970)
Sweden					
^{51}Cr ads.	0.036	Sand	36	Swedish coast, Baltic Sea, Island Makläppen, 1957	Cf. Courtois (1967)
United Kingdom					
^{46}Sc inc. glass	4	Ground glass	0.085	Thames estuary, 1954–1957	Allen and Grindley (1957)
	29	Ground glass	0.845	Thames estuary, 1954–1957	
^{140}(Ba + La) ads. pebbles	0.018	Pebbles	1200 pebbles	Scolt Head Island beach, 1956	Kidson et al. (1958), Smith and Eakins (1958)
^{46}Sc inc. glass	1.2	Ground glass	0.060	Coast of Norfolk, 1957	Cf. Courtois (1967)
^{46}Sc inc. glass	2.1	Ground glass	0.200	Bay of Liverpool, 1958	Cf. Courtois (1967)
^{140}(Ba + La) in holes in pebbles	0.219	Pebbles	±200.000 pebbles	Orford Ness, Suffolk, 1957–1962	Cf. Courtois (1967)
^{46}Sc	20	Ground glass	1100	Firth of Forth, 1961	Smith and Parsons (1965, 1967)
^{46}Sc	130	Ground glass	1140	Firth of Forth, 1964	Smith and Parsons (1965, 1967)
^{140}(Ba + La)	40	Ground glass	550	Firth of Forth, 1965	Smith and Parsons (1965

United States					
^{198}Au ads.	—	Natural sediment	—	Bay of San Francisco, 1959	Cf. Courtois (1967)
^{32}P, irradiation of nat. sand	—	Natural sand	0.860	California, 1957	Cf. Courtois (1967)
^{133}Xe	—	Sand	—	Cape Kennedy, Florida; Surf, Calif. Point Conception, Calif.	Acree et al. (1969)
^{198}Au	—	Sand	—	Oceanside Harbor, Calif.	Case et al. (1970b)
Fallout labeling	—	Natural sediment	—	San Francisco Bay	Klingeman and Kaufman (1965)
^{59}Fe ads.	5 Ci/10^6 gal.	Sewage sludge	—	Water res., Centre Ada, Okl.	Scaff et al. (1968)
^{198}Au ads.	5 Ci	Natural sediment	—	Cape Fear River, 1962, navigation channel	Duke et al. (1965)
^{51}Cr, ^{65}Zn waste nuclides	—	Natural	—	Marine sediment derived from Columbia River	Gross and Nelson (1966)
U.S.S.R.					
^{59}Fe fixation with agar-agar	0.03	Sand	10	Caspian Sea, Krasnovodsk, 1956	Cf. Courtois (1967)
Natural ^{32}Si	Few mCi	Natural sediment glass	—	Sea bottom, shore	Makowski and Grissener (1967)
^{24}Na activated	—				
Na glass, some ^{59}Fe	—				
Venezuela					
^{14}C (by dating)	—	Dredged natural sediment	—	Recycling of spoil, Baie d'El Tablazo	Tamers (1969)
Yugoslavia					
^{51}Cr ads.	—	Sand	—	Velika Morova River, 1965	Vukmirović (1965)

[a] From Duursma (1972).
[b] See source for references.

while the color of luminophors must be changed to permit their use in the same area.

Similar to the situation that occurs in other studies we have discussed, the radionuclide should have a high gamma energy and a short half-life to assure environmental safety; in addition, when the element or radionuclide is incorporated into glass, a radionuclide of a high specific activity or a stable element with a large neutron-capture cross section must be used in order that neutron activation be effective. Duursma's discussion of labeling methods is an excellent summary of the subject. He comments that an ideal labeled sediment would be one in which the distribution of radioactivity is known for all grain sizes of the natural sediment. The problem is that finer sediments may absorb a disproportionate amount of the radionuclide. The activation of stable elements in the sediment has been considered, but according to Duursma, the yield is generally too low and a disproportionate amount of the activated element may be associated with different grain sizes. He discusses the use of an artificial sediment that contains particles equal in size and proportion to those of the natural sediment and also with the same specific weight. One example is ground glass into which the stable element has been incorporated during manufacture of the glass and activated after the glass has been ground. Although this procedure permits safe handling of the substance, in special cases the radionuclide has been introduced directly during manufacture of the glass. An important consideration is that the radionuclide not be dissipated during the sediment transport by abrasion or dissolution. The probability that this will occur is smallest when the radionuclide is incorporated into an artificial matrix, e.g., glass.

Understanding the movement of seashore material has very practical implications. Consequently, considerable effort has been expended on investigations involving various tracer techniques. Brunn (1962), in a brief discussion, commented on conventional methods as well as those that involve a radioactive or luminescent tracer. He stated that use of luminophors has some advantages over radionuclides, e.g., safety aspects, ease of preparation, and less expense. It should be noted that public opposition to the introduction of a radioactive substance into the environment would probably be greater. Brunn also believes that radionuclides may be better suited for studies in deep water and luminophors for those on beaches and within the surf zone.

Fallout radionuclides have been used in studying lake sediments. On the assumption that ^{137}Cs would have a distribution in lake sediments similar to that found in rain and airborne particles, Pennington et al. (1973) studied the levels of ^{137}Cs in sediments at various depths in five lakes in the English Lake District, assuming that the relationship to rain and airborne particles would be valid if there was no transfer by biota or mixing by diffusion in the sediment. They believed that they had strong evidence for the absence of vertical movement of

^{137}Cs. They assumed that the peak deposition observed was a result of the maximum deposition following nuclear weapons testing in 1963 and that another less precise appearance was correlated with the first detection of "significant levels" of ^{137}Cs in the atmosphere in 1954. All sediments above these horizons were considered to have been deposited following these dates.

7.3. Water Movement

The application of radionuclide techniques in studying water movement in oceans, streams, and lakes is considered in the references cited in Section 7.1. In addition, Ellis (1967) prepared a review of the literature relevant to stream gauging with radionuclide methods. The study of water movement includes techniques that utilize fallout radionuclides, radionuclides released during operation of a nuclear facility, and direct introduction of a radionuclide by the investigator. In reference to the sea, Duursma (1972) tabulated some investigations of water movement using radionuclide tracers (Table 12).

D.M. Nelson *et al.* (1970) determined the concentrations of the fallout radionuclides ^{95}Zr, ^{106}Ru, and ^{144}Ce in samples of Lake Michigan water with the purpose of utilizing the data to study water-mixing and of evaluating the technique in general. Since these radionuclides had a uniform horizontal distribution, these investigators concluded that the nuclides had value as tracers of vertical transport in the Great Lakes. Since most ^{3}H was deposited in Lake Michigan in the mid-1960s during the period of major nuclear-weapons testing and because it was observed to be uniformly distributed with depth, Nelson and his associates concluded that uniform mixing to a depth of at least 130 m occurred in 5 years or less.

Operation of the production reactors at Hanford on the Columbia River, with the consequent release of radionuclides via cooling water into the river, provided a unique opportunity to study sediment deposition behind impoundments on the river below Hanford as well as the rate of water movement downstream and its subsequent dispersal into the ocean. J. L. Nelson *et al.* (1966) utilized ^{24}Na, which was released at a constant rate, and ^{131}I, which was released instantaneously into the river, to study the "flow times" downstream from the plant area (Figure 42a). Since ^{24}Na has a short half-life, 15.0 hr, the decay of this radionuclide is used as a basis for determining flow, while the use of ^{131}I, with a half-life of 8.070 days, involved following a particular release of activity (Figure 42b). Osterberg *et al.* (1965) used the ^{51}Cr released during plant operations to delineate the plume of the river water in the sea (Figure 43). They concluded that the technique was best used during winter months when river flow is at a minimum and the "salinity pattern is confused." This conclusion

Table 12. Investigations Using Radionuclides to Study Water Movements[a]

Radionuclide	Quantity	Area	Purpose of investigation	References[b]
^{125}I, ^{131}I together at different ratios	0.5–3 μCi/m³ oil	Sea, Sweden	Oil pollution from ships	Carlson et al. (1970)
In, with subsequent activation analyses after sampling	71.5 g In/liter and discharge of 0.42 liters/hr	Sea, Trondheim, Norway	Dilution and current in and around the harbor	Dahl et al. (1970)
^{82}Br, compared with other radionuclides	0.3 Ci	Sea, United Kingdom	Dispersal of sewage in the sea	Eden and Briggs (1967), Barett et al. (1968)
^{82}Br	7 Ci	Mediterranean, coastal water, Israel	Sewage dilution from outflow into the sea	Gilath et al. (1970)
^{131}I	1.5 Ci	Mediterranean, Menton coast, France	Sewage dilution from outflow into the sea	Guizerix et al. (1967)
^{82}Br	1.2 Ci	Mediterranean, Nice coast, France		Guizerix et al. (1967)
^{82}Br	± 1 Ci per experiment	Sound, Denmark, Sweden, Dakar, Senegal	Sewage engineering ± 130 experiments	Hansen (1970), Harremoës (1966, 1967)
^{131}I	—	Ocean in general	Determination of low velocities by the deep-water isotopic current analyzer	Johnston (1966)
^{84}Rb, ^{86}Rb	—	Sea, 0–500 m, U.S.S.R.	Determination of average direction and speed of transport, and turbulent diffusion at greater depths	Shirei (1964)
^{60}Co	—	Ocean, India	Determination of pattern and extent of eddy diffusion	Srivastava (1963)

[a] From Duursma (1972).
[b] See source for references.

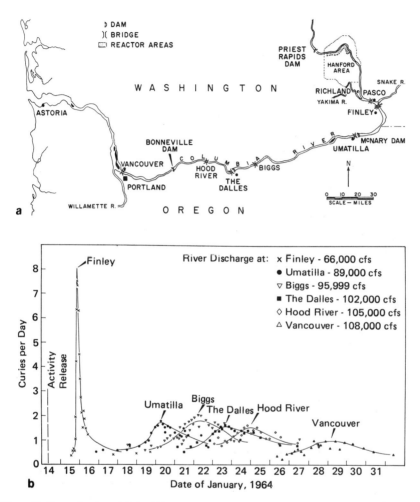

Figure 42. Determination of Columbia River flow times using radionuclide tracers released by the Hanford reactors. (a) Site map of Columbia River from Priest Rapids to mouth. (b) ^{131}I in Columbia River samples from six locations. From J. L. Nelson *et al.* (1966).

was the result of the plume's losing its identity as a result of wind action and floodwaters from coastal streams.

W. S. Broecker, an acknowledged authority on ocean mixing, has authored a review paper, "Radioisotopes and large-scale oceanic mixing" (Broecker, 1963), and another with associates, "Geochemistry and physics of ocean circulation" (Broecker *et al.*, 1961). In the first paper, he states:

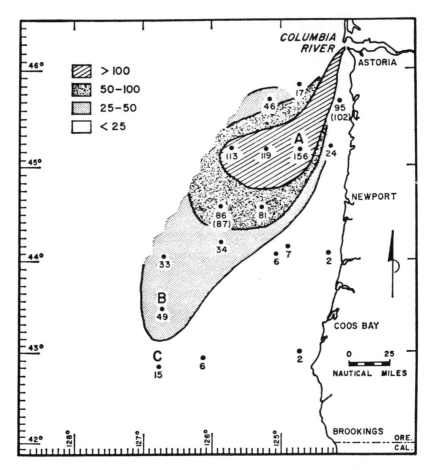

Figure 43. Chromium-51 (cpm/100 liters surface sea water), corrected to date of collection, June 26 to July 1, 1965. ( ) Duplicate samples. The cpm/100 liters can be converted to pC/liter by multiplying by 0.861. The greatest velocity of water movement was between points A and B. From Osterberg *et al.* (1965). Copyright 1965 by the American Association for the Advancement of Science.

To be suitable for large-scale oceanic mixing studies, an isotope should have the following ideal characteristics: (1) it should be present in measurable quantities in all parts of the ocean, (2) differences in concentration well outside the limits of measurement error should exist, (3) the mode and rate of injection of the isotope into the system must be known both as a function of time and of space, (4) the isotope should move with the water acting as an infinitely soluble salt, and (5) contributions of natural and artificial production of the isotope should be distinguishable.

According to Broecker, serious consideration for circulation studies has been given to only four natural radionuclides: ^{3}H, ^{14}C, ^{32}Si, and ^{226}Ra. The low production rate, short half-life, and artificial production of ^{3}H are disadvantages for using natural ^{3}H in circulation studies. The direct measurement of ^{32}Si, which has a half-life of a 650 years, is costly and time-consuming, since the levels in sea water are low and the biological cycling of silicon in diatom tests introduces another problem. Radium-226 is introduced into sea waters primarily from deep-sea sediments, and according to Broecker, little is known about its release rates, but there is some basis for assuming a constant influx with time at a specific location, and additional information is needed to evaluate transport in various solid phases, other than as calcium carbonate. He attributes great importance to the fact that radium, as contrasted to carbon, is not released to and transported by the atmosphere. Natural carbon has received more attention than the radionuclides mentioned above in studies of ocean circulation, and Broecker emphasized the use of this element in his paper, commenting that fallout radionuclides ^{90}Sr, ^{137}Cs, and ^{14}C " . . . should resolve the problem of the vertical mixing rates for the upper 1000 m of the ocean." It is regrettable that space does not permit a more extensive discussion of this interesting subject. The reader is referred to the cited papers of Broecker as well as to the additional readings for more information on the subject.

One study that involved the introduction of a radionuclide tracer directly into an aquatic system to study water movement was that of Likens and Hasler (1962). Since relatively little was known about the movement under lake ice, the investigators introduced ^{24}Na into a small Wisconsin lake and followed its movement as a tracer. The ^{24}Na was in a HCl and alcohol solution prepared to the specific density of the lake water at the release point. A device was developed to crush the shipping bottles that contained the solution while they were in the lake, in order to reduce turbulence and facilitate handling. Prior to being crushed, the bottles were kept immersed in the lake so that the solution would reach thermal equilibrium with the lake water. A sodium iodide crystal, scintillation detector, and scaler were used to monitor the movement of the radionuclide. The detector was waterproofed and lowered into the water through holes in the ice at various locations. Some of the results of the investigators' 2-year study are presented in Figure 44. The significance of these observations and of others is discussed by the authors.

7.4. Soil-Moisture Determination

Applications of ionizing radiation to determine soil density and moisture content are widely used in the agricultural sciences. Although the techniques have ecological implications, we have relegated these to a minor role in this

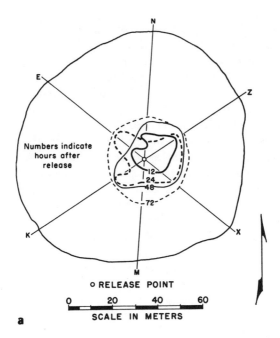

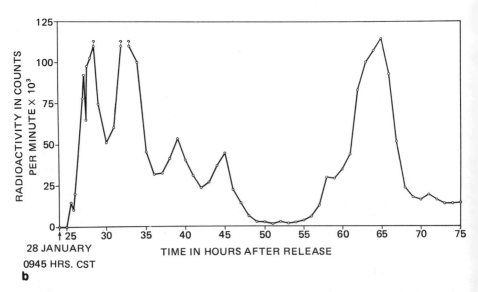

Figure 44. Movements of ^{24}Na within an ice-covered lake. (a) Outlines of the maximum horizontal displacement of ^{24}Na in Tub Lake following its release at a depth of 5 m on January 25, 1961. (b) Fluctuations in radioactivity at the 5-m depth along radius N [see (a)], 10 m from the release point, during the 1960 experiment. From Likens and Hasler (1962).

book and will restrict our comments to a description of the method as paraphrased from Shilling and Shilling (1964). Neutron moderation by soil moisture is the basis for this measurement. Fast neutrons are released from a source, such as a mixture of radium and beryllium, and when they collide in the vicinity of the source with light atoms, such as hydrogen, energy is lost, while in collision with heavier atoms, the fast neutrons are merely scattered without significant loss of energy. As a result of loss of energy, some of the fast neutrons become slow neutrons, which are measured by a probe sensitive to slow neutrons. These data are used to determine the amount of hydrogen and thus of water in the soil, since the major source of hydrogen in soil is in soil moisture. Soil density may be determined by gamma-ray scattering, somewhat analogous to neutron scattering. Another method of determining soil density is by means of gamma-ray trans- mission, a method whereby the source and detector are separated by the soil under investigation, as contrasted to the measurements described above.

8

Physiological Studies

8.1. General Comments

The application of radionuclides to physiological studies of "wild" organisms can be classified into either of two categories based on the reason for the use of the radionuclide: (1) interest is not in the radionuclide *per se,* but only as it serves the purpose of identifying a labeled compound, e.g., tritiated water; and (2) interest is in the specific radionuclide or its stable form, e.g., the study of the biological half-life of the fission product ^{137}Cs.

In this chapter, we will consider use of radionuclides for the first purpose and refer the reader to the abundant literature on applications in studies that are not ecological or do not involve "wild" organisms. For example, Haber (1968), in an article entitled "Ionizing radiations as research tools," discusses applications to plant physiology and related subjects. Studies that deal with the second purpose will be treated in Chapter 10.

8.2. Terrestrial Organisms

8.2.1. Plants

A very common label of organic compounds is ^{14}C, since all organic compounds contain carbon. Many compounds have been labeled with this radionuclide, and undoubtedly thousands of studies have been conducted by biologists using this tracer. We will mention only two of these. Coulson and Peel (1971), studying the effect of temperature on the respiration of sugars in willow *(Salix viminalis)* stems, used ^{14}C-labeled sugars. Leaves of cuttings were grown in control chambers and permitted to assimilate $^{14}CO_2$, which was generated by adding ^{14}C-labeled Na_2CO_3 to a solution of lactic acid. [^{14}C]carbon dioxide was produced by stem phloem respiration of labeled sugars. The increase of radio-activity, measured with a liquid scintillation counter, was observed in the sieve tube sap as reflected in the aphid honeydew and was then compared with respiratory $^{14}CO_2$ from stems.

In a more ecologically oriented paper entitled "A physiological and mathematical study of the growth and productivity of a *Calluna–Sphagnum* community. III. Distribution of photosynthate in *Calluna vulgaris* L. Hull," Grace and Woolhouse (1973) described the use of $^{14}CO_2$ in a laboratory study that was part of a much broader study. *Calluna* plants collected in the field were brought into the laboratory and placed in a closed gas circuit chamber associated with a gas analyzer for determination of CO_2. The $^{14}CO_2$ introduced into the chamber was prepared from a lactic acid solution of ^{14}C-labeled $NaHCO_3$. After a period of time, the total sugar was determined in the soluble fraction of leaves and wood by measuring the labeled sugar produced.

Another radionuclide commonly used in physiological studies is the isotope of hydrogen known as tritium and symbolized by ^3H or T. Tritiated water (HTO) is used in studies of plant tranpiration. HTO is used as a tracer of H_2O and measured with a liquid scintillation counting system. Kline and his associates have published several papers on the application of this method in the study of transpiration in trees. Of these, we have selected one that concerns coniferous trees and also includes considerable theoretical discussion (Kline *et al.*, 1972). HTO is introduced by injection into the base of the tree in an attempt to introduce it into the water pool of the tree. Following injection, the labeled water is followed by studying the activity of foliage and small branches as a function of time. These data are used in the study of transpiration. Biomass determinations also require the mean residence time of water and the mean moisture content of the tree. Figure 45 illustrates a typical response curve relating tritium activity to time.

Woods and O'Neal (1965) used HTO in a study of water uptake by small oak trees (*Quercus laevis, Q. incana,* and *Q. stellata*) in the sandhills of South Carolina. Pipes were driven into the ground at three depths (5, 35.5, and 66 cm), and labeled water was placed within these pipes. Sample plants were at an average distance of 2.1–2.4 m from these pipes. Plastic bags enclosing the ends of branches were used to collect transpired water that was counted for tritium by the liquid scintillation method.

8.2.2. Animals

Radioactive iodine has been used in thyroidectomy to measure metabolism and to label compounds of interest. Iodine-131 was injected intraperitoneally into Oregon juncos (*Junco oreganus*) by R. E. Bailey (1953) to thyroidectomize

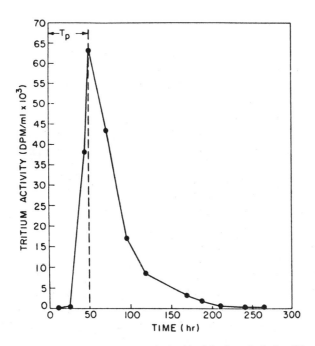

Figure 45. Typical activity–time response curve obtained by injecting a jack pine *(Pinus banksiana)* tree with HTO and sampling twigs as a function of time for tritium content. (T_p) Peak arrival time. From Kline *et al.* (1972).

the birds physiologically. The ^{131}I accumulates in the thyroid, where, at sufficiently high levels, it destroys by irradiation the thyroid cells without destroying the parathyroid and surrounding tissues. Since important phenomena such as fat deposition, feather molt, and pigmentation are associated with the thyroid, the scientist interested in these phenomena has a useful tool at his disposal. In a comparative study of responses of two salamanders to thyroid-stimulating hormone, Lynn and Dent (1961) injected ^{131}I intraperitoneally into mature specimens of *Triturus v. viridescens* and *Desmognathus f. fuscus* and periodically measured the radioactivity of the thyroid and heart regions with a scintillation counting system. In addition, histological investigations of thyroid sections were conducted.

In a study by O'Farrell and Dunaway (1967), wild-caught cotton rats *(Sigmodon hispidus)*, housed individually in cages, were provided the thymidine analogue ([131]IUDR) or ^{131}I-labeled sodium iodide *ad libitum*. In addition, each animal was injected intraperitoneally with 1 µCi of the material at a specific time. Whole-body counts were made at 0 time and at 12-hr intervals to 48 hr

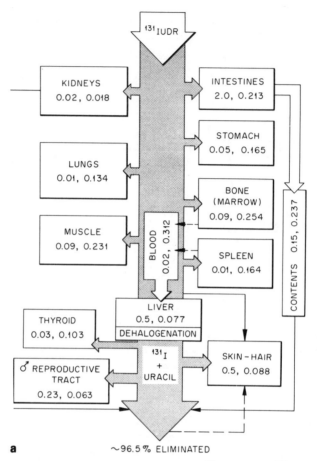

Figure 46. Preliminary models of the tissue distribution of ^{131}IUDR and Na^{131}I in the cotton rat *(Sigmodon hispidus)* 48 hr postinjection. (a) ^{131}IUDR; (b) Na^{131}I. From O'Farrell and Dunaway (1967).

postinjection with a well-type scintillation detector. Tissues and organs were taken from animals sacrificed periodically and assayed for radioactivity. In this study, the investigators were interested in the incorporation and tissue distribution of the thymidine analogue. Tissue distribution of the analogue and Na^{131}I at 48 hr postinjection time are illustrated in Figure 46.

Animals subjected to environmental stresses make physiological adjustments within their range of capability. In homeotherms, the thyroid influences thermoregulation and cell metabolism; therefore, a measure of thyroid activity

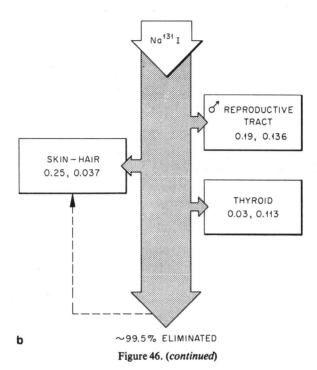

b   ~99.5% ELIMINATED

Figure 46. (*continued*)

would be useful to study the reaction of homeotherms to their environment. A useful technique is to study the release rate of ^{131}I from the thyroid. Kodrich and Tryon (1973) studied the seasonal variation in release rates of ^{131}I by free-ranging adult eastern chimpmunks *(Tamias striatus)* in northwestern Pennsylvania. An intraperitoneal injection of a solution containing 3 μCi ^{131}I was given to trapped animals that had been marked by toe-clipping. The animals were released at the trap site, and once a day for at least four successive recaptures, with an average of 2 days between recaptures, the whole-body and thyroid radioactivity levels were determined. Whole-body counts were made by use of a NaI scintillation counting system. A surgical scintillation probe was used to determine externally the thyroid activity along the ventral side of the neck. The investigators stated: "Iodine-131 thyroid release rates are sensitive enough to provide valuable data in comparing relative thyroid activity under different experimental treatments in free-ranging animals."

In a study of thyroid function in desert ground squirrels (*Citellus tereticaudus* and *C. leucurus*) with different daily activity patterns, Hudson and Wang (1969) used ^{125}I turnover rates in the species to study the regulation of basal metabolism by the thyroid. A dose of 4–8 μCi ^{125}I was injected intraperitoneally, and the radioactivity of the thyroid was measured periodically at the neck region of the animal. Counting was accomplished with a 1×1 inch NaI(Tl) crystal placed over the neck region of the animal while the animal was moved back and forth until a maximum reading was obtained. The rate of decrease of protein-bound ^{125}I was studied in *C. leucurus* from which blood samples obtained by cardiac puncture were analyzed for protein-bound [125]I (Figure 47a). The authors also presented ^{131}I comparative unpublished data for other species (Figure 47b). Regrettably, we have not done justice to this excellent research and suggest that the interested reader consult the paper in its entirety.

Another radionuclide that has been commonly used in physiological studies of terrestrial animals is tritium. As stated in Section 8.2.1, water can be labeled as HTO and the compound used to study the water pool in plants. Somewhat similarly, total body water and water turnover in mammals can be studied. Longhurst *et al.* (1970) utilized HTO to compare water kinetics in winter and summer Columbian black-tailed deer *(Odocoileus hemionus columbianus)* and domestic sheet *(Ovis aries)*. The animals were injected intravenously with 8 mCi HTO, and blood samples were collected periodically and examined for radioactivity with a liquid scintillation counting system. In a water-turnover study in mule deer *(Odocoileus hemionus)*, Knox *et al.* (1969) also used HTO and observed that the biological half-life of HTO differed in animals maintained in a 0.9×1.5 m metabolism stall from that in the same animals maintained in a 4.6×5.8 m room.

Two reindeer *(Rangifer tarandus)* were placed in stalls located within controlled environment chambers, and 100 μCi HTO was injected into their jugular veins. Periodically, blood samples were inspected for radioactivity. This study of body-water volume and turnover was conducted using 12 different combinations of diet and temperature. A comparison of water-flux rate, as determined with HTO, to measured water input showed a linear relationship (Figure 48). The investigators (Cameron *et al.*, 1976) concluded that the tritium water dilution technique provided accurate determinations of total-body-water flux over the wide range of experimental conditions in reindeer.

In a study involving eight species of rodents, Yousef *et al.* (1974) used HTO to study water flux in a fashion similar to that in the investigation described above. They were interested in estimating the flux in rodents from different habitats and in correlating this with ecological distribution, phylogeny, and metabolic rate.

Bullard (1964) used ^{86}Rb as a tracer to study regional blood flow and volume during arousal from hibernation of thirteen-lined ground squirrels *(Citellus tridecemlineatus)* that had been captured in the wild, maintained for at least 2 months in the laboratory, and then placed in a cold room at 5°C to induce hibernation. After entering hibernation, the animals were implanted with a venous

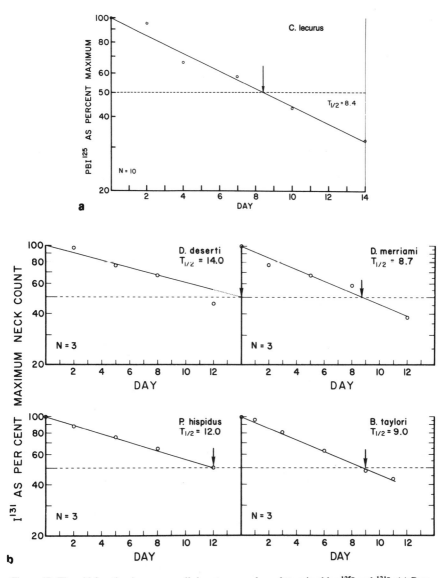

Figure 47. Thyroid function in some small desert mammals as determined by ¹²⁵I and ¹³¹I. (a) Rate at which plasma protein-bound ¹²⁵I is lost in *Citellus leucurus* during the period of rapid loss. Each point represents an average of data from 10 animals. (↓) Point at which radioactivity declined to 50% (T₁/₂). (b) Biological half-life of ¹³¹I released from the neck region of four species of rodents *(Dipodomys merriami, D. deserti, Perognathus hispidus,* and *Baiomys taylori)*. Each point is the average of data from three animals used in each group. (↓) Point at which radioactivity declined to 50% (T₁/₂). From Hudson and Wang (1969).

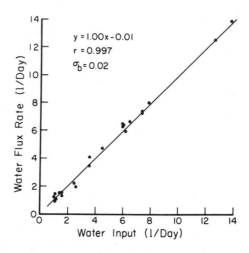

Figure 48. Relationship between water flux determined by HTO dilution and the total water input, i.e., the sum of measured water intake plus calculated metabolic water production (trials A–K). From Cameron *et al.* (1976).

catheter. Rubidium-86, which distributes itself into intracellular spaces, was injected via the implanted catheter at the desired physiological state. Following a period of 200 heartbeats after introduction of the radionuclide, the animal was sacrificed, and selected tissues and organs were assayed for radioactivity. The period of 200 heartbeats was determined by electrocardiogram to be the partial arousal state. The technique assumes that the fraction of the activity injected that is observed in a tissue or organ will be equal to the fraction of the total cardiac output reaching the tissue (Figure 49).

An extensive literature exists on the use of radionuclides in physiological studies of terrestrial and aquatic insects. Consequently, we will refer the reader to O'Brien and Wolfe (1964b) for studies that the authors classify as "Digestion and absorption," "Uptake and distribution of inorganic materials," "Elemental turnover," "Permeability of the central nervous system," and "Miscellaneous studies."

8.3. Aquatic Organisms

8.3.1. Plants

Research on physiological processes of aquatic higher plants using a radionuclide tracer is unknown to us. If such research has been conducted, we are reasonably sure that it is not common.

8.3.2. Animals

We will now consider the use of radionuclide labels in physiological studies of aquatic invertebrates and vertebrates. Of those that involve invertebrates, we will consider a study of coral, sea urchin, and water fleas, while studies that involve vertebrates are represented by those investigating processes in rainbow trout.

The uptake of glucose by solitary coral *(Fungia scutaria)*, collected in Hawaiian waters, was studied by Stephens (1962). The coral was placed in marine laboratory aquaria containing ^{14}C-labeled glucose. Glucose movement was studied by determining activity of ambient water and suitable animal extracts with a thin-window Geiger–Müller tube. In addition to ^{14}C-labeled glucose, the author studied other ^{14}C-labeled compounds: tyrosine, lysine, aspartic acid, glycine, and lactate.

Hsiao and Boroughs (1958), studying the physiology of calcium accumulation by sea urchin *(Tripneustes gratilla)* eggs, with particular attention to the role of the jelly cover of the eggs, mixed a solution of ^{45}CaCl$_2$ with sea water in which the researchers placed normal eggs of the urchin and those from which the jelly coat had been removed. Following various incubation periods, the eggs were separated from the incubation medium, and an aliquot of the medium and eggs was counted with a thin-window GM counter. Figure 50 shows some of the results of this experiment.

A study of the uptake and release of inorganic phosphorus by the plankton crustacean, *Daphnia magna,* was conducted by Rigler (1961). Groups of the organism were immersed for various periods of time in artifically prepared water

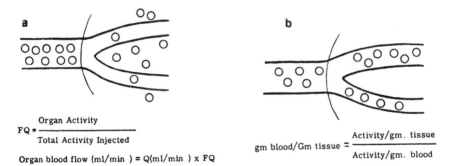

$$FQ = \frac{\text{Organ Activity}}{\text{Total Activity Injected}}$$

Organ blood flow (ml/min) = Q(ml/min) x FQ

$$\text{gm blood/Gm tissue} = \frac{\text{Activity/gm. tissue}}{\text{Activity/gm. blood}}$$

Figure 49. Method of measuring organ or regional blood flow with ^{86}Rb and ^{131}I. (a) Method of measuring organ or regional blood flow by ^{86}Rb distribution. The label has a large volume (intracellular and extracellular) in which it can be distributed. The fraction of the total activity delivered and distributed in a tissue will, for a given period of time, equal the fraction (F) of the cardiac output (Q) delivered to that tissue. (b) Method of measuring organ or regional blood volume by ^{131}I-tagged albumin. The label remains in the bloodstream. From Bullard (1964).

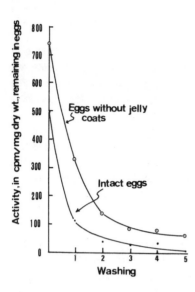

Figure 50. Decrease in radiocalcium in sea urchin eggs after washing with detergent solution (Sterox SK). From Hsiao and Boroughs (1958).

containing ^{32}P, and the uptake of inorganic phosphorus was computed from the following equation:

$$\frac{\text{Avg PO}_4 \cdot \text{P in solution } (\mu g/ml) \times P^{32} \text{uptake } (cpm/animal/hr)}{\text{Avg } P^{32} \text{ in solution } (cpm/ml)}$$

Rigler commented that this equation was satisfactory, since the P^{32} in solution was almost constant and that the uptake by the organism, as well as the change of $PO_4 \cdot P$ in the water, was linear. Chemical analysis of the water was used to determine the net loss of inorganic phosphorus by the organism. Figure 51 shows the results of using filtered and autoclaved river water and compares the uptake by sterile and nonsterile *Daphnia magna*.

The use of the rainbow trout *(Salmo gairdneri)* as a laboratory animal to study physiological processes in fish is common practice. Hunn and Fromm (1964) studied the iodine metabolism of the species by using ^{131}I-labeled NaI that was carrier-free. The tracer in distilled water was injected intraperitoneally. At 24 hr after injection, samples of blood, lower jaw, and gill were obtained

---

→

Figure 51. Uptake and release of inorganic phosphorus by *Daphnia magna*. (a) Uptake of ^{32}P by *Daphnia magna* from filtered and from filtered and autoclaved Ottawa River water. (b) Uptake of inorganic phosphorus by nonsterile and sterile *D. magna* from Ottawa River water, and by nonsterile individuals from artificial Ottawa River water (AW) calculated from uptake of ^{32}P. The average percentage of the ^{32}P in suspended solids in each case was: nonsterile, 0.9; sterile, 0.3; nonsterile in 'AW' 2.2. From Rigler (1961).

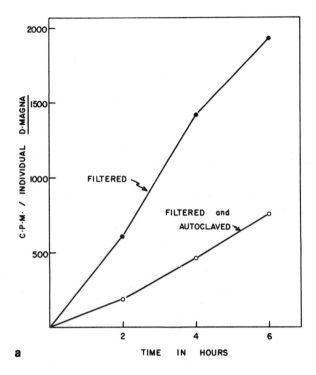

a

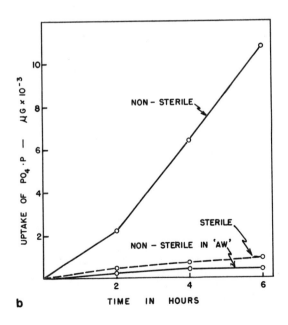

b

from anesthetized fish. The samples were ashed and counted, using a 2-inch NaI(Tl) crystal. The portion of the study concerned with routes of excretion of iodine utilized fish that had been in distilled water containing Na^{131}I for 24 hr and also fish that had been injected intraperitoneally with the compound. Figure 52 illustrates the apparatus in which the anesthetized fish were placed. The activity of the exchange resin, of urine collected while the fish were in this apparatus, and of the blood plasma, from samples collected after the urine and resin samples, was determined.

Interest in effects of thermal effluents from power plants on fish has stimulated research along this line, using radionuclides. Dean and Berlin (1969), in

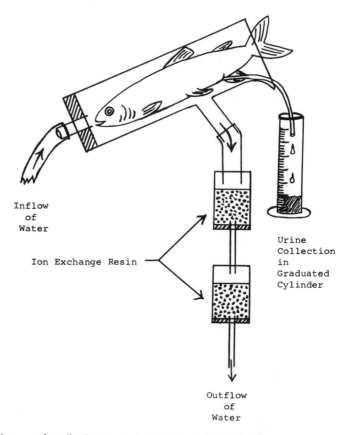

Figure 52. Apparatus for collecting samples from anesthetized fish. Distilled or tap water was pumped over the gills of the experimental fish in the chamber, flowed out the side arm into the two columns, each containing 10 g ion-exchange resin (IRA 400). The cannula delivered urine into a 10-ml graduated cylinder. To secure the animals in position, damp cotton was tucked in around the tail of the fish. From Hunn and Fromm (1964).

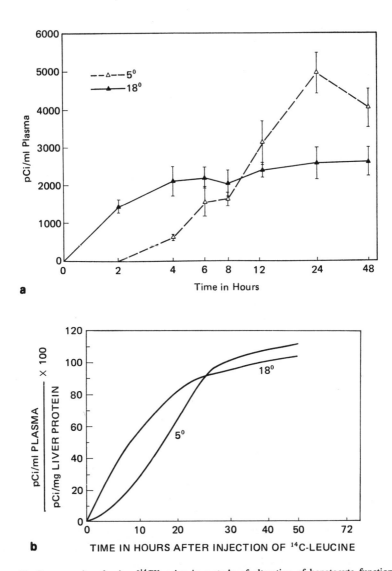

a

b

Figure 53. Some results of using [¹⁴C]leucine in a study of alteration of hepatocyte function of thermally acclimated rainbow trout *(Salmo gairdneri)*. (a) [¹⁴C]Leucine incorporated into plasma proteins of warm-acclimated (18°C) and cold-acclimated (5°C) rainbow trout. Results shown are means ± 1 S.E. and are expressed as pCi/ml plasma. (b) Ratio of labeled plasma protein to labeled liver proteins from 0 to 48 hr after injection with [¹⁴C]leucine. From Dean and Berlin (1969).

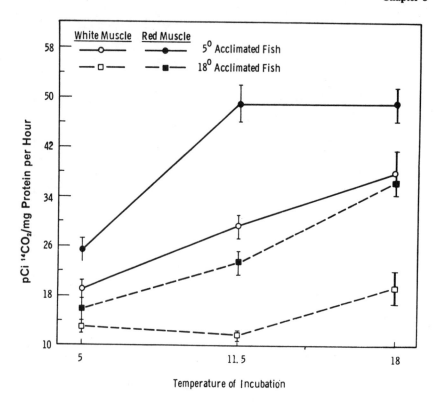

Figure 54. Conversion of acetate-1-[^{14}C] to $^{14}CO_2$ by red and white muscle tissue of warm- and cold-acclimated rainbow trout *(Salmo gairdneri)*. Values shown are means ± 1 S.E. Number of samples at 5, 11.5, and 18°C, respectively: (○) 11, 11, and 12; (●) 11, 11, and 11; (□) 6, 16, and 7; (■) 6, 9, and 7. From Dean (1969).

a paper entitled "Alterations in hepatocyte function of thermally acclimated rainbow trout *(Salmo gairdneri)*," described a portion of the study involving leucine incorporation in which they used ^{14}C-labeled leucine injected intravenously in the dorsal aorta. Blood and liver samples were collected from various postinjection groups and, after treatment, counted by liquid scintillation. Some results are presented in Figure 53. In another study of thermal acclimation of the rainbow trout concerned with metabolism of tissues, Dean (1969) acclimated fish at 5 and 18°C and homogenized samples of tissue. The tissue was centrifuged and the supernatant fraction incubated with acetate-1-[^{14}C] and palmitate-1-[^{14}C]. Following suitable incubation time, the $^{14}CO_2$ evolved was counted with a liquid scintillation counting system. Some results are presented in Figure 54.

Other radionuclides have been used in physiological studies of rainbow trout: Kerstetter *et al.* (1970) used ^{22}Na in a study of mechanisms of sodium ion transport in irrigated gills; Schreck (1973) injected [^{3}H]testosterone intramuscularly to study accumulation and retention of androgen by various tissues and organs of this trout; and Bilinski and Jonas (1973), in an investigation of effects of cadmium and copper on oxidation of lactate by rainbow trout, studied the oxidative activity of trout gill filaments, measuring the production of $^{14}CO_2$ from Na-lactate-3-[^{14}C].

Primary-Productivity Determination

9.1. General Comments

Whether it be in terrestrial or aquatic environments, primary production, the base of the food web, relates to the production of organic compounds from inorganic carbon and water through the process of photosynthesis. In aquatic systems, investigators are concerned with community composition and dynamics of primary producer communities, the green algae and higher aquatic plants that through the process of photosynthesis form sugar from light energy and carbon dioxide plus water.

Primary productivity and its measurement in aquatic systems are discussed in most textbooks on hydrobiology. Further, the International Biological Program (IBP) has produced two excellent volumes on the subject: (1) *A Manual on Methods for Measuring Primary Production in Aquatic Environments* (Vollenweider, 1969) and (2) *Primary Productivity in Aquatic Environments* (Goldman, 1966). In addition, the Fisheries Research Board of Canada sponsored the bulletin of Strickland (1960), *Measuring the Production of Marine Phytoplankton*. Since it was proposed by Steemann Neilsen, the method of measuring primary productivity with ^{14}C has stimulated considerable interest and research. Although other methods of measuring productivity are of interest, it is to the ^{14}C method that we will direct our comments. Beyers and Beyers (1974) have prepared an extensive listing of publications on measuring primary productivity in aquatic ecosystems for those readers interested in a detailed information source.

9.2. Carbon-14

Excellent discussions of the ^{14}C method are available in the publications of Schwoerbel (1970), Steemann Nielsen (1963), and Strickland (1960) and in papers by various contributors to the manual edited by Vollenweider (1969). It is from these sources that the following comments have been obtained. Application of the method must rest on a sound biological knowledge of the organism and the ecosystem of which it is a part as well as a knowledge of statistical sampling procedures and analytical sampling error. Assuming that these aspects have been considered in developing the experimental design, the basic steps in the method are: (1) collect a water sample from the site of interest; (2) determine the total carbon in the sample; (3) add a known amount of ^{14}C to the sample; (4) allow a period of time to pass; (5) filter the sample contents; (6) count the ^{14}C in the residue; and (7) calculate the assimilated carbon by the following formula:

$$^{12}C \text{ assimilated} = \frac{^{14}C \text{ assimilated}}{^{14}C \text{ available}} \times {}^{12}C \text{ available} \times K$$

where K is a constant that adjusts for time, dimension, and aliquot volume. Elaboration of this equation is available in Vollenweider (1969, pp. 72–73).

Although the technique as described is relatively simple, interpretation of the results is not. Strickland (1960) regrets that initial efforts were directed toward collecting data rather than toward a critical evaluation of the technique. He believed that the evidence to 1960 indicated that the method results in a measure of photosynthesis between net and gross production, but closer to the former.

We will now comment on the various steps of the procedure as applied to phytoplankton. Admittedly, our comments are oversimplified and incomplete, but they should serve to clarify some aspects of the technique. Readers interested in a more comprehensive discussion are referred to the publications cited above.

Water samples should be collected from the area of interest (e.g., depth) with clean, nonmetallic sampling bottles, and the filled bottle should be free of bubbles. The material from which the bottle is made is an important consideration. Although Pyrex or glassware of a similar quality is satisfactory for most purposes (Vollenweider, 1969), the fact that light absorption by glass is different from that by natural waters must be taken into consideration. This varies with the quality of the glass and the depth at which the bottles are placed. Quartz bottles are the most satisfactory, but are expensive; therefore, bottles made of Plexiglas, which has optical properties similar to those of quartz, might be an appropriate substitute. The sampling bottles should be cleaned frequently with 50% HCl to prevent accumulation of ^{14}C and should be washed with a detergent to prevent growth of bacteria (Strickland, 1960).

The total inorganic carbon in the sample is obtained from tables of total carbon based on pH and alkalinity such as those published by Schwoerbel (1970, p. 139). A known amount of ^{14}C-labeled sodium carbonate in a dilute solution is added to the sample. The amount to be added is dependent on the phytoplankton content of the water under study. The labeled sodium carbonate solution can be prepared from commercial solutions of a high specific activity or from solid ^{14}C-labeled barium carbonate, or it can be purchased directly in ampules of the desired strength. Preparation and standardization of the sodium carbonate solution are discussed in detail in Vollenweider (1969). It is recommended that to prevent growth of bacteria, the solution be autoclaved and, if it is to be used in marine studies, NaCl be added to adjust to the salinity of the sample water. Strickland (1960) does not think the addition of NaCl is necessary if 1 ml of carrier-free standardized solution is added to 200–500 ml of sample seawater. Although there is a lower limit to the amount of the ^{14}C-labeled sodium carbonate added to the water sample, there is no upper limit except as influenced by cost, co-incidence counting errors, and public-health hazards (Strickland, 1960). Strickland also comments with respect to marine studies: "In general, there would seem to be little point in using more than 50 microcuries of activity in an experiment and addition of only one to two microcuries would be preferable." He presents a working formula of the amount to be added based on the counting efficiency of the equipment used, anticipated uptake of carbon over a period of time, and the desired counts per minute from the radioactive residue being counted. In the manual edited by Vollenweider (1969), it is suggested that 1 µCi/100 ml of "moderately productive water" would give sufficient counting statistics after exposure to 4–6 hr of "optimum light."

If interest is in determining primary production at various depths in the sea, lake, or pond, water samples are obtained from these depths and the experiment is conducted. In the case of studies conducted on the open sea, inoculated samples are placed in temperature-controlled incubators and exposed to artificial or natural light, while in lakes, ponds, or bays, the sealed bottles are returned for a period of time to the depth at which the samples were obtained. One of two bottles containing water obtained from the same location is blackened to prevent light penetration and, consequently, photosynthesis. Paired bottles, one blackened and one clear, are then incubated as described above for both open-sea and lake investigations. The dark-bottle technique was developed in an attempt to correct for the fact that there occurs in the dark an exchange of CO_2 ("dark fixation") that is not related to photosynthesis and that ^{14}C may thereby be introduced into the phytoplankton organic matter. Steemann Nielsen (1963) remarked that dark fixation of $^{14}CO_2$ by a culture of algae is neglible as contrasted with fixation due to photosynthesis at light saturation, but added:

> In ordinary ^{14}C-experiments for measuring organic production in the sea other organisms are present in addition to autotrophic algae. Nevertheless, in experiments lasting 4 h, the dark fixation in water from the photic layer is usually only a few (1–3) per cent of the fixation at light saturation. In water with a very low production, preferably from the lower boundary of the photic layer, dark fixation may be relatively higher. . . . The same is true in polluted water with a high stock of bacteria. Whenever possible, dark bottles

should be employed in addition to the ordinary clear bottles and the dark fixation rates should be subtracted from the ordinary measurements. In experiments of short duration, dark fixation is usually of minor importance only. In experiments of long duration, however, a very pronounced growth of bacteria takes place. . . . It cannot be repeated often enough that the enclosure of a water sample in a bottle is severe interference. The duration of experiments must be kept short!

The longer the incubation period, the more pronounced the undesirable features of the method become, so it is desirable to use short exposure of no longer than a few hours; furthermore, in very productive waters, even 1 hr may result in problems such as supersaturation of oxygen and raised pH (Vollenweider, 1969).

After a suitable period of incubation, the water sample and its contents are filtered through a membrane or Millipore filter to separate the labeled material from the liquid. The filters are placed onto counting planchets and placed in a desiccator. Before the activity of the filters is counted, the inorganic carbon must be removed, and this can be accomplished with HCl after the filters have been dried.

Labeled organic material may be counted with any of three types of detectors, which are, in decreasing order of detection efficiency: windowless, thin-window, and thick-window. The detection efficiency of the windowless detector is accompanied by complications such as a decrease in counting rate resulting from the possible development of static charges on the filters (Vollenweider, 1969). According to Strickland (1960), it is undesirable to have counting times exceed 5–10 min in routine work. Consequently, the filter activity should exceed 200–330 cpm and preferably be 1000 or greater. Unless a coincidence curve for the instrument is determined, he recommends a counting rate not exceeding 5000 cpm, since appreciable "coincidence errors" occur with Geiger–Müller detectors at higher counting rates. Strickland further states that is is common practice to use either an end-window or a windowless gas-flow detector; the latter increases counting efficiency, but the former is simpler to handle and easier to decontaminate. Since beta radiation will be absorbed to some degree by the material being counted, it is necessary that "self absorption" be considered. The loss of carbon through respiration may be considerable in long-term experiments; thus, the photosynthesis measured by the ^{14}C technique measures net production rather than gross production. Steemann Nielsen (1963) discussed a method for determining the rate of respiration for phytoplankton using the ^{14}C method.

Suitability of the ^{14}C method of measuring primary productivity for autotrophs other than phytoplankton has been investigated. Wetzel (1966) summarizes the literature for the use of this method with periphyton and higher aquatic plants. He discusses applications in both the field and the laboratory. It is obvious that determination of primary productivity in periphyton and higher aquatic plants is more difficult than in phytoplankton.

Cycling Studies

10.1. General Comments

For many years, ecologists have been interested in the uptake, retention, and excretion of stable elements by organisms as well as the total pattern of mineral cycling within and among ecosystems. The availability of radionuclide tracers as a tool in studying stable elements has stimulated research and provided knowledge previously not available. Although the subject of cycling could have been considered in our discussion of physiological studies in Chapter 8, we have elected to present it as a category by itself. This is justified by the enormity of the subject and by the special interest of radiation ecologists in the cycling of man-made radionuclides that find their way into the environment.

We have organized this chapter in three primary sections: (1) general comments, (2) the organism, and (3) the ecosystem. Ingestion, biological uptake, and excretion of nuclides by terrestrial and aquatic organisms will be discussed, as will the techniques developed with nonmetabolic tracers to study these subjects. In discussing the ecosystem, we have emphasized the food web and the complete system with aquatic and terrestrial examples. Obviously, the various parts of the system are interrelated, and references cited in one section might appropriately have been considered in another. Since the literature abounds with papers on the topic of cycling, we have restricted the number of selected references and have attempted to stress the diversity that exists in radionuclide techniques.

Since a single reference source on design of experiments in the cycling of radionuclides is available only to the marine biologist, the terrestrial or freshwater ecologist must review the literature in his field of interest to search for assistance in designing experiments. However, the document available to the marine biologist, *Design of Radiotracer Experiments in Marine Biological Systems* [International Atomic Energy Agency (IAEA), 1975c], provides an excellent starting point, particularly for the freshwater biologist. This technical report of the IAEA includes discussions on laboratory and field experiments and also integrated field–laboratory experiments. Included are supporting papers on experiments with phytoplankton, zooplankton, benthic algae, benthic invertebrates, molluscs, and marine fishes, and also subcellular techniques, modeling, and comparison of field and laboratory techniques. Recommendations from this report include:

1. Whenever releases of radioactivity into the marine environment take place, they should be utilized as fully as possible for studies on transport, distribution and behaviour of the radionuclides to obtain information that is difficult to derive from laboratory experiments.
2. The influence of other contaminants and effects (e.g., organic matter, heavy metals, increased siltation, elevated temperature) on radioecological parameters in field studies should be carefully considered for possible synergistic effects.
3. Radioecological experiments in quasi-natural field conditions (e.g., in enclosed marine areas) should be encouraged because they represent an important step between laboratory and field conditions.
4. Emphasis should be placed on the use of modelling to analyze results of radioecological experiments in order to predict the behaviour of radionuclides and stable elements in nature.
5. Consideration should be given to comparing the methodology of marine radioecological experiments to achieve comparability of results from different laboratories. For full interpretation, all flux results should be expressed on a total element basis when chemically possible. Furthermore, sometimes experiments with the same or closely related organisms should be used to clarify discrepancies not otherwise solvable.

During the three-day coordination meeting held on May 29–31, 1972, in Monaco at which the establishment of a panel to prepare the document cited above was agreed on, the following general recommendations in reference to marine experiments, which are also essential considerations for terrestrial and freshwater experiments, were made (Renfro and Fowler, 1973; IAEA, 1975c):

(1) Depending upon the purpose of the experiment, it is necessary to know (and describe) the physico-chemical forms of the radioactive tracer, the carrier solution, and any contaminant present.
(2) Models of laboratory or field systems should conform to the conditions of the system, hence, it is necessary to know the number of compartments in the system and whether the system is "open" or "closed" with respect to the elements considered.
(3) For convenience and avoidance of confusion, notations and symbols such as used in the report to the *International Commission on Radiation Units* by Brownell, G. L., Berman, M. and Robertson, J. S. (1968), Nomenclature for tracer kinetics, *International Journal of Applied Radiation and Isotopes*, 19, 249, should be considered for use as standard terms for turnover models.
(4) In general, when using a radioisotope as a tracer, laboratory experiments should commence only after insuring that isotopic equilibrium exists. If isotopic equilibrium cannot be attained (in all the existing physico-chemical forms of the element), the dis-

equilibria must be described. In addition, the experimental conditions should be closely monitored. For these reasons, consideration should be given to designing carefully controlled experiments of long duration.

(5) Physiological parameters which could influence tracer experiments should be controlled or measured (to be taken into account in analysis of the results). Included among these factors are: (a) behaviour of the organism under laboratory conditions, (b) size and age, (c) growth, (d) feeding rate, (e) reproductive status, osmoregulatory and ion regulatory ability of organisms, (f) changing elemental composition, (g) moulting patterns, etc.

(6) Physical or chemical conditions which could influence radiotracer experiments should be controlled or measured (to be taken into account in analysis of the results). Included among these factors are: (a) temperature, (b) light, (c) salinity, (d) radiotracer specific activity, (e) sorption of radiotracer or stable elements contaminating the system, etc.

10.2. The Organism

10.2.1. Ingestion

The broad spectrum of topics associated with cycling of stable elements and radionuclides includes studies on biomass production and energy flow, which, in turn, are related to the nutrition of animals and plants. The use of radionuclide tracers in the study of the nutrition of animals is a common research practice. Sorokin (1968) discusses the use of ^{14}C in nutritional studies of aquatic animals in which he includes topics on labeling the food, ingestion, respiration, and assimilation.* Calow and Fletcher (1972) present a new technique for studying assimilation in two species of freshwater gastropods in which they measured ^{14}C and ^{51}Cr in food and feces. Food intake can be calculated from the total radioactivity of the animal and its feces as well as by other methods. Edmondson and Winberg (1971) discuss the advantages and disadvantages of methods that involve tracers in reference to secondary productivity in fresh water. They illustrate the methods as follows:

Method 1: Zooplankton feeding on labeled algal cells. The radioactivity of particulate matter in a known amount of water is measured before introduction of zooplankton into the media and after they have been allowed to feed for a period of time.

Method 2: Algal cells labeled and fed on by the marine copepod, *Calanus finmarchicus*. The radioactivity of the algal cells in a given volume of media and that of the copepod, eggs and feces are determined.

---

* The use of the term "assimilation" may be confusing to the reader. Rigler, in Edmondson and Winberg (1971), stated that it is used by physiologists ". . . to mean the conversion of digested food into the structural materials of the animal."

Method 3: Similar to Method 2 but the copepod would be measured again after a feeding period too short to produce radioactive pellets.

The feeding rates of terrestrial invertebrates have been studied by many investigators. Hubbel *et al.* (1965) discussed a study of the ingestion and assimilation rate of an isopod *(Armadillidium vulgare)* in the field and laboratory in the vicinity of San Francisco, California. They used a technique of soaking food of the isopod in a solution of ^{85}Sr. This radionuclide was selected because these isopods readily assimilate strontium and the turnover rate is low. This gamma emitter had the added advantage of eliminating the problem of self-absorption such as one would have with a beta emitter when making whole-body counts. The experimental procedure in the laboratory included feeding the animals on nonradioactive food for 5 days followed by feeding them on the same food tagged with ^{85}Sr of a known amount. The total feeding period was 96 hr, but after the first 48 hr, the radioactive food was replaced with fresh radioactive food. In another experiment in which ingestion was studied by the gravimetric method, radioactive food was made available to the animals for 48 hr, and the amount of food consumed was determined by subtracting the weight of the remaining food from the initial weight. A somewhat similar study was made in the field to compare the two methods, with the radioactive food placed in a plastic bucket sunk into the ground. In both field and laboratory, the radionuclide technique involved determining the amount of food consumed by calculating the difference between initial activity and final activity of the food. Radioactivity loss in an isopod after it was taken off radioactive food in the laboratory is shown in Figure 55 and that in a field enclosure in Figure 56. The investigators concluded:

> . . . this investigation presents a convincing demonstration of the feasibility of using radiotracers to obtain accurate estimates of feeding and assimilation rates of animal populations in the field. But it has been shown, also, that experimental analysis of the parameters involved in determining radionuclide turnover may be essential in such a study. In particular, assumptions about the assimilation fraction, a, and the rate constant for radionuclide elimination, k, should be made with caution. These parameters are usually amenable to empirical analysis, and such a study should accompany experiments measuring feeding rate with tracers.

In a study of insect–plant relationships at Oak Ridge National Laboratory, Crossley (1963) utilized a field nuclear waste site containing ^{137}Cs. *Chrysomela knabi* beetle larvae were collected on leaves from willow trees *(Salix nigra)* growing on White Oak Lake bed. This lake was formerly a low-level waste disposal site at the laboratory, and the sediments contained various radionuclides, including ^{137}Cs. Consequently, the leaves of the willow tree contained ^{137}Cs

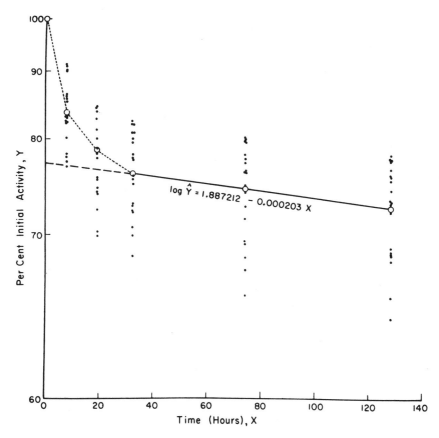

Figure 55. Loss of radioactivity from isopods *(Armadillidium vulgare)* containing ^{85}Sr in the laboratory. Time 0 was the end of the feeding period. (•) Percentage activity remaining in the different experimental groups; (○) the average loss of unassimilated material during the first 2 days; (—) loss by elimination of assimilated ^{85}Sr and by physical decay, a least-squares estimate of the regression calculated from observations made at 32, 74, and 128 hr. From Hubbell *et al.* (1965). Reproduced from *Health Physics* **11**:1485–1501 (1965) by permission of the Health Physics Society.

resulting from uptake from the sediments. The feeding rate of this 3rd-instar larva was calculated by determining the activity of the larva per gram of dry weight (72.9 ± 14.6 pCi), which was the steady-state equilibrium value, A_q, and the biological half-life (8 hr), which was calculated from laboratory data based on retention of ^{134}Cs (Figure 57a). The elimination constant, k, was computed (2.08/day) based on an exponential decrease. This is illustrated in Figure 57b for a grasshopper *(Melanoplus differentialis)*. It should be noted that

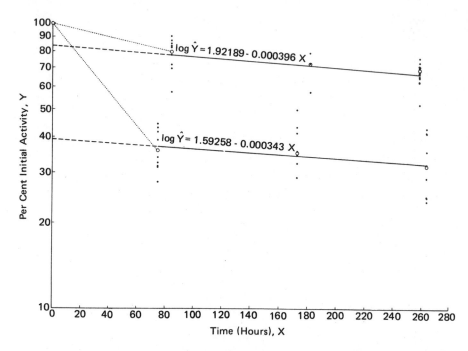

Figure 56. Loss of radioactivity from isopods *(Armadillidium vulgare)* containing [85]Sr in a field enclosure. Upper curve based on counts of color-marked individuals; lower curve based on counts of groups of animals (20 in each) collected from the enclosure; (——) least-squares estimates based on the last three count times in each case. For an explanation of the different x = ○ intercepts, see Hubbell *et al.* (1965). From Hubbell *et al.* (1965). Reproduced from *Health Physics* **11**:1485–1501 (1965) by permission of the Health Physics Society.

an exponential decrease with time plots as a straight line on semi-log paper. Using these values, one can compute the feeding rate as defined by Crossley, of the larva, in μCi/day by inserting them within the equation that Crossley developed:

$$\text{``Feeding rate''} = kA_q$$

where k and A_q are as defined above. Thus, in this case, his "feeding rate" = (2.08)(72.9) = 151 pCi/g beetle per day. We prefer to define feeding rate in g/day rather than μCi/day.

The feeding-rate equation can be utilized when more than one species is involved. Crossley discussed its application and commented that some sort of weighted average of k for all insects must be computed. Since it is not practical to compute k for possibly hundreds of species in an area, he suggested that the relationship of body weight to biological half-life (see Figure 57c) be used. He concludes: "These radioisotope techniques are fulfilling their initial promise as an uncomplicated technique for specifying rates of movement of materials along food chains, and thus quantifying the relationships of herbivorous insect populations to plants and of predators to prey."

In a study of microarthropod ingestion rates of pine mor detritus, Kowal and Crossley (1971) used a method in which the organism ingested ^{45}Ca-tagged pine mor and the gain in ^{45}Ca due to ingestion and excretion was observed. The arthropods were maintained at various temperatures in containers with one of four layers of pine mor that had been tagged by soaking with ^{45}Ca. Every 5 days for 60 days, the organisms were identified, weighed, counted, and measured for radioactivity, and the mor in the container was weighed and counted for radioactivity. The investigators concluded that the experiment resulted in "rough estimates of the fluxes of dry organic material from the detritus to saprovores, and from the saprovores to the predators in the pine-mor microarthropod food web." An interesting discussion of the development of the mathematical model is presented. This model is similar to the one discussed above (Crossley, 1963) and discussed by Reichle (1969). Comprehension of the mathematical model development presented in these three papers should provide a good base for understanding papers on the cycling of radionuclides.

Fallout ^{137}Cs associated with forage of big-game animals has been used to estimate forage intake rates. Alldredge *et al.* (1974) utilized data on ^{137}Cs content in muscle of free-ranging mule deer *(Odocoileus hemionus)* and the content of forage from the animals' range (Figure 58) to estimate forage-intake rate as related to season and deer age. The mathematical model is derived in their paper. A similar model with stochastic properties was applied by Hanson *et al.* (1975) in a study of forage-intake rates of free-ranging caribou *(Rangifer arcticus)* in northern Alaska. The data included concentrations of fallout ^{137}Cs in *Cladonia* lichen and caribou flesh over a period of years (Figure 59).

In addition to their use in measuring ingestion in terrestrial organisms, radionuclide techniques for measuring ingestion by aquatic animals have been developed. Reference was made above to methods described by Edmondson and Winberg (1971) for secondary producers in fresh waters. An early historical paper on the general subject for marine animals is that of Chipman (1959), in which he discussed filter-feeding of tagged algae to molluscs and included minor comments on fish.

Feeding rates and food utilization of a caddisfly *(Neophylax concinnus)* were studied by Sedell (1973) using the tracers ^{14}C and ^{60}Co. Caddisfly larvae were collected from a small stream in Pennsylvania and maintained in the laboratory on rocks. The rocks were placed in a solution containing ^{60}Co to tag the

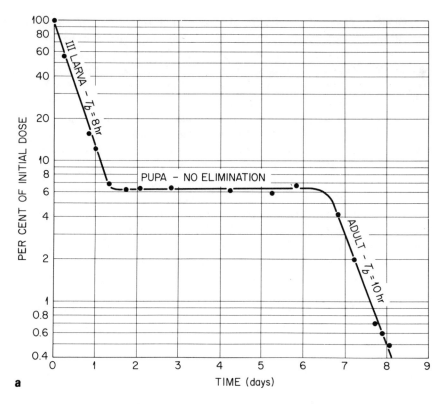

a

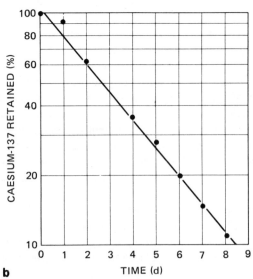

b

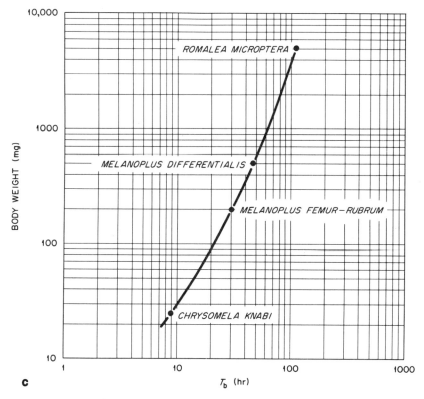

Figure 57. Some results of a study on insect–plant relationships utilizing radioactive tracers. (a) Retention of ^{134}Cs by an individual beetle *(Chrysomela knabi)*. Third-instar larva, pupa, and adult stages are shown. (b) Retention of ^{137}Cs by a single grasshopper *Melanoplus differentialis*. (c) Relationship of insect weight to biological half-life of cesium. From Crossley (1963).

aufwuchs (periphyton attached to the rocks) and the organic debris on them with the radionuclide, removed and washed with filtered stream water, and placed in shallow pans. The caddisfly larvae were then placed on these rocks for a period of time, removed, and counted. Samples of the periphyton were collected and counted prior to introduction of the larvae and following their removal. The amount of food ingested was calculated.

Sedell used ^{14}C and ^{60}Co in a study of assimilation rates by placing rocks in a solution containing [^{14}C]bicarbonate and [^{14}C]glucose and exposing them to constant light for a period of time, washing and placing them in a ^{60}Co solution for 1–3 hr, and rinsing them again before placing larvae on them. The quantity of food consumed was then calculated. Following the initial count to determine the amount of food ingested, the organisms were placed on untagged food and

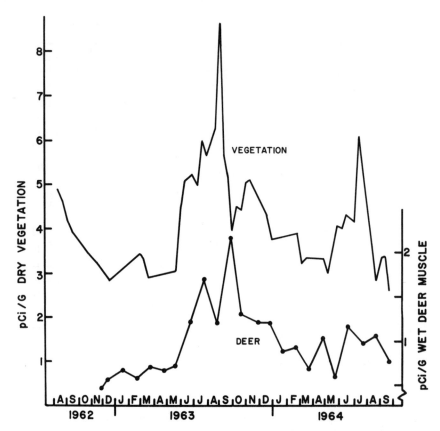

Figure 58. Cesium-137 concentration in mule deer *(Odocoileus hemionus)* muscle and dietary cesium concentration curve generated for deer wintering on the middle winter range. From Alldredge *et al.* (1974).

monitored until they eliminated the ^{60}Co (Figure 60a). The larvae and samples of aufwuchs were processed for radioactivity. Assimilation rates were determined from the ^{14}C tag using the same equation. Ingestion rates determined from the ^{60}Co experiment were not significantly affected by the types of organisms on the rocks (Figure 60b).

Filtering rates of molluscs have been determined by the reduction in numbers of tagged unicellular algae in an aquarium containing the mollusc of interest. Rice and Smith (1958) studied the filtering rate of the hard clam *(Venus mercenaria)* by this procedure. Single and mixed cultures of four species of planktonic algae were fed to the clam. The algae were tagged by placing them in seawater containing carrier-free ^{32}P for a period of time, the filtrate containing the tagged algae was counted, and the number of cells per given volume was determined. By utilizing the total-number data, media containing a specific number of algae could be prepared. The researchers commented that by incorporating a sufficient amount of ^{32}P in the cells, a small change in the number of cells in suspension could be determined, even at levels considerably smaller than those that occur in nature. Clams were placed in battery jars containing the algal culture, and the solution was continuously stirred. Periodically, 10-cc samples of the suspension were collected, filtered, and counted, and the filtering rate was computed from Jørgensen's formula.

Malone and Nelson (1969) estimated the feeding rate of the freshwater stream snail, *Goniobasis clavaeformis,* by allowing the snail to feed on the surface of rocks that had been soaked in a ^{60}Co solution. The procedure was similar to that of Sewell (1973), so it will not be discussed in further detail.

Two papers concerning the use of a radionuclide technique in studying feeding rate of fish will be discussed, that of Kevern (1966) for yearling carp *(Cyprinus carpio)* collected from White Oak Lake, Oak Ridge National Laboratory, and that of Kolehmainen (1974) for bluegill *(Lepomis macrochirus)* from the same lake. The studies involved determination of the amount of ^{137}Cs required to be ingested to maintain an equilibrium body burden in both species. The

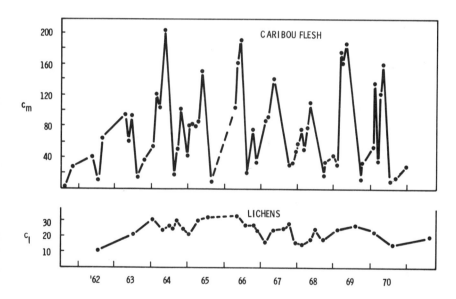

Figure 59. Fallout ^{137}Cs concentrations in lichens (C_l) and caribou flesh (C_m) at Anaktuvuk Pass, Alaska, during the period 1962–1970. Units of C_l and C_m in $pCi^{137}Cs/g$ standard dry wt. From Hanson *et al.* (1975).

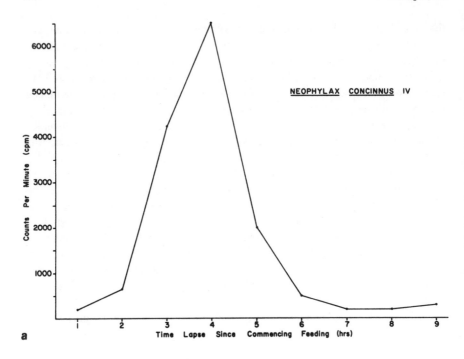

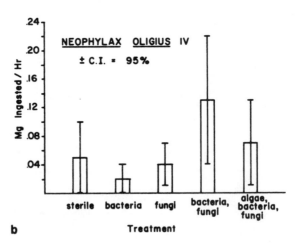

Figure 60. Some results of utilizing ^{60}Co in a study of feeding rates and food utilization of stream caddisfly larvae (*Neophylax* spp.). (a) Rate of passage of ^{60}Co-tagged food through the digestive tract of *N. concinnus* IV. Feces were collected en masse from 30 larvae at 1-hr intervals for a 9-hr period. (b) Ingestion rates of *N. oligius* IV when feeding on various types of microorganisms tagged with [60]Co. From Sedell (1973).

procedure was similar to that of Crossley (1963) in his study, described previously, on insects from the lake bed. Values for body burden, biological half-life, and assimilation factors were used. It was assumed that the body burden was at equilibrium with the ^{137}Cs in the food. Since the fish must have spent their life in the lake for the equilibrium assumption to be reasonable, Kevern (1966) prepared autoradiographs of fish scales that revealed radioactivity throughout the scales, indicating that the fish had been there since hatching. Laboratory experiments at two different water temperatures were conducted in a study of the biological half-life of ^{134}Cs in carp. The biological half-lives computed were used together to obtain a single value of the elimination constant, k. The assimilated fraction of the ingested ^{134}Cs was determined from fish measurements before and after elimination of the tag. The large variability in ^{137}Cs concentration in samples of algae, on which carp feed, resulted in a wide range of estimated feeding-rate values; however, Kevern (1966) believed that the results were valuable as a first approximation and as an illustration of the method. He also commented that general application of the technique depends on sufficient levels of ^{137}Cs in the environment and that, based on the literature, levels appeared to be sufficient in some areas, especially in northern latitudes. As a result of relatively little atmospheric nuclear-weapons testing since the signing of the limited test ban treaty by some nuclear powers, it is unlikely that levels of ^{137}Cs still exist in the general environment that would make the technique of general applicability. However, some specific areas do exist that contain sufficient amounts of ^{137}Cs for this purpose.

The technique of Kolehmainen (1974) is somewhat more sophisticated in that it is suitable for determining daily feeding rates and ^{137}Cs intake for the nonequilibrium state. The nonequilibrium-state calculations utilized measures of fish growth and seasonal fluctuation of ^{137}Cs in the fish as well as the relationship of temperature to elimination rate (Figure 61).

10.2.2. Biological Uptake and Retention

We will now consider radionuclide techniques utilized in studies of biological uptake and retention within the organism. First, studies will be reviewed that are concerned with the nutritional aspects of essential elements. These will be followed with studies of radionuclides associated with the nuclear age, such as fission and neutron-activation products.

For years, there has been a natural curiosity as to the morphological and physiological characteristics of antler growth. Since phosphorus is an important constituent of the skull and antler, the mineral metabolism of phosphorus is of interest. Rerabeck and Bubenik (1963) studied this mineral using ^{32}P with red deer *(Cervus elaphus),* fallow deer *(Cervus dama dama),* and roebuck *(Capreolus*

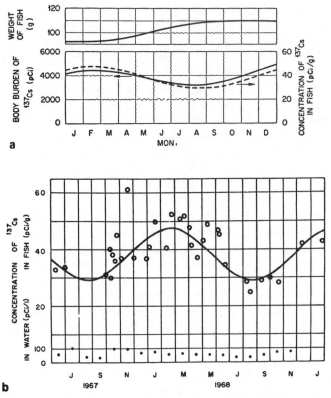

Figure 61. Daily feeding rates of bluegill *(Lepomis macrochirus)* determined by a refined radionuclide method. (a) Daily average weights of 74 bluegill during 1967–1968 (upper solid line) calculated from a derived equation presented in Kolehmainen (1974) and concentrations of ^{137}Cs [pCi/g wet wt. of fish (- - - -)], represented by a sine function; concentrations of ^{137}Cs in fish (lower solid line) calculated by multiplying the average concentration of the radionuclide in fish at time t by the weight of the fish at time t. All values are calculated for average-size White Oak Lake bluegill that were 4 years old in the summer. (b) Monthly concentrations of ^{137}Cs in White Oak Lake bluegill (pCi/g wet wt.), and of ^{137}Cs in the water, June 1967–January 1969. (—) Sine wave calculated with a least-squares method based on 33 samples totaling 206 fish. From Kolehmainen (1974).

capreolus) and iodine with ^{131}I in the roebuck. One experimental procedure was to inject ^{32}P as an inorganic phosphate into the marginal ear lobe vein and another was to feed the animal a baked dough loaf on which drops of ^{32}P-labeled inorganic phosphate had been placed. The animals were maintained in a metabolic stall (Figure 62), and the feces and urine were collected, although the latter incompletely. Distribution of ^{32}P in the antlers was studied by means of audioradiography and by samples of tissues and excreta that were counted using a

Geiger–Müller (GM) tube. The specific activity of ^{32}P in a growing antler of a fallow buck is shown in Figure 63. In another experiment, the researchers obtained phosphorus bound in the plant by spraying growing bean plants with a solution of ^{32}P. After a period of time, the plants were rinsed to remove the nonincorporated ^{32}P, counted, and fed to a deer. In still another study, the

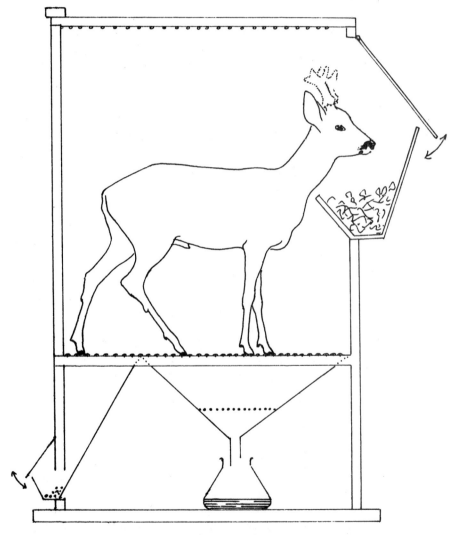

Figure 62. Holding pen used in a study that utilized radionuclide tracers of the metabolism of phosphorus and iodine in deer. From Rerabek and Bubenik (1963).

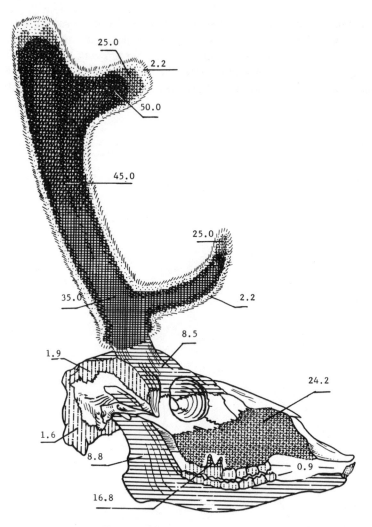

Figure 63. Specific activity of ^{32}P in growing antler tissue of fallow buck *(Cervus dama dama)* in mCi $\times$ 10^{-5}/g. From Rerabek and Bubenik (1963).

investigators used a "gardening type of duster" to spray growing alfalfa plants, then rinsed, counted, and fed the alfalfa. In addition, a minor study involving the injection of ^{131}I into a roebuck was conducted.

In a study of calcium and strontium metabolism as related to age and antler growth of white-tailed deer *(Odocoileus virginianus)*, Cowan *et al.* (1968) maintained deer in metabolism cages after injecting the deer intravenously with ^{45}Ca and [89]Sr. Feces and urine were collected over a period of time and counted. The sternum, various ribs, and vertebrae were also counted.

Mineral metabolism of various types of aquatic organisms has been studied. McEnery and Lee (1970) used ^{14}C, ^{32}P, ^{35}S, [45]Ca, and ^{90}Sr in a study of mineralization and cycling in two species of foraminifera. Bryan (1968), in a study of stable zinc concentration in tissues of 18 species of decapod crustaceans (shrimps, prawns, lobsters, crayfish, hermit crab, crabs), injected the crab *Maia squinado)* with carrier-free [65]Zn and placed the animal in seawater containing 100 μg/liter of zinc to see whether zinc was lost via the feces. The animal was fed, and the resulting feces were collected from the holding tank. Figure 64 shows the results of this study.

The uptake of sodium in freshwater turtles has been thought of as occurring via food, but recent investigations indicate that a significant amount of sodium may be obtained from the environment via active transport (Dunson, 1969).

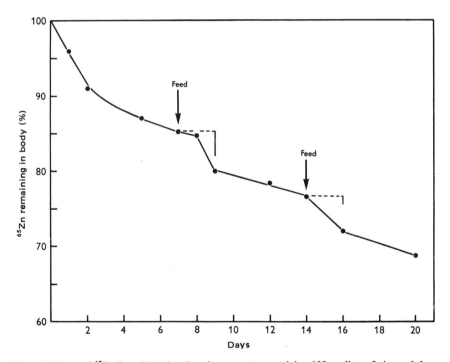

Figure 64. Loss of [65]Zn from *Maia* into inactive seawater containing 100 μg/liter of zinc and the effect on this of two periods of feeding with the worm *Arenicola*. The broken line represents the period during which feces were collected; the vertical line represents the amount of [65]Zn in the feces. From Bryan (1968). Courtesy of Cambridge University Press.

Dunson used hatchling slider turtles *(Pseudemys scripta)* in sodium flux studies. The turtles were placed in a sodium chloride solution containing ^{24}Na, and the body burden was determined with a scintillation counting system for the turtles with the cloaca open and closed. On the basis of these studies on intact animals and of *in vitro* membrane studies, it was concluded that transport was localized in the cloacal and oral regions.

Studies on marine zooplankton element-elimination rate were conducted with zooplankton labeled with tracers and with fallout radionuclides (Kuenzler, 1969). The animals were placed in nonradioactive seawater, and after a period of time they were removed and the radioactivity of the water was determined. The tracer-labeled zooplankton were obtained by placing zooplankton in carrier-free solutions of $Na^{131}I$, $^{58}CoCl_2$, or $^{65}ZnCl_2$, retained in the solution until labeled adequately, washed, and placed in another container to study elimination.

Although we have directed most of our discussion toward animals, numerous studies of mineral metabolism in plants have also been conducted using tracer techniques. Methods used in labeling plants will be considered in Chapter 11. The radionuclides ^{32}P and ^{45}Ca were used by Woods and Brock (1964) to study interspecific transfer of phosphorus and calcium by root systems of various plants in a mixed hardwood forest in North Carolina. Red maple trees *(Acer rubrum)* 2–3 inches in diameter were cut, and the radionuclides, in a solution of water, were placed in cups formed with modeling clay around the tops of the stumps. The stumps were covered with plastic bags to prevent movement of the radionuclide off the stumps. In one case, the ^{32}P was introduced into the tree with a hypodermic syringe under the bark with results similar to those for the cup procedure. Leaves of plant species surrounding the tagged tree were collected and counted. The authors observed that 19 species up to 24 ft from the tagged tree contained detectable ^{32}P.

In another study of root extension of trees, Brown and Woods (1968) tagged surface soils in a hardwood forest by applying ^{131}I with a NaI carrier to plots that had been treated with methyl bromide to kill roots at the application point. Autoradiographs were made to determine the volume of soil treated with the radionuclide. They were made by inserting "no-screen medical X-ray film, sealed with polyethylene and plastic tape" into vertical slits at the point of application from 4 to 8 weeks after application of the radionuclide solution. In addition, the film was placed on the surface of the ground to study horizontal distribution of the radionuclide. The detection equipment is illustrated in Figure 65, and some results are presented in Figure 66.

The redistribution of calcium in dogwood trees *(Cornus florida)* was studied over three growing seasons by Thomas (1970), who inoculated trees with ^{45}Ca. Water was placed in troughs around each tree, cuts were made under water into the xylem, and an amount of ^{45}Ca proportional to estimated tree weight was introduced into the water on May 4, 1966. During the fall of that year, a sample

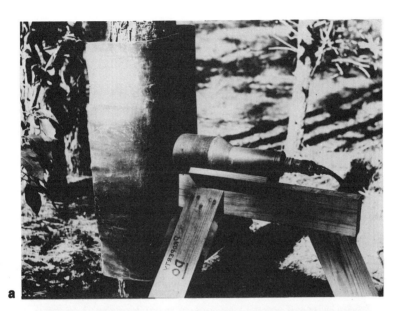

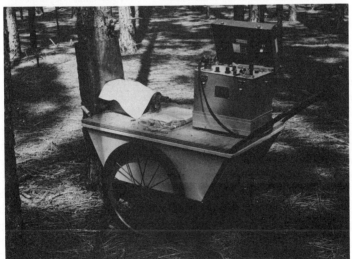

Figure 65. Detection equipment and accessories for measuring ^{131}I in stems. (a) Lead shield and scintillation probe in position. (b) Portable scaler in position for taking measurements. Courtesy of F. W. Woods.

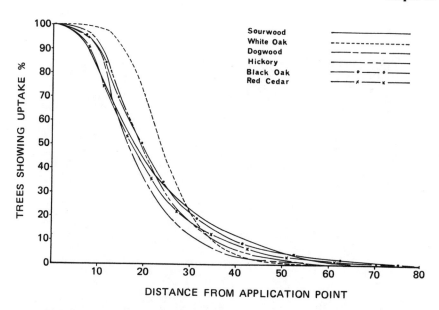

Figure 66. Expected percentage of trees showing uptake with distance from ^{131}I application spot for sourwood *(Oxydendrum arboreum)*, the white oak group *(Quercus alba, Q. stellata)*, dogwood *(Cornus florida)*, hickories *(Carya* spp.), the black oak group *(Q. velutina, Q. falcata, Q. coccinea, Q. rubra, Q. marilandica)*, and red cedar *(Juniperus virginiana)*. Based on probit analyses. From Brown and Woods (1968).

of the tagged trees was cut, and the distribution of [45]Ca within wood tissues was determined. Additional trees were cut during the fall of 1967 and 1968 for the same purpose. Leaf samples were collected each month they were available after the initial inoculation and were also counted.

The loss of [45]Ca via fall and decomposition of leaves from deciduous and evergreen trees was studied by Monk (1971), who inoculated tree stems. He observed that the difference in leaf fall between the two groups was also reflected in loss of calcium, with greater retention observed in evergreen species.

Many studies have been conducted on the biological uptake and retention of fission and neutron-activation products in organisms, including man and domestic plants and animals. We will consider a limited selection of studies using wild organisms to illustrate this use of tracer technology.

Zinc-65, a strong gamma emitter produced by neutron activation in water-cooled reactors such as those at Hanford, was of interest to radiation ecologists. We have discussed the tagging of waterfowl by this nuclide and ^{32}P-tagging in waterfowl in the Columbia River at Hanford (Hanson and Case, 1963) in Chapter 6 (Section 6.3.3). The biological uptake and retention of [65]Zn by mallard ducks

(Anas platyrhynchos) was studied by Curnow *et al.* (1967), who either force-fed the ducks every 2 days for a 30-day period with gelatin capsules containing ^{65}Zn absorbed into food granules or placed the ducks in a tank with water containing ^{65}Zn so that the animals became tagged by drinking the water or through body absorption. After contamination, this latter group of birds was divided into two groups, one allowed free access to treated and untreated water and the other limited to untreated water only in a study of retention of surface ^{65}Zn. Whole-body counts were made throughout the experiment, and tissue assay was performed at the end of whole-body counting. It was observed that the biological half-life of ^{65}Zn was similar for the two methods of tagging birds where the birds had limited access to water.

A fission product of considerable interest to radiation ecologists is ^{137}Cs. The cycling of this radionuclide in natural systems has undergone considerable investigation. In addition, controlled laboratory and field studies have been conducted wherein plants and animals have been tagged with the radionuclide.

In conjunction with an extensive study of fallout ^{137}Cs in a mule deer *(Odocoileus hemionus hemionus)* population, Hakonson and Whicker (1969) investigated the biological uptake and elimination of ^{134}Cs in deer placed in metabolic cages ($3 \times 4 \times 6$ ft) as well as others confined in large outdoor holding pens of various sizes. The study was designed to study effects of sex and age, elevated dietary potassium, and dietary crude fiber on uptake and elimination. After a week of dietary adjustment, the deer were given an acute oral dose of carrier-free $^{134}CsCl$ by placing the radionuclide in water and allowing the deer to drink it after being water-starved for 24 hr. Some of Hakonson and Whicker's data are presented in Figure 67.

Radioactive tungsten has been observed to occur in significant quantities following detonation of certain nuclear devices; consequently, the study of its biological uptake and retention by organisms and its cycling within ecosystems is justified. Reed and Martinedes (1973) designed a study of the uptake and retention of ^{181}W by the crayfish *(Cambarus longulus longerostris)* by placing them in containers with a solution of the radionuclide for 7 days, then removing them and placing them in a container of flowing spring water. The animals were then whole-body-counted daily for a period of days using a single-channel analyzer with a NaI(Tl) well crystal. Tissues of sample crayfish were also counted, and the highest concentration was observed in the exoskeleton. The whole-body retention curve is shown in Figure 68.

The metabolism of ^{90}Sr and its biological analogue, ^{45}Ca, has been studied. The uptake of the former, which is an important fission product, is related to the amount of calcium available to an organism. The distribution of these tracers in various tissues of the guppy *(Lebistes* sp.) has been reported by Rosenthal (1957). The fish were maintained in glass aquaria with water containing the

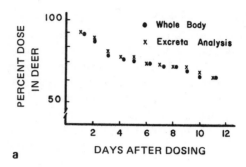

a

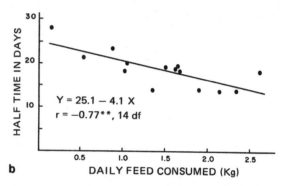

b

Figure 67. Uptake and elimination of [134]Cs by mule deer *(Odocoileus hemionus hemionus)*. (a) Cesium-134 retention curve in deer as derived by whole-body counting vs. exreta analysis. (b) Cesium-134 half-time of slow component in deer as a function of daily feed consumption (kg). (c) Cesium-134 half-time of slow component in deer as a function of body weight (kg). (d) Effect of "fasting" on [134]Cs retention in deer. From Hakonson and Whicker (1969).

radionuclide and were sacrificed periodically for tissue-counting with a gas-flow windowless counting system (Figure 69).

The biological uptake of cesium has been studied in trees under field conditions. In a study of cesium cycling in white oak trees *(Quercus alba)* at Oak Ridge National Laboratory, Witherspoon (1963) inoculated trees on four contrasting soil types. Cesium-134 was introduced into the trees as a chloride in a weak acidic solution via Mauget feeders that were attached to the tree trunk 1 m above the ground. Leaves from these trees and adjacent soil and litter samples were counted during the growing season. In an investigation of movement of the radionuclide from litter to vegetation, leaves tagged with [134]Cs were placed on the ground around white oak saplings, and release of the radionuclide and

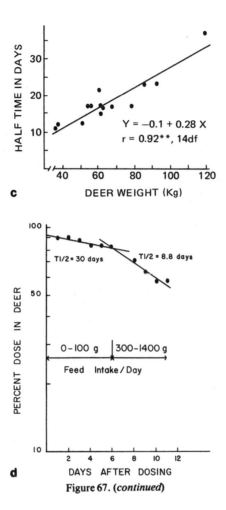

Figure 67. (*continued*)

uptake were compared with the uptake by trees growing on a plot on which aqueous solutions of the radionuclide had been placed (Figure 70a). The uptake and losses of ^{134}Cs are shown in Figure 70b.

10.2.3. Excretion

Radionuclide techniques have been used to measure the rate of food passage through an organism by determining the rate of appearance of the radionuclide in feces. Such techniques have been used in studies of metabolism, since the rate of elimination of a substance is related in some fashion to metabolic rate. Tracer techniques have been developed specifically to study a process, while

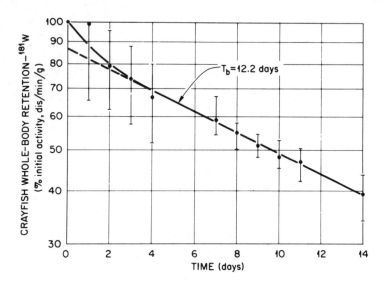

Figure 68. Crayfish *(Cambarus longulus longerostris)* whole-body retention of [181]W after 7 days of radionuclide uptake from water. The points through day 4 are means of 5 animals ± 1 S.E.; those from days 7–14 are the means of 2 animals ± 1 S.E. From Reed and Martinedes (1973).

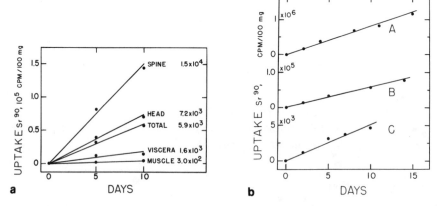

Figure 69. Uptake of ^{90}Sr by the guppy *(Lebistes* sp.) (a) Uptake of ^{90}Sr by various tissues of the male guppy vs. days in water containing 9×10^4 cpm/ml. Values for each tissue represent rate of uptake of ^{90}Sr in terms of cpm/100 mg per day. Each point represents 6 values. (b) Uptake of ^{90}Sr by male guppies vs. days in water containing the radionuclide. Each point represents 2–4 fish. Water activity for the curves (in cpm/ml): (A) 1 times 10^6; (B) 1.7×10^5; (C) 1.1×10^4. From Rosenthal (1957).

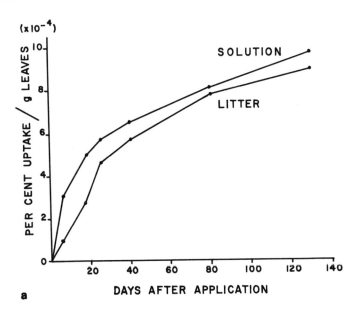

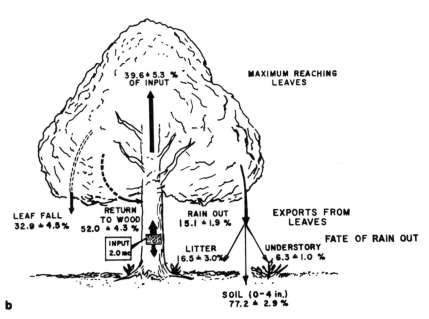

Figure 70. Cycling of ^{134}Cs in white oak *(Quercus alba)* trees. (a) Percentage uptake of ^{134}Cs by sapling leaves from tagged litter and solution applied to Landisburg soil. (b) Cycle of ^{134}Cs in white oak. Average of 12 trees at end of growing season. (a) From Witherspoon (1964). (b) From Witherspoon *et al.* (1962).

others have been directed to studying the radionuclide itself. The latter is of concern to the radiation ecologist and has been discussed to some degree in Section 10.2.2. In this section, we will restrict our discussion to the use of tracers in studying food-passage rate in animals.

Various techniques have been developed to study the rate of food passage through the digestive tract, such as use of dyes, rubber pellets, and beads that have been introduced into the food prior to ingestion. The radionuclide technique involves selection of a radionuclide that is totally or almost totally excreted, rather than absorbed. Such an inert radionuclide is ^{51}Cr, which has a physical half-life of 27.8 days and decays by gamma emission. According to Shilling and Shilling (1964), ^{51}Cr is used extensively in medical diagnosis and in the study of red blood cells. It has been used in food-passage-rate studies of birds by G. E. Duke *et al.* (1968) and Gasaway *et al.* (1975) and in mammals by Petrides (1968), Mautz and Petrides (1967), and Mautz (1971). The radionuclide method has the advantage over other methods in being more sensitive.

Food metabolism and passage-rate studies using the inert tracer ^{51}Cr have been conducted on the ring-necked pheasant *(Phasianus colchicus)* by G. E. Duke *et al.* (1968) wherein the ^{51}Cr was applied to food. In single-dose studies, the ^{51}CrCl$_3$ solution was placed on a food pellet with a pipette. Excreta were counted with a scintillation counting system. Food consumption and total excreta data permitted computation of a metabolism coefficient:

$$\left[1 - \frac{\text{weight of total excreta}}{\text{total weight of food}} \right] \times 100$$

The labeled foods enabled the investigators to associate excreta with specific foods assuming that the nuclide adheres tightly to a specific food in the gut. Continuous-dose studies utilized food that had been mixed uniformly with ^{51}Cr and fed to test animals for one to several days. In these studies, the metabolism coefficient was equal to

$$\left[1 - \frac{\text{cpm}^{51}\text{Cr/g feed}}{\text{cpm}^{51}\text{Cr/g excreta}} \right] \times 100$$

which should be equal to the values obtained from the previous equation. The investigators stated that the equations did not give similar results. Passage rate was determined in the single-dose studies from the time the ^{51}Cr was first detected in the feces following feeding to the time it disappeared. Figure 71 shows the results of a continuous feeding study.

In a study of movement of digesta in the intestine and cecum of the rock ptarmigan *(Lagopus mutus)*, Gasaway *et al.* (1975) used ^{133}BaSO$_4$, [^{51}Cr]-EDTA, and ^{144}Ce as single-dose markers delivered into the esophagus by means of a

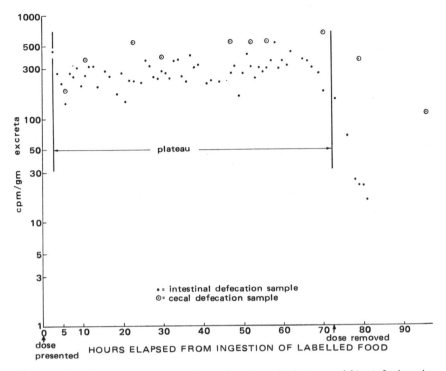

Figure 71. Defecation rate and pattern for a ring-necked pheasant *(Phasianus colchicus)* after ingestion of a continuous dose of ^{51}Cr on turkey breeder pellets. From G. E. Duke *et al.* (1968).

syringe to which was attached a ⅛-inch plastic tube. The excreta was separated into portions of cecal and intestinal origin, dried, and counted with a NaI(Tl) crystal connected to a pulse-height analyzer. In quantifying label concentrations in multiple isotope experiments, a gamma-ray spectrum stripping technique was used. Calculations were as follows:

> Rates of passage of water and DM [dry matter] were determined from accumulative excretion curves of ^{51}Cr-EDTA and Ce-144, respectively. The accumulation of 5, 50 and 95% of the marker were used to compare flow rates through the intestine, cecum and entire gut.
>
> The amount of water and DM entering the cecum, expressed as fraction of water and DM entering the hindgut, was calculated from the respective recoveries of ^{51}Cr-EDTA and Ce-144 in cecal droppings compared with total droppings.
>
> The fraction of cecal contents emptied per cecal defecation was calculated by assuming that the cecum was dosed by the marker and subsequently uniformly distributed in cecal contents. However, perfect mixing probably does not occur, hence this is a source of error. The total dose of marker entering the cecum was estimated by summing the marker contained in individual cecal droppings. The percentage of cecal fill expelled in each dropping was calculated as follows:

% of cecal fill emptied in first dropping = 100 × (μCi marker in first dropping) / (Sum of μCi marker excreted in cecal feces)

% of cecal fill emptied in second or succeeding droppings = 100 × (μCi marker in 2nd or succeeding droppings) / [(Sum of μCi marker excreted in cecal feces) − (μCi in 1st or sum of preceding droppings)].

The accumulation of two of the tracers is illustrated in Figure 72. The investigators used [^{51}Cr]-EDTA as a water or liquid marker and ^{144}CeCl$_3$ as a particulate marker. The study of G. E. Duke *et al.* (1968) assumed that ^{51}Cr was a particulate marker. Gassaway *et al.* (1975) discussed this assumption and questioned its validity. They cited research indicating that ^{51}CrCl$_3$ behaves more as a liquid marker. The ^{133}BaSO$_4$ was used to calculate the average percentage of cecal contents emptied per cecal defecation. The investigators presented a very interesting discussion of their procedures and results in a more detailed fashion than our summarization.

Petrides (1968) reported preliminary investigations of ^{51}Cr as a label of ingested foods in the cotton rat *(Sigmodon hispidus)*, bobcat *(Lynx rufus)*, opossum *(Didelphis virginiana)*, domestic goat *(Capra hircus)*, and a millepede *(Julus* sp.); however, only data on the opossum were reported (Figure 73) that disclosed

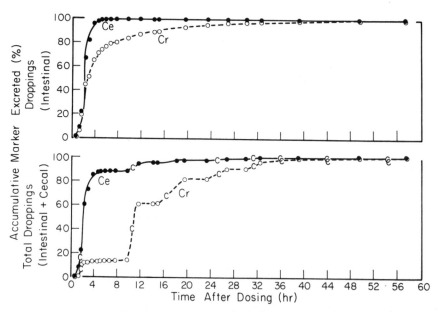

Figure 72. Cumulative percentages of markers [^{51}Cr]-EDTA and ^{144}Ce recovered in intestinal and total excreta of rock ptarmigan *(Lagopus mutus)* No. 2. Cecal defecation during a collection period is indicated by a "C" on the total excreta curves. From Gasaway *et al.* (1975).

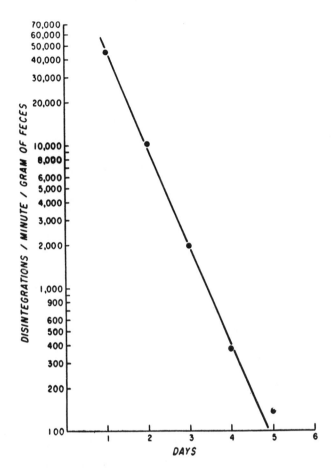

Figure 73. Defecation of ^{51}Cr by an oppossum *(Didelphis virginiana)*. From Petrides (1968).

an exponential relationship between the parameters, implying good mixing in the gut. Tagging of food was accomplished by placing a single small dose of ^{51}Cr on a food item, usually dried on the food. In a passage-rate study of white-tailed deer *(Odocoileus virginianus)*, Mautz and Petrides (1967) used ^{51}CrCl$_3$ as a food marker. Both single-dose and continuous-dose studies were conducted using labeled food. Single-dose studies utilized food that had been tagged directly with a pipette and dried. A tray of food used for the continuous-dose experiments was sprayed with an atomizer containing the label and dried. Feces were collected from the time of ingestion until the label was no longer detectable in the feces. Chromium-51 was not detected in the urine or tissue samples collected from sacrificed animals following termination of fecal collection. Figure 74 illustrates

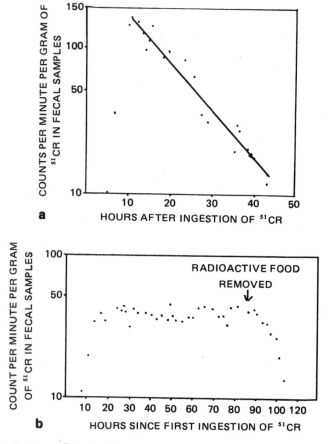

Figure 74. Defecation of ^{51}Cr by white-tailed deer *(Odocoileus virginianus)* on different tagged diets. (a) Defecation pattern for a deer fed a single 9.2-μCi dose while on a lamb-finisher diet. July 1966. (b) Defecation pattern for a deer fed a continuous dose while on a lamb-finisher diet. August 1966. From Mautz and Petrides (1967).

some of the observations. The investigators concluded that the technique provides a useful indicator of many digestive characteristics of deer and that if only passage-rate determinations are to be made, single-dose experiments are faster than continuous-dose experiments. An extension of the results in this paper was presented by Mautz (1971).

A food-passage-rate study in the pinfish *(Lagodon rhomboides)* was conducted by Peters and Hoss (1974) using ^{144}Ce-labeled food. Cerium was selected as a tag because it is "poorly assimilated." Peters and Hoss commented that other elements of the rare earth series should also serve as suitable tags and those elements that occur primarily as hydroxides attach readily to particles by adsorption, thus facilitating tagging. The investigators compared the radionuclide technique with a conventional method of measuring evacuation time. The food items, small fish and shrimp, were either labeled by individual injection with a syringe or mass-tagged by holding the animals for 12 hr in a tank containing $^{144}CeCl_3$ in seawater. The pinfish were denied food until their gastrointestinal tract was free of food, and they were then offered tagged food. Whole-body counts of the fish were made periodically in a scintillation counting system, and feces were examined for radioactivity. Also, some fish were sacrificed, food was removed from the gastrointestinal tract, and sagittal sections of the tract were measured to detect residual ^{144}Ce. A desirable feature of this study was the investigation of individual variation, a matter not stressed by other investigators, perhaps because of the relative ease of replication in fish in contrast to the animals others studied. However, some investigators did study variability within an animal. The authors concluded that the ^{144}Ce technique gave results similar to a conventional method of serial slaughter, but required fewer fish for the same precision. In addition, more than one determination could be made per fish. A comparison of the data is presented in Figure 75. The investigators further commented that the technique could also be used to study digestibility of foods.

10.3. The Ecosystem

10.3.1. General Comments

Previous discussions have been concerned with the behavior of nutrients in individual organisms in both laboratory and field settings. Although such studies are valuable, the ultimate interpretation of the ecological cycling of nutrients must be based on observations in the real world—the natural ecosystem. This is not to imply that laboratory investigations of the organism or artificial ecosystems are useless, since many specific parameters under investigation may be impossible to study in the field, e.g., when various environmental parameters must be controlled. Both types of investigations are often conducted simultaneously to justify the extrapolation of laboratory results to field situations. Except for very unusual situations, an ecosystem is extremely complex and is impossible to study in all its biotic and abiotic aspects. There are, however, certain basic principles and properties of this dynamic system that have been studied extensively and are still being investigated. The cycling of nutrients and trace elements in food webs; the previously discussed subjects of ingestion, biological uptake, and retention; excretion and other ecological processes associated with the dynamics of the system; intra- and interspecies competition and aspects of population growth such as birth and death rates and immigration and emigration—all

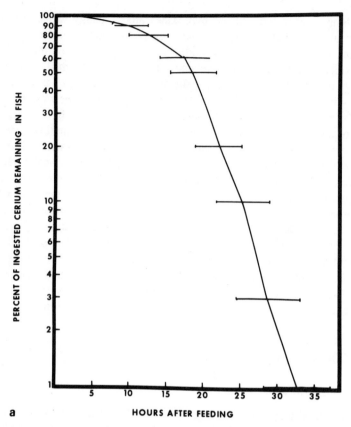

a   **HOURS AFTER FEEDING**

Figure 75. Food-evacuation time in the pinfish *(Lagodon rhomboides)* measured with ^{144}Ce. (a) Retention of ^{144}Ce at 24°C. Standard errors are shown ($n = 5$). (b) Gastrointestinal evacuation of commercial food at 24°C using the serial slaughter method. Log $y = 1.037 - 0.033 (x - 2)$; where $y = \log_{10} (1 + \% \text{ dry body wt. in GI tract})$; and $x = $ hours since feeding (except $x - 2 \geq 0$). From Peters and Hoss (1974).

these topics have been discussed in a multitude of ecological textbooks and monographs. Many of these processes can be fruitfully investigated with radioactive tracers.

An initial step in the study of nutrient cycling in an ecosystem is the preparation of a diagram or model of the system or subsystem under study showing the various pathways of nutrient movement in the system. A common objective of the ecologist is to associate transfer rates with these pathways and determine their magnitude and relative importance. Development of a realistic

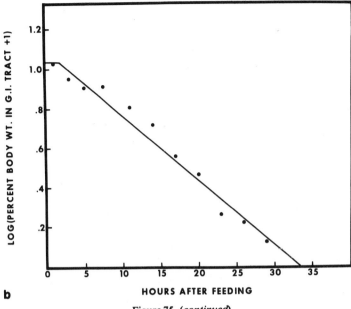

b   **HOURS AFTER FEEDING**

Figure 75. (*continued*)

model requires considerable knowledge of the system, a fact not obvious to many persons who have not been actively engaged in ecological research. The initial model of an ecosystem would be of rather broad scope, e.g., like that proposed by T. W. Duke and Rice (1966) for an estuary (Figure 76), with a second-stage development of a trophic structure such as that developed by Wiegert *et al.* (1970) for a soil–liter subsystem in reference to food resources in general (Figure 77) and that developed by Reichle and Crossley (1967) for a study of the cycling of radiocesium in an herbivorous food web (Figure 78). With the advent of the computer and development of the discipline of model-building in relatively recent years, these schematic diagrams have been translated into mathematical models such as briefly described for compartment models by Olson (1968) in his paper on radionuclide techniques in the study of biogeochemical cycling and Conover and Francis (1973) for transfer studies in aquatic food webs.

One subject that is of considerable interest is the productivity of a system, considered as the total amount of organic material or energy produced by a specific system or population of a specific species in time and space. Golley (1967) has written an excellent summary of methods of studying energy flow as related to secondary productivity in wild terrestrial vertebrate populations,

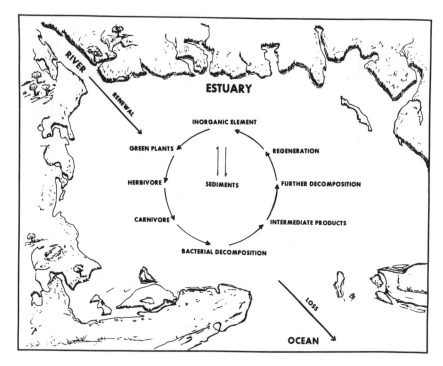

Figure 76. Simplified schematic diagram of a nutrient cycle in an estuary. From T. W. Duke and Rice (1966).

including application of radionuclide techniques. In an early paper on measurement of energy flow in natural populations, E. P. Odum and Golley (1963) reviewed radiotracer methods used with autotrophic and heterotrophic organisms with examples of studies of invertebrates and fish. They stated:

> To obtain a complete picture of energy flow rates, two distinctly different kinds of measurement must be made: (1) the rate of organic production, or "growth" per unit of time, and (2) the rate of respiration, or the maintenance cost of the average standing crop per unit of time. Both measurements, at best, are very difficult to make in the field. To date, it has usually been necessary to base estimates, in part at least, on data obtained in the laboratory or field enclosures. Transference of such data to completely open nature is nearly always open to question in one aspect or another. Radioactive tracers offer a number of possible aids, even though they alone cannot solve all problems. . . . At ecological levels of study (i.e., populations, communities, and ecosystems) three distinct kinds of labels have great potential, namely: (1) *individual labels* where it is desired to clarify activity, dispersal, dispersion, or behavior of individual organisms in the population, (2) *population labels* where whole populations, or samples of the population, may be labeled to determine mortality rates, density by labeling–recapture procedures, etc., and (3) *metabolic labels* where it is desired to measure some specific rate of function.

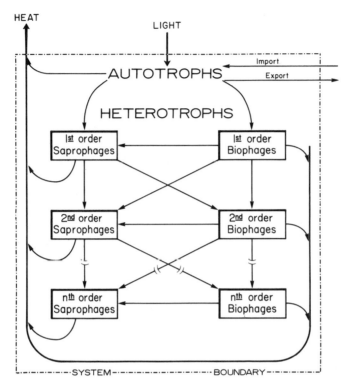

Figure 77. Modified trophic model for the soil–litter subsystem with two parallel pathways of food resources. From Wiegert *et al.* (1970).

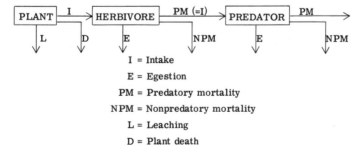

Figure 78. Model of the distribution and exchange of radiocesium among the trophic compartments of an herbivorous food chain. At steady-state conditions, determination of the loss parameters allows quantification of the I terms. Predatory I is, in effect, equivalent to NPM of herbivores. Standing crop of a compartment plus mortality represents the gross production by that trophic level. From Reichle and Crossley (1967).

In their Summary they stated:

> Radionuclides as tracers provide tools of major importance in environmental research when used in conjunction with other ecological approaches, and provided careful laboratory and/or field-enclosure experiments designed to determine mechanisms accompany extensive field applications.

As mentioned above, studies of nutrient and trace-element cycling in ecosystems have included laboratory and field studies. Field studies of radionuclide cycling include those in natural areas contaminated by wastes from nuclear facilities, such as the Irish Sea, the Columbia River, and White Oak Lake and its bed. Broader areas such as those in the South Pacific and the Arctic have also been studied from the standpoint of cycling of fallout constituents resulting from nuclear-weapons testing. Although these studies are very valuable in the understanding of the cycling of waste products of the nuclear age, we have not to any great extent included a discussion of them in this book. Rather, we prefer to discuss those studies wherein known amounts of radionuclides were introduced into the environment to study the cycling of an essential stable element or a specific radionuclide or ecological process.

As a result of possible health hazards associated with introduction of radionuclides into the environment, such studies have been restricted to the use of specific radionuclides at low levels of application on areas poorly accessible to the public or to government-controlled areas, particularly onsite areas of the U.S. Atomic Energy Commission (AEC) (now the Department of Energy) such as Oak Ridge National Laboratory, where radiocesium cycling has been investigated in a forested area. This study has been briefly described by Auerbach *et al.*(1964) and by Olson (1968).

10.3.2. The Food Web

An expression used to describe the linkage of animals by food—or, in other words, the food relationship among animals—is the "food chain." The base of the food chain is the autotrophs, which are organisms capable of producing organic material from inorganic materials and energy received from sources other than organic material. The set of interconnecting food chains of an ecosystem is known as the "food web" or "trophic web." Trophic levels of a food web have been organized into four levels: (1) primary producers, (2) herbivores, (3) carnivores, and (4) decomposers. In our discussion, we will utilize the expression "food web" as interchangeable with "food chain," and we will speak of trophic levels of the food web.

We have selected a sample of the many papers utilizing radionuclide-tracer investigations of the food web that have appeared in the literature. As before, we have selected these papers on the basis of diversity to illustrate procedures that have been used, rather than on the basis of results of the tracer experiments.

Phosphorus-32 has been used commonly in food web studies, since it is an essential nutrient with a relatively short physical half-life (14.3 days) and has a considerably longer biological half-life [1155 days in bone (Shilling and Shilling, 1964)]; it has an effective half-life of 14.1 days (Shilling and Shilling, 1964); further, it is a pure beta emitter with a relatively high energy that results in desirable counting characteristics. The short physical half-life is desirable, since it ensures a short period of environmental contamination.

Dr. R. C. Pendleton, who was one of the earliest ecologists in the field that is now known as "radiation ecology," made many contributions to the cycling of radionuclides within the food web. In a study of insect–plant relationships, Pendleton and Grundmann (1954) introduced ^{32}P into a thistle plant (*Cirsium undulatum*) that was heavily infested with aphids (*Anuraphis* sp.). Following inoculation, samples of aphids, ants, and other insects were collected daily, either on or off the plant, ashed or desiccated, and counted for radioactivity with a GM detector. The ants (*Formica sanquinca puberula* and *Camponotus novaboracencis*) were collected as they used plant honeydew. The plant was inoculated with 1mCi ^{32}P in 3 cc distilled water that was placed with a hypodermic syringe in a cavity formed by making a cut in the side of the plant and removing a small amount of pith. The researchers concluded that the radiotracer technique was more accurate than direct observation in establishing phytophagous insect–predator complex and plant pollinator relationships.

In a field study involving more than one plant individual and species, E. P. Odum and Kuenzler (1963) used ^{32}P as a tracer to delineate food webs in an old-field ecosystem at the U.S. AEC's Savannah River Plant, near Aiken, South Carolina. Three large quadrats (81, 100, and 100 m^2) containing different plant dominants were established at considerable distances apart. All individuals of the different dominant plants (*Heterotheca subaxillaris, Rumex acetocella,* or *Sorghum halepense*) in each quadrat were labeled. The first two species, which are broadleaved plants, were labeled by using a squeeze bottle containing the radionuclide in water together with a wetting agent. The total mixture was divided into a number of aliquots corresponding to the number of subplots established within the major plot. Application of a fine spray to the crowns of the plants was conducted on a calm, sunny day. It was observed that 90% of the material was absorbed by the vegetation. Over 90% of the leaves collected a week after application contained enough tracer to be detectable in insects feeding on the leaves. Since sorghum is a grass, a different technique was used to apply the tracer. A small pipette attached to a syringe was used to place two drops of a concentrated solution of ^{32}P between the base of a leaf and the stem about halfway up the shoot (Figure 79). To facilitate labeling, this quadrat was also marked off into subquadrats. In this quadrat, all the labeled plants were marked

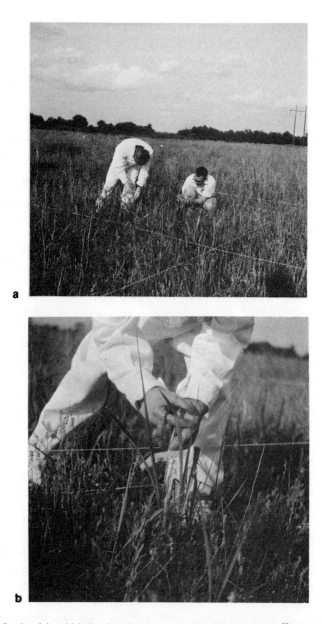

Figure 79. Quadrat 3 in which *Sorghum halepense* plants were labeled with [32]P. (a) General view of the quadrat on the day the plants were labeled. (b) Method of applying drops of ^{32}P solution in axils of leaves. Note the three stalks of *Sorghum* grass and the several other species in the stand that are not labeled. (a) Courtesy of E. P. Odum. (b) From E. P. Odum and Kuenzler (1963).

with plastic tape for identification. The authors concluded that this latter method was better than the squeeze-bottle method, since each plant was labeled with the same amount of ^{32}P and none of the solution was lost to the ground or other surfaces. A very important aspect was that this method virtually assured that insects and adjacent plants were not inadvertently labeled. Odum and Kuenzler (1963) stated:

> When concentration of the tracer per unit of biomass (milligrams of wet weight) was plotted against time, a clear graphic separation of certain trophic and habitat groups was evident in all three quadrats. . . . The trophic position of two of the most common species, whose exact food source in nature was previously unknown, was rather clearly established by comparison of their uptake curves with those of species whose food was known. . . . The experiments demonstrated that labeling with radiotracer of single species of producers can aid in the isolation or "untangling" of food chains, as well as aid in determination of the energy source being utilized by specific heterotrophic populations in nature.

In a study of an isopod (*Armadillidium vulgare*) in California, Paris and Sikora (1965) tagged the forbs, *Vicia sativa*, *Silybum marianum*, and *Picris echioides*, each in separate plots, with $H_3{}^{32}PO_4$ in leaf axils with a capillary pipette. Periodic samples of plants and isopods were collected and analyzed for radioactivity with a GM detector. The investigators concluded that it was feasible to use radiotracers in a study of trophic relationships in these cryptozoans.

Following the study of Odum and Kuenzler (1963) of consumers in an old-field ecosystem in South Carolina, Wiegert *et al.* (1967) studied the forb–arthropod food chain in a field in the same area 1 year following cultivation. Two quadrats (10 × 20 m) were established in which the horseweed (*Erigeron canadensis*) and camphor weed (*Heterotheca subaxillaris*) grew, with one more abundant in one plot than in the other. Individual plants were labeled by placing ^{32}P in water contained in wells constructed around the plant stem base (Figure 80a). The plant was well labeled within a few minutes on hot, dry days. The investigators stated:

> Results of this study have verified and extended the suggestion made in previous radioisotope food chain studies . . . that the shape of the uptake curves [Figure 80b] can be indicative of the trophic position of a population of consumers in the field. Thus, populations known to be strictly herbivorous reach a peak of radioactivity very soon after the primary producers have been labelled, while known predators such as spiders show delayed uptake at lower levels. Intermediate patterns could then be interpreted as indicating feeding from more than one trophic level.

Other radionuclides have been utilized in food web studies. Coleman and McGinnis (1970) used ^{65}Zn in an attempt to quantify the fungus–small arthropod food chain in a broomsedge stand (*Andropogon* sp.) at the Savannah River Plant.

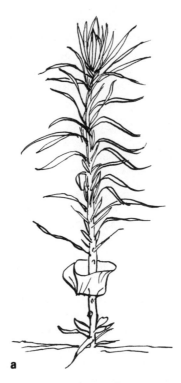

a

Figure 80. Forb–arthropod food chains studied with ³²P. (a) Sketch showing method of labeling plants with ³²P. Plastic sealing compound was used to form a "well" at the base of the stem. After introduction of tracer, the upper edges of the well were pinched together to close the cavity so as to prevent direct contamination of animals. (b) Phosphorus-32 uptake curves for selected species and groups of organisms. Except for the plants, the lines connect the mean activity density values for the entire sample on the indicated dates. Phosphorus-32 levels in the plants are indicated by moving averages drawn through the data points. From Wiegert *et al.* (1967). Copyright 1967 by The Ecological Society of America.

Fungal mycelia (*Geotrichum* sp.) isolated from old-field soil were labeled by growing them in a soil-extract medium containing ⁶⁵Zn. Portions of the rinsed mycelia were placed at several 2- to 3- cm deep locations in the broomsedge stand. A control area was inoculated with the sterilized medium containing ⁶⁵Zn. At 2, 4, 6, and 8 weeks later, core samples were taken adjacent to the sites containing the labeled mycelia and sterilized medium. Microarthropods were removed from the core, identified, and counted with a NaI(Tl) well crystal. Results are illustrated in Figure 81.

In another study using ⁶⁵Zn, Mason and Odum (1969) studied the effect of feces ingestion on retention and bioelimination of the radionuclide by the detritus-

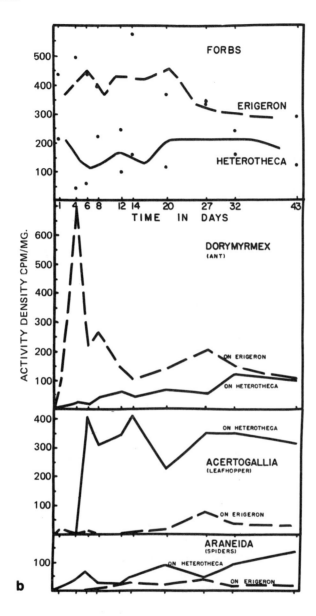

Figure 80. (*continued*)

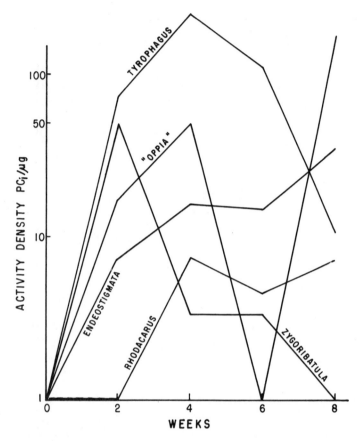

Figure 81. Activity densities (pCi/μg) of mites extracted from cores of litter–soil every 2 weeks for 2 months. Cores were taken near sites inoculated with ^{65}Zn-labeled fungus. *Amblyseius* sp. was omitted due to limitations of space. From Coleman and McGinnis (1970).

feeding horned passalus beetle (*Popilius disjunctus*). Small pieces of wood on which the beetle fed had been soaked for 15 min in tap water containing ^{65}ZnCl$_2$. After being labeled, the wood was fed to the beetles. Both wood and beetles were placed in glass dishes for 24 hr. The beetles were then placed in containers in which their feces were either available or not available to them. The body weight and whole-body radioactivity were determined for a 12-day period. It was observed that at the end of the 12-day period, the beetles that had access to feces had a higher body burden of ^{65}Zn than those to which feces were not available. In addition, the mean body weight over the 12-day period showed little change in the feces-available group, while for the other group it declined rather drastically. In fact, continuation of the experiment for an additional 12 days resulted in the death of the beetles that had no access to feces. Thus, it was demonstrated that the consumption of feces was an important link in the food web of this species.

Rubidium-86 and ^{32}P were stem-inoculated into milkweed plants (*Apocynum cannabinum*) with a syringe by Williams and Reichle (1968) in a study of energy turnover in the chrysomelid beetle (*Chrysochus auratus*). Direct inoculation was fast and eliminated the possibility of indirect contamination of insects from tag residues on the plant. Disposable syringes were used by inserting the needle (22- and 24-gauge Huber type) into the pith of the plant and injecting 160 and 275 μCi ^{32}P and ^{86}Rb, respectively, and sealing the injection site with a gum. The individual plants in the field were then enclosed in cages containing four or five beetles. Rubidium-86 was counted with a 3-inch NaI(Tl) crystal, and a nuclear gas-flow counter was used to count the ^{32}P body burden of the beetle and plant material. The effective half-lives of the radionuclides were determined in the laboratory with beetles fed labeled leaves for a period and then fed nonlabeled leaves. This procedure has been discussed in a previous section (10.2.1). The whole-body retention of ^{86}Rb is shown in Figure 82.

In a short but interesting paper, Wiegert and Odum (1969) discussed the use of radiotracer measurements in studies of food web diversity and utilized the data from the study discussed above (Wiegert *et al.*, 1967). They stated: "We feel that radionuclide tracers can simultaneously serve to identify the actual, as opposed to the merely possible trophic interactions, and tell us something about the quantitative importance of a given pathway."

The terrestrial food web studies discussed above have used radionuclides as tracers. Now let us consider studies concerned with the cycling of a specific nuclide through terrestrial food webs, e.g., ^{137}Cs, a fission product. In Section 10.2.1, the study of Crossley (1963) on insect–plant relationships utilizing the natural tagging of willow leaves with ^{137}Cs on White Oak Lake bed was discussed. Another paper by Crossley (1969) discussed an investigation in the same area on the comparative movement of ^{60}Co, ^{106}Ru, and ^{137}Cs in arthropod food webs. Previous studies of invertebrate and vertebrate food webs on the lake bed were concerned with ^{90}Sr and ^{137}Cs. Crossley commented that food-web studies of ^{106}Ru were not pursued because the concentration of the radionuclide was quite variable over the bed. Ruthenium-106 reached the lake bed via seepage from liquid waste pits near the lake bed; consequently, high concentrations of the radionuclide were localized in a small portion of the contaminated area. Further spreading of ^{106}Ru was apparently limited to this area when a balance between input and radioactive decay was reached. In the summer of 1964, line transects were established in the seep area (Figure 83), and samples of soils, vegetation, and predaceous and herbivorous arthropods were collected and analyzed for ^{60}Co, ^{106}Ru, and ^{137}Cs (Table 13); it was noted that ^{106}Ru was consistently detected and exceeded concentrations of ^{137}Cs in the arthropod food

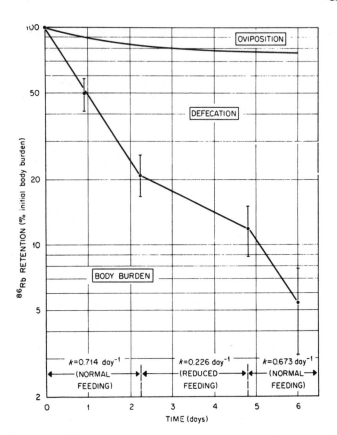

Figure 82. Fate of ^{86}Rb body burden in *Chrysochus auratus*. Decreasing body burdens are plotted as the mean ± 1 S.E. (n = 6 beetles). Rubidium-86 loss-rate coefficients (k) are given for the three experimental periods: normal feeding, food supply exhausted (reduced feeding); and resumption of normal feeding. Areas of the graph represent, respectively, the percentage of initial radioactivity (body burden) remaining in beetles, lost through defecation, and transferred to eggs (oviposition). From Williams and Reichle (1968).

web. Crossley (1969) commented that although the chemical form of the ruthenium isotope from this site was different from that in fallout, the study illustrated the potential for [106]Ru movement in ecological systems and possible concentration in excess of ^{137}Cs at the ends of food chains (Table 13). He stated:

> The net effect of passage through arthropod food chains was a significant rearrangement of relative abundances of the three radionuclides. Concentrations (pCi/mg) of ^{137}Cs, [106]Ru and ^{60}Co in soils were of the order of approximately 14:28:5. At the predator trophic level these had been rearranged to approximately 0.1:2.1:0.1. All three radionuclides

showed greatly reduced concentrations. Ruthenium-106 exceeded the other two radionuclides in predators by an order of magnitude. . . . For each radionuclide, concentration
factors always increased in this vegetation–arthropod food chain.

For public-safety reasons, the introduction of a long-lived radionuclide in
tracer quantities into a natural ecosystem for experimental investigation must be
restricted to areas of rigidly controlled access. The only investigation of this type
in the United States was initiated at Oak Ridge National Laboratory in May
1962. A second-growth stand of tulip poplar (*Liriodendron tulipifera*) was studied
by tagging trees of various species, mostly tulip poplar, in a 20 × 25 m portion
of a forest. A description of the area and technique is presented by Auerbach
et al. (1964), Olson (1968), and others in many papers describing research in
the area. Figures 84–86 illustrate the tagging procedures. Figure 86 shows a
tulip poplar being tagged. A trough or well was formed around the tree with a
malleable sealing compound that was covered with aluminum foil. To the im-
mediate right of the tree J. S. Olson is shown using a chisel to cut slits 5 cm
apart into the inner bark around the tree. D.L. Nelson at left, poured diluent

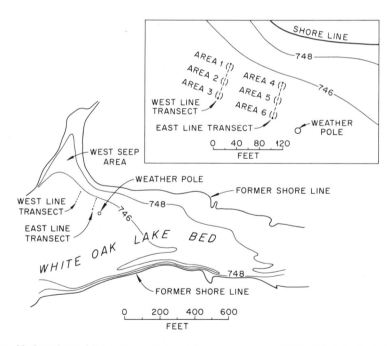

Figure 83. Locations of line transects and sampling areas on upper White Oak Lake bed. From
Crossley (1969).

Table 13. Arthropod-Food-Chain Distribution of ^{137}Cs, ^{106}Ru, and ^{60}Co on White Oak Lake Bed[a]

| Trophic level | pCi/mg air-dry wt | | | | | |
	West line transect	East line transect	Grand mean	Standard error	Number of samples	Concentration factor[b]
Cesium-137						
Soil	11.03	17.23	14.13	0.617	48	—
Vegetation	0.240	0.514	0.377	0.0391	48	0.027
Herbivore	0.086	0.133	0.110	0.0388	16	0.29
Predator	0.113	0.090	0.101	0.0119	13	0.92
Ruthenium-106						
Soil	28.5	28.1	28.3	2.477	48	—
Vegetation	1.525	1.956	1.741	0.200	48	0.062
Herbivore	0.990	0.451	0.721	0.186	16	0.41
Predator	3.091	1.175	2.059	0.453	13	2.86
Cobalt-60						
Soil	4.11	5.02	4.57	0.160	48	—
Vegetation	0.219	0.312	0.265	0.0257	48	0.058
Herbivore	0.133	0.095	0.114	0.0228	16	0.43
Predator	0.137	0.108	0.122	0.0166	13	1.07

[a] From Crossley (1969). Samples were from two line transects taken during an 8-week period in the summer of 1964. The standard error and the number of samples are shown for the grand mean only.
[b] Concentration factor = grand mean for level/grand mean for preceding level.

into the trough continuously while H. Wallen (kneeling) prepared the radionuclide tag to be placed into the trough by diluting with water a known amount of the radionuclide placed in a vial in the laboratory. The radioactivity was monitored by S.I. Auerbach (also kneeling). The amount of ^{137}Cs per tree was proportional to the mass of the tree. A total of about 467 mCi ^{137}Cs was applied to this plot.

Crossley and Reichle (1969) studied the behavior of ^{137}Cs in saprophagous arthropods that fed on the litter containing tagged leaves that had fallen from the tagged tulip trees. In the laboratory, leaves tagged with ^{134}Cs were fed to a saprophagous arthropod, a millipede (*Dixidesmus erasus*), to determine the loss coefficient for the arthropod. As a consequence of wetting to maintain high humidities required by the millipede, the ^{134}Cs was leached from the leaves. Figure 87 shows the ^{137}Cs fluctuation in leaf litter and in two types of arthropods during the fall and winter of 1964–1965. The authors discussed a differential equation and its solution relating the change in ^{137}Cs concentration with time as well as their estimates of the various parameters. They stated:

Although developed in conjunction with radioisotope tracer experiments, these descriptions have broad application in studies of the trophic dynamics of animal communities. Functional interpretation of trophic level exchanges can similarly be made for the cycling of important nutrient elements, dry matter, and energy flow. Particularly valuable is the ability to predict the transient concentrations of such substances in successive trophic levels and the characteristic response times of interdependent populations to fluctuations elsewhere in the trophic structure.

In another aspect of their endeavors in this forest, Reichle and Crossley (1969) investigated trophic-level concentrations of ^{137}Cs and stable sodium and potassium, all of which are alkali metals. The radiocesium concentration was

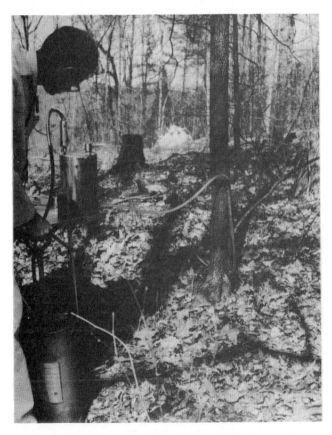

Figure 84. A garden pressure-pump pressure tank being used by J. S. Olson to hasten movement of tracer mixture from Tygon tubing into a pipe threaded into the bole of a flowering dogwood tree *(Cornus florida)*. From Olson (1968).

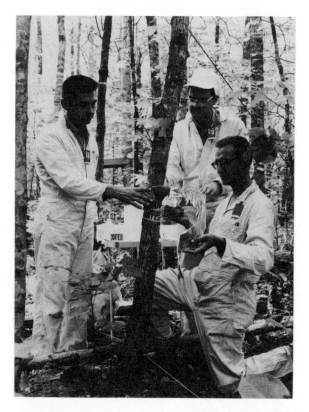

Figure 85. Preparation of troughs for tagging a tulip tree *(Liriodendron tulipifera)* forest (left to right: H. Waller, J. S. Olson, and D. L. Nelson). Malleable perma-gum pipe-sealing compound was formed into a trough around plastic tape over smoothed bark and then supported by aluminum foil and wire. From Olson (1968).

determined as before with a NaI(Tl) well crystal. The stable elements, Na and K, were used in oral-dose laboratory experiments to study the biological half-lives and assimilation efficiencies of these elements in the cricket, *Acheta domesticus*, for a comparison of the biological uptake and retention of the three elements in arthropods.

In a laboratory investigation of trophic structure and feeding rates of forest-soil invertebrates, McBrayer and Reichle (1971) collected soil-core samples at Oak Ridge National Laboratory in a forest dominated by second-growth tulip poplar from an area cleared of litter down to the mineral soil. The background radioactivity in organisms in a subsample of these cores was determined. Litter 8 months old was collected from the forest, homogenized, and soaked in a solution of ^{137}Cs. The tagged litter was applied evenly to the surface of the soil cultures, and at intervals to 84 days, animals were extracted from sacrificed cultures. Because of the low concentration and small size of the animals, it was necessary to assay the invertebrates on a low-background, thin-window, gas-flow beta detector. The investigators stated:

> Radionuclide uptake kinetics effectively distinguished among the various trophic levels of the decomposer fauna. Due to the variety of food chains present and the resultant differential rates of trophic transfer, only the fungivores could be distinguished on the basis of a single parameter—the characteristic spike in the uptake curve. Predators and saprophages having access to the surface litter were readily distinguished on the basis of the time lag before initial radionuclide uptake.

Study of food webs in marine and freshwater ecosystems by radiation ecologists have been concerned primarily with cycling of fallout and nuclear waste

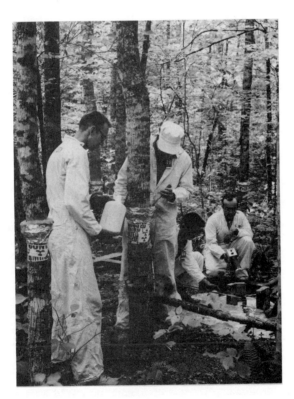

Figure 86. Water being poured into the trough while chisel cuts are being made every 5 cm around the tree, to keep the xylem from being blocked by air until the ^{137}Cs was removed from the lead shield and poured in, and followed by rinse water (left to right: D. L. Nelson, J. S. Olson, H. Waller, and S. I. Auerbach) From Olson (1968).

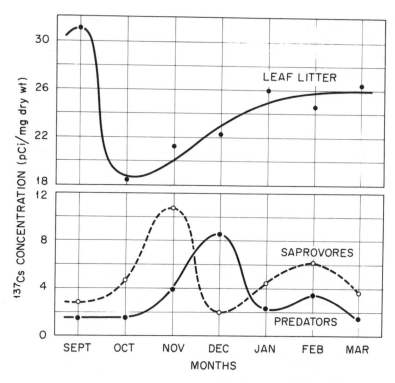

Figure 87. Seasonal fluctuation of ^{137}Cs concentration in leaf litter and in saprophagous and pre-daceous arthropods in a tulip tree *(Liriodendron tulipifera)* stand experimentally tagged with ^{137}Cs. The leaf-litter content of radiocesium increased in September following autumnal leaf drop, but then decreased due to leaching. The higher trophic levels of arthropod consumers also show the changing concentrations of ^{137}C, which reflect changes in their food bases. The relative amplitudes of the curves illustrate the decrease in ^{137}Cs concentrations through arthropod food chains. From Crossley and Reichle (1969).

products in natural systems. The vastness of such systems, the difficulty of confining the introduced radionuclide tracers within a confined area restricted from public access, and the fact that humans consume aquatic organisms greatly limit the type of study that can be conducted. It is only the rare investigation that involves experimental addition of tracer amounts of a radionuclide to an aquatic system, and such a study is further restricted to specific radionuclides such as ^{32}P. Controlled experiments of aquatic food webs are for the most part restricted to laboratories or simulated natural systems.

Cross *et al.* (1975) discussed methodology associated with investigations of radionuclide cycling in marine food webs. Reviewing the complexities of marine food chains, they discussed the various types of studies that have been conducted, including field studies associated with the nuclear testing program of the United States in the central Pacific, those of the distribution of radionuclides from the Hanford Operations in the Columbia River estuary and adjacent ocean, and releases from Windscale into the Irish Sea. As contrasted to investigations in the United States, most of the work in the Irish Sea was prompted by concern about human radiation exposure. Following a discussion on field investigations, Cross *et al.* (1975) considered laboratory research and commented that the prime reason for such research is to be able to assess the role of a single variable, which cannot be done in the field. These considerations were followed by comments on the use of specific activities and concentration factors in marine food-web studies. Following a consideration of the dynamic processes in a marine ecosystem they commented:

> Accurate descriptions of these dynamic processes will demand that comprehensive studies be conducted on specific marine ecosystems. To supplement these field studies, laboratory experiments will have to be done to understand which environmental parameters control the processes. . . . Experimental designs in radioecological foodchain studies must bring nature into the laboratory to a greater degree than has been done in the past. Experimental foodchains and feeding rates must be realistic. In experiments involving radioisotopes specific activities need to be measured wherever possible and experiments may have to be conducted for relatively long periods of time to ensure equilibration between the radioisotope and its stable isotopes. Larger and more complex experimental ecosystems such as large tanks or outdoor ponds must be established to allow marine organisms to exercise more natural behaviour patterns under experimental conditions. Increased knowledge of food selectivity, feeding rates, biomass levels, etc. of marine organisms will aid in the design of radioecological foodchain experiments.

A radiotracer laboratory experiment was conducted by Hargrave (1970) to study the utilization of benthic microflora by a freshwater benthic amphipod, *Hyalella azteca*. In the radiotracer experiments, the amphipod food items were cultured from surface-sediment samples and were tagged as follows: (1) algae—*Navicula* sp., *Anabaena* sp., *Mougeotia* sp., and *Chlorella* sp.—were cultured with a medium containing $NaH^{14}CO_3$ and (2) bacteria—*Pseudomonas* (Group I), *Flavobacter* sp., and *Vibrio* sp.—were cultured anaerobically on a medium containing [^{14}C]glucose. Details concerning the procedures are presented by the investigator. The labeled food items were added to sterilized sediment, and the sediment was placed in a vial to which were added sterilized lake water and a single amphipod. Each vial had a lid containing a filter disk soaked with hyamine hydroxide to absorb the respired $^{14}CO_2$. An air-tight seal was accomplished by using stopcock grease on the vial lids. The sealed vials were shaken gently for 3–6 hr while kept at 15°C at constant light; the amphipods were then transferred to nonradioactive sediment for 30 min of feeding. Feces were collected, weighed, and counted. The sediment and amphipods were also weighed and counted with a scintillation counting system. The radiotracer in the water over the sediment and on the disks in the lids was filtered through a Millipore membrane, and counted. It was assumed that the filtered material remaining was dissolved organic compounds. These data were used to compute assimilation efficiency and sediment ingested. Assimilation efficiency was also determined by the gravimetric method and by a chemical procedure comparing organic matter in potential food and feces. In a comparison of the three techniques, Hargrave (1970) stated:

> In all experiments, assimilation was determined more by the type of diet, that is the species composition of microflora and the proportion of living and non-living organic matter, than by the technique used. Thus, while criticisms of some of the techniques used to measure assimilation . . . may have a physiological basis, it appears that differences in digestion of various food sources are so great that they cannot be attributed to the method used.

In another laboratory experiment (perhaps the first on food relationships), Pendleton and Smart (1954) used ^{32}P to label food items of the least chub (*Iotichthys phlegethontis*) in a study of food relationships of this fish. Fish collected in the field were transported to the laboratory in specially prepared experimental tanks that later contained the tagged food and fish during the experimental exposure period. The food items included water fleas (*Hyalella knickerbockeri*), ostracods (*Herpetocypris chevreuxi*), and mosquito larvae (*Aedes niphadopsis*) that were labeled by placing each species in gallon jars containing ^{32}P in solution for 24 hr and then removed, washed and counted until counts were no more than 10% above background. As a composite sampler, 20–25 individuals were ashed and counted. The number of counts per individual was used to determine the number of prey consumed in the experiment. The labeled food species and fish were placed together in the specially built tank for a period of 24 hr. The fish were then removed, ashed, and counted. Commenting on the method, the investigators stated:

> Although brief and incomplete, our findings indicate that the labelling of suspected food species with P^{32} or other beta-emitting radionuclides is practical in research on food chains of fishes. Also, preliminary results of such work can be obtained in the field with suitably sensitive portable counters.

Lee *et al.* (1966) reported on using radiotracers in a study of predator–prey relationships among littoral foraminifera. These investigators tested more than 50 axenic species of unicellular organisms as potential food for different foraminifera, including *Allogromia* sp. (NF), *A. laticollaris, Ammonia beccarii,*

Quinqueloculina spp., *Rosalina floridana*, *Anomalina* sp., *Elphidium* sp., *Spiroloculina hyalina*, *Globigerina bulloides*, and *Globorotalia truncatulinoides*. In previous feeding studies, many difficulties occurred and the investment of considerable man-hours was involved in testing potential food items. Using tracer techniques, the investigators concluded that " . . . it is now practical to analyze the predator–prey relationship among the foraminifera despite there being more variables than we had anticipated" and that "application of tracer techniques to the feeding of foraminifera in the laboratory has been a major contributing factor toward solving rearing problems . . . ." The labeled food items included diatoms, dinoflagellates, chlorophytes, chrysophytes, cyanophytes, rhodophytes, bacteria, and yeasts. These organisms were cultured in appropriate media to which had been added ^{32}P or ^{14}C. The slower-growing organisms were inoculated into nonradioactive media, with the radionuclide being added when the organisms showed logarithmic growth. Centrifugation of the organisms was followed by washing them in sterile seawater, and an aliquot sample was counted on a hemocytometer or Coulter counter. The desired concentration of the food item was then obtained by dilution. Each foraminifer was placed with the labeled food item for a period of time, removed, cleaned, placed in a vial and counted for radioactivity with a liquid scintillation counting system. On the basis of the amount of radioactivity observed, the investigators estimated the number of food items consumed. Competition experiments between two foraminifers were conducted by presenting to them two different food items, each with either a ^{32}P or a ^{14}C tag.

Baptist and Lewis (1969) designed an experiment to study the transfer of ^{65}Zn and ^{51}Cr through an estuarine food chain that involved transfer of assimilated and unassimilated radionuclides through four trophic levels. They described their study as that of an " . . . unnatural and simple but reproducible food chain and uniform, controlled environmental conditions to facilitate comparisons between the experiments." Their stepwise experiments are illustrated in Figures 88 and 89. The use of ^{65}Zn and ^{51}Cr was not in the function of tracers, since the investigators were interested in these specific radionuclides that have been introduced into the marine environment by man's activities. The authors commented that limiting experimental conditions probably resulted in lower concentrations than might be expected in the natural environment. They stated:

> To determine the maximum concentration of radionuclides that can be transferred through an experimental food chain would require (1) equilibrium between the radioactivity in the organisms and in their environment before they were fed to the next trophic level and (2) sufficient radioactive food organisms to satisfy the needs of predator organisms in each trophic level.

They considered these conditions impractical for their four-step design.

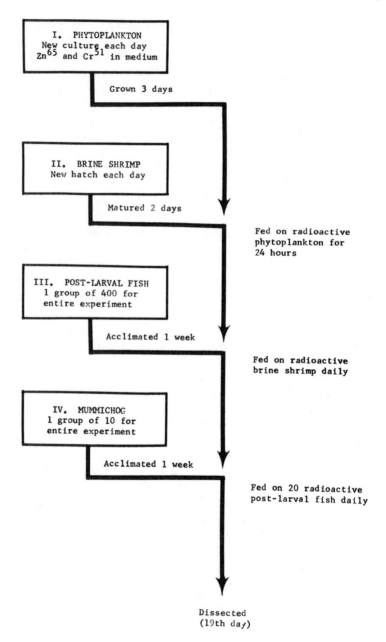

Figure 88. Experimental procedure for an estuarine food chain designed to follow the transfer of ^{65}Zn and ^{51}Cr from daily feeding of radioactive food. From Baptist and Lewis (1969).

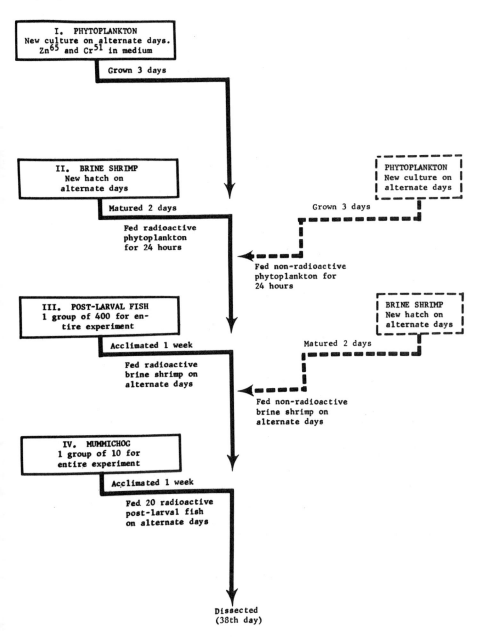

Figure 89. Experimental procedure for an estuarine food chain designed to follow the transfer of ^{65}Zn and ^{51}Cr from alternate-day feeding of radioactive food and nonradioactive food. From Baptist and Lewis (1969).

10.3.3. The "Complete" System or Subsystem

10.3.3.1 General Comments

In our general comments on the experimental study of mineral cycling (Section 10.1), we stressed the complexity of the natural ecosystem and the futility of attempting to develop a complete study in nature. Such efforts are limited by prior knowledge concerning the system, measurement techniques, and the dynamic nature of the system. To conduct comprehensive studies has been the desire of ecologists for years, and out of this desire evolved the International Biological Program (IBP). Although radiotracers have played a limited role in cycling studies, they have not played a dominant role such as that envisioned for the tulip poplar forest study at Oak Ridge National Laboratory and associated studies of White Oak Lake bed. Admittedly, a complete ecosystem was not studied at either of these sites, yet what might be termed "subsystems" have been investigated. Similar comments might be made concerning aquatic systems, which we will discuss. Obviously, the many studies discussed previously might have been included in this section; however, we preferred to consider them in other sections to preserve continuity in our discussion. In particular, Section 10.3.2 is intertwined with discussions of complete-system or subsystem studies, but it seemed to us that the endeavors concerned with techniques used in elucidation of the food web and describing some of its properties deserved a section by itself. It is our plan to discuss tracer techniques used in terrestrial and aquatic ecosystems that have been associated with studies somewhat broader than those discussed in the previous sections on cycling studies. Here again, our aim is not to discuss results of specific experiments, but to discuss techniques and to show their diversity. To say the least, we are not completely satisfied with our allocation of papers to the subsections, but we hope that our decisions will be accepted by the reader to illustrate points within the scope of this book.

Various aspects of mineral and nutrient cycling in terrestrial systems are, generally speaking, more easily studied in plant and invertebrate populations than in the more mobile, lower-density populations of vertebrates, particularly the higher forms of vertebrates. Consequently, the literature stresses the former, and this will be reflected in our discussions.

10.3.3.2. Terrestrial Studies

In western Washington, Riekerk and Gessel (1965) conducted a study with radiotracers of the movement of minerals through soil in a 40-year-old stand of Douglas fir *(Pseudotsuga menziesii)*. The study was conducted in cooperation with the Fern Lake study, which is discussed in Section 10.3.3.3. Study plots (Figure 90) were selected so that each contained a central dominant tree not near

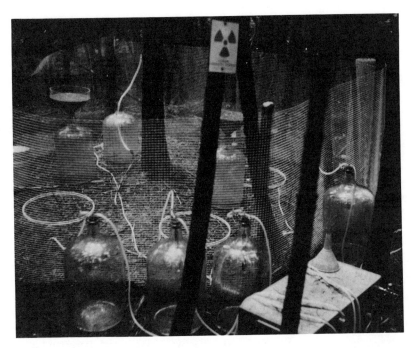

Figure 90. A study plot used in an investigation of mineral cycling in a stand of Douglas fir *(Pseudotsuga menziesii)* with radionuclides. Courtesy of H. Riekerk and S. P. Gessel.

other dominants. A single tracer was applied to each plot. Chosen for study were three contrasting minerals, P, Ca, and K, and their tracers, ^{32}P, ^{45}Ca, and ^{86}Rb, respectively. Known concentration of these radionuclides with carrier were applied by spraying the forest floor. Tension lysimeters installed at two depths collected the soil solutions, one beneath the forest floor and another 6–8 inches below the soil surface. Young midcrown foliage was sampled periodically from the dominant tree by researchers using a steel tower. In addition, fallen leaves were collected in troughs and "rainwash" was collected in a rubber channel around the tree stem. The flow of these solutions was passed through resin columns and monitored by flowmeters, and rainfall onto the forest stand was measured with rain gauges on towers. Radioactivity of solutions in the lysimeter was recorded continuously with "throughflow" GM tubes. Background radioactivity was monitored in a control plot. An interesting innovation was the spraying of the tracer directly onto the mineral soil by using a board to separate the mineral soil from the forest floor. The forest floor was replaced after the mineral soil was sprayed. Periodically, solutions, exchange resins, and crown leaves were sampled, processed, and counted. Among the interesting observations was that radionuclide uptake from that applied to the soil surface was considerably less than for uptake of all three radionuclides applied to the forest floor.

The cycling of nutrients and their pathways is of particular interest to ecologists working in tropical ecosystems. In a discussion of the subject, Stark (1973) refers to

> . . . the direct nutrient cycling hypothesis which states that on the poorest soils in the tropics and possibly on other soils, nutrients are removed from dead organic matter by mycorrhizal fungi and are transported through rhizomorph tissue to living roots, thus bypassing the soluble and leachable phase of nutrients in the soil.

There are several possible pathways of nutrient cycling, of which direct nutrient cycling is one. In his studies in a tropical rain forest in Puerto Rico and in an associated laboratory study, Stark (1973) used radionuclide tracers to relate soil organisms to the nutrient cycle and to study the subsurface depth of nutrient uptake by climax and second-growth vegetation. Phosphorus-32 was used in the subsurface uptake study by introducing it into the soil at various depths via Tygon tubes that had been placed in holes dug with a soil auger. A solution of ^{32}P and water was poured into a funnel at the end of the tubing, washed with additional water, and allowed to drain for 15 min. Surface application was made by pouring the solution over 10×10 cm areas. Using a cork-borer and rubber stopper, the researchers collected planchet-sized leaf disks from test trees daily for 20 days and measured radioactivity of samples. Samples of soil and fungi were also collected on a planchet and counted. The nutrient pathway study involved tagging fresh leaves, seedlings, and rolls of humus-root mat with 100 μCi ^{59}Fe, ^{75}Se, and ^{65}Zn. The labeling procedure was conducted by partial submersion in a solution containing the radionuclides, with the mat being soaked in the solution, the leaves tagged via the petiole, and the seedlings via roots. After being tagged, the materials containing the identical label were made into litter that was placed on the forest floor over the root system of the saplings. Periodically, samples of litter, humus, soil, roots, rhizomorph tissue, and living leaves were collected and analyzed for radionuclides with a 400-channel gamma counting system. Sodium-22 was used to label sterile organic litter for greenhouse tests involving fungi and higher plants. The experiment involved paired flasks connected with flexible tubing, with one of the flasks containing the labeled litter and the other containing sterile sand and "surface-sterilized seeds." Litter–fungi mixtures and several strains of various mycorrhiza-forming fungi were introduced into the flask containing the labeled litter. Since both these inoculants are cellulose digesters and because it was assumed that transport of the radionuclide to the seedlings that developed from the seeds in the second flask must be through the fungi or other soil organisms, it was possible to study direct cycling of ^{22}Na.

Since the laboratory investigation was conducted utilizing labeled litter placed over the living root system of a tree, it was impossible to determine whether or not the radioactivity picked up by roots came from the soil solution, fungi, or organic matter. Commenting on the leaching of ^{65}Zn, the investigator notes the increase in leaching when the label was applied by dipping a plant in ^{65}Zn solution as contrasted to labeling via the petiole or root. According to Stark (1973), demonstration of the leaf–fungi–root-type cycling requires that the researcher:

1. Show that the radionuclide is combined in organic compounds in living plant material. Radionuclide which adheres to the surface or is in soluble form may leach out when living material is converted to litter and exposed to rain.
2. Show that a suitable level of radionuclide is present in the dead litter for easy detection.
3. Show that radionuclide is present in fungal tissue, which is also a proven mycorrhizal associate of the higher plant being tested and is in physical contact with the labeled litter and living roots.
4. Show that the radionuclide appears in the root in a reasonable time sequence with points 1–3 above, and that the roots contain the mycorrhizal fungus.

He states further:

The final proof of the pathway of radiotracer movement may come from radioautography of soil sections, where fungi and soil particles can be seen separately.

Heterotrophic productivity in insect populations associated with the ^{137}Cs-tagged tulip poplar stand at Oak Ridge National Laboratory was discussed in an excellent paper by Reichle and Crossley (1967) that summarized their research on the subject. Although we have cited several papers by these authors that include some of these investigations, we are citing this paper again because of its wealth of information. The authors commented on the forest study area, sampling and analytical procedures, radionuclide tracer methods, radiocesium turnover by insects and its distribution in the "canopy food chains," primary productivity in the forest, food consumption, and a model of secondary production. One technique they discussed that we have not mentioned involves a laboratory study of ^{134}Cs retention by the common bean aphid (*Aphis fabae*) maintained at three temperatures. Radioactivity concentration was determined by counting a group of aphids occurring on a single plant by placing the entire plant seedling within a counting chamber. Elimination of radioactive cesium as measured by percentage of initial body burden was determined for mothers and their young as group and for mothers alone by removing the young. This design permitted estimation of loss due to bioelimination by the adult as well as that due to transfer from mother to young.

In a study of turnover of radionuclides and energy flow of four species of terrestrial isopods (*Armadillidium vulgare, A. nasatum, Cylisticus convexus, Metoponorthus pruinosus*), Reichle (1967) utilized ^{134}Cs in a study that related uptake, body burden equilibria, and rates of elimination to temperature. This study was unique in that the investigator related turnover rates to units of energy utilization. Oxygen-consumption measurements were obtained from a group of organisms held in a respirometer placed in a Warburg apparatus. A Parr adiabatic oxygen bomb calorimeter was used to determine caloric equivalents of isopods and their food. Isotopic methods for estimating ingestion, assimilation, and elimination have been discussed previously in Section 10.2; however, Reichle presents an encompassing summary of isotopic principles in measuring pertinent parameters. Since the levels of various salts in the diet have an effect on cesium behavior and because alkali metals are noted for their mobility in vegetation and leach easily, the detritus on which isopods feed may be deficient in these elements. Consequently, Reichle (1967) conducted a study of the effect on ^{134}Cs retention of adding K, Na, and Cs to the diet of the isopods. He observed that the supplemented diet had no effect on ^{134}Cs elimination rates. In studies of assimilation, the investigator marked lettuce with a tracer and also with a red dye. The red dye was used to detect visually the appearance of tagged excrement. Reichle observed that food-turnover time was longer when the dye-tag technique was used than when the radioactivity method was used. In an effort to compare field and laboratory results, the investigator placed ^{134}Cs-tagged isopods in enclosures open to soil that contained litter. Turnover rates for these animals were compared with those in the laboratory. In a concluding statement, Riechle said:

> Although temperature is a paramount factor to be considered in extrapolating laboratory turnover rates of radiocesium to the field, there may be other more subtle environmental influences which will require additional study before more precise estimates can be made. Potentially, however, radioisotope technology offers the ecologist a valuable tool for the study of ecosystem energetics.

The cycling rate of elements is influenced by the rate of litter breakdown and leaching from litter with the subsequent release of elements to the ground surface. The use of radiotracers incorporated in the litter offers a means of studying this rate of transfer. Olson and Crossley (1963) tagged living leaves of trees using the trough method discussed in section 10.3.2 and cited from Auerbach *et al.* (1964) and Olson (1968); this method was illustrated in Figures 85 and 86. Olson and Crossley used several millicuries of the radionuclide applied to trees 2–5 inches in diameter. The investigators observed a relatively high uptake of ^{134}Cs and usually lower and more variable amounts of ^{45}Ca, ^{59}Fe, ^{60}Co, ^{65}Zn, ^{89}Sr, ^{90}Sr, and ^{106}Ru. Factors that affected translocation variability were season of tagging, weather, techniques, and location of the radionuclide in the tree. Litter bags 1 dm^2 were constructed of fiber-glass curtain material, and the tagged leaves were placed in these bags. The bags were then placed on the forest floor and were periodically sampled. Radioactivity was measured by placing the litter bag in a plastic sandwich box that was in turn placed on a scintillation crystal. Three methods of collecting periodic samples were described by the authors. Observations on the change in radioactivity of the litter merely measured that lost to the litter. The amount of radioactivity remaining in the soil surface beneath the litter was studied by cutting 1-dm^2 pieces of ground surface and placing this material in a box containing holes on the bottom and sides, covering this with the litter bag, and placing the entire combination in the field. During the counting period, the litter box and its contents were placed in a plastic bag and inverted so that the forest floor material was flush with the counting crystal. Standardizing the counting geometry offered some problems that are discussed by the investigators. In one experiment, the standard geometry was accomplished by adjusting the material with a cellulose sponge. Figure 91 illustrates the procedure as described above. In addition, results of radionuclide retention are presented in Figure 92.

In another study of litter decomposition, D.R. Gifford (1967) grew Scots pine (*Pinus silvestris*) seedlings in a closed atmospheric chamber containing $^{14}CO_2$ during the period of shoot elongation. The labeled carbon dioxide that replaced the nonlabeled gas was generated from $Na_2^{14}CO_3$ by adding HCl and then introducing it into the chamber from which CO_2 had been removed by passing the air through KOH and washing. On completion of growth in late autumn, plants were dried and the current year's litter was retained for experimental use. The labeled litter was placed on the ground, and at a later date, a "circular core cutter" was used to sample the area. The fauna in these samples was extracted with a high-gradient extractor. The core was sliced into 1-cm-thick pieces and the amount of activity determined in these pieces and the fauna with a liquid scintillation counting system after oxidation of the sample and absorption of the carbon dioxide in hyamine hydroxide. This was the same compound used by Hargrave (1970) to collect $^{14}CO_2$ in his study of the utilization of benthic microflora by a freshwater benthic amphipod (See Section 10.3.2).

Utilizing many of the techniques discussed above, Crossley and Gist (1973) prepared a paper, "Use of radioisotopes in modeling soil microcommunities," that is recommended to the mathematically inclined reader.

In concluding our discussion of terrestrial ecosystems, it seems appropriate to quote from Reichle and Crossley (1967) on the radionuclide model for secondary production:

> The application of radioisotopes to the measurement of food consumption and energy flow in food chains involves the dynamic flux of tracer materials between and within

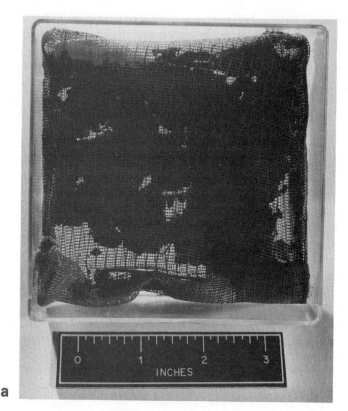

a

Figure 91. Litter bag used in a tracer study of the breakdown of forest litter. (a) Bag of fiber-glass curtain material containing leaves subject to apparently normal breakdown, except for restricted removal of large particles by large animals. (b) Close-up of old forest floor and humus material undergoing decay underneath the litter bags in the litter boxes. (c) Combination of litter bag nestled in position over litter box. (d) Bottom view of litter box, showing fiber-glass window-screen material that supports the slab of forest floor material, and holes providing access for movement of small forest animals. The plastic bag maintains moisture and nuclides in the sample during handling. (e) Litter box inverted in cardboard positioner, ready for counting over a scintillation crystal in a large lead shield. The sandwich box containing the litter bag is at left, the standard with cellulose sponge at upper right, and the cellulose sponge for slight compression of loose litter at lower right. From Olson and Crossley (1963).

trophic levels. The balance and loss concepts and transfer kinetics vital to such an approach have led to the development of a preliminary model for the movement of radioisotopes through food chains. . . . In graphical form . . . there are three basis trophic levels or compartments in the model—plant, herbivore, and primary predator [see Figure 78]. The energy and material flow between compartments occurs through consumption of vegetation and the feeding of predators upon herbivores. Predatory intake, in effect, is equivalent to the predatory mortality of herbivores. By using isotopic tracers, the standing crop of

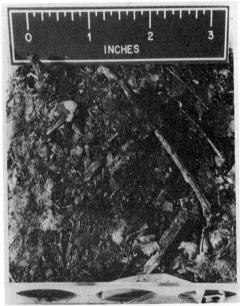

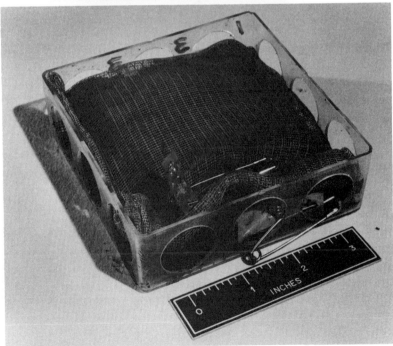

Figure 91. (*continued*)

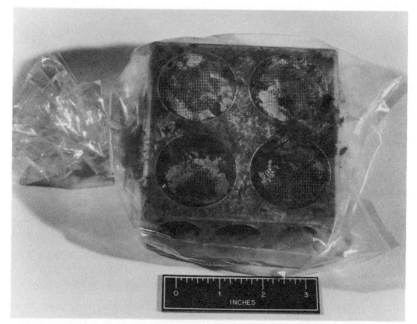

d

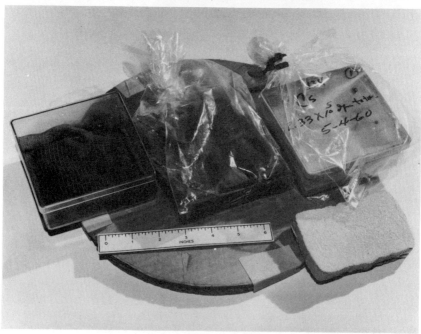

e

Figure 91. (*continued*)

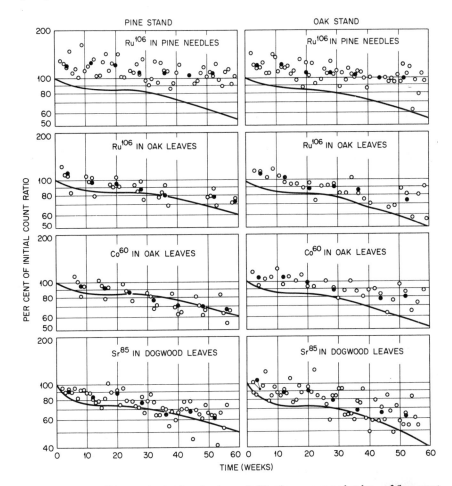

Figure 92. Radionuclide retention by decaying leaves in litter bags, expressed as $\log_{10}$ of (bag count ratio/standard count ratio), as a function of time. (○) Individual measurements; (●) averages for 8-week cycles; (—) weight loss plotted on a semi-log scale. The lines were fitted by eye. From Olson and Crossley (1963).

predator biomass can be used to estimate predatory mortality (grazing) of the preceding (herbivore) compartment.

Productivity cannot be interpreted separately from other phenomena of the food chain. Standing crops, rates of feeding, total energy intake, and energy utilization for maintenance are all variables which ultimately affect productivity. Radioactive tracers are among the new tools which are being used to measure phenomena associated with food chains. When animals feed upon plants containing certain radioisotopes a steady-state condition is attained. At equilibrium concentrations the daily intake of radioisotope is balanced by daily elimination. In the food chain model . . . intake is through feeding alone, while there are three principal pathways of elimination or loss: (1) egestation, which encompasses bioelimination and non-assimilated isotope, (2) non-predatory mortality, and (3) predatory mortality. If mortality is excluded (as in short-term field or laboratory experiments), radioisotope input to either of the animal compartments can be predicted from egestion measurements and compartmental concentrations of radioisotope. Under field conditions the losses due to mortality may result in a reduction in size and radioisotope content of the herbivore or predator compartment. If mortality is balanced by production, however, the compartment size is maintained.

10.3.3.3. Aquatic Studies

In one of the early papers on the subject, Foster (1959) summarized the available data at that time and discussed the use of a radiotracer to study movement of an essential element in an aquatic ecosystem. His emphasis was on ^{32}P, perhaps because of the amount of literature available and the extensive research at Hanford on this radionuclide that was associated with the discharge of ^{32}P into the Columbia River from plutonium production reactors. This paper should be required reading for aquatic biologists interested in radiotracer techniques who wish to get an overview of the subject before studying the literature in depth. Foster stresses the difficulty of duplicating natural situations in the laboratory and the fact that the "true measure" of the dynamics of these systems requires field work. However, he realized the complexity of the natural system and comments that only through controlled laboratory experiments, in conjunction with field research, can the relationships within the system become clear.

Since ^{32}P has been used extensively in aquatic research at an ecosystem level in the field and in a simulated field system, we will consider a selected set of papers in which investigators used this radionuclide. Two aquarium studies of interest are those of Kkmeleva (1959) and Whittaker (1961). The objectives of investigations by the former were to clarify the distribution of phosphorus within a body of water treated with inorganic fertilizers containing only P or a combination of C, N, P, and K. Aquaria were constructed of wood and lined with paraffin. The aquaria contained either a substrate of washed sand and phytoplankton or a substrate of washed sand, waterweed, zooplankton, and phytoplankton. Fertilizer containing ^{32}P was placed in the aquarium of substrate and phytoplankton, and only ^{32}P was placed in the other aquarium containing other components. It is not clear how the plankton were introduced into the systems. Phosphorus-32 was introduced as a dilute sodium acid phosphate. Samples of the various components, including bacteria, in each of the aquaria were sampled periodically and counted. The "coefficient of accumulation" was calculated by

$$(cpm/g \text{ wet wt. of sample})/(cpm/ml \text{ filtered water})$$

In a series of seven exploratory experiments involving aquaria and an artificial pond, Whittaker (1961) investigated the transfer and concentration of ^{32}P. He described in considerable detail his experimental design and the mechanics of the experiments. However, we will only describe some of the procedures in broad generalities and quote the investigator concerning difficulties he encountered in his investigation. In this study, 60-gal indoor aquaria equipped with controls for variable illumination and temperature were used. Glass plates 8.9 cm wide were placed along the walls of the aquaria to collect organisms adhering to the sidewalls. Sampling of bottom organisms and sediment was by means of movable trays 2 cm deep and 8.7×11.1 cm in area in which the sediment had been placed or by four microscope slides used to collect adhering organisms. A special device was fabricated to remove the trays without the previously observed loss of organisms or sediment as a result of water currents. Macroscopic animals were removed with nets and plankton were filtered from water samples, and the filtered water was also collected for counting. A dose of 100 μCi ^{32}P/ 200 liters of water was introduced with the carrier H_3PO_4. An interesting method of establishing a time schedule for sampling was established. Since the uptake of ^{32}P is geometric, Whittaker established a geometric time schedule, e.g., 1, 2, 4, 8, . . . hr. The periodic samples of "plankton" or seston were collected by filtering 2 liters of water with a Foerst centrifuge. Aliquot samples of the filtered water and filtrate were dried and counted. The glass plates placed along the side of the aquarium were taken out, and algae and other organisms were removed from both sides by scraping with a razor. In addition, the plates were washed and cleaned with warm nitric acid to remove the ^{32}P that was more closely bound to the plate surface. Trays that had been placed at the bottom of the aquarium were processed by taking them from the aquarium and removing algae on the glass slides by scraping with a razor blade. Filamentous algae on the mud mat were removed with a scapel from a circle 2.5 cm in diameter. Mud samples were also taken within the circle where possible. All samples were processed and counted with a GM counting system.

A circular concrete basin was used as an outside pond. The basin was 9.5 m in diameter and 92 cm deep at the perimeter, sloping to a maximum depth of 107 cm in the center. Waterworn Columbia River rocks were placed in the bottom of the pond and were later sampled for adhering organisms. Glass plates were also placed along the sidewalls, similar to the laboratory study. A dose of 20 mCi ^{32}P was introduced into the pond, and samples were collected on a geometric schedule. Macroscopic animals consisted of various insects and a breeding fish population of guppies (*Lebistes* sp.). Seven experiments were "Movement of P^{32} in oligotrophic aquaria," "Movement of P^{32} in eutrophic aquaria," "Effect of phosphate levels on P^{32} movement and concentration," "Surface uptake in living and dead aquaria," "P^{32} movement in aquaria at different temperatures," "Uptake and loss of P³² by *Daphnia* and fish," and "P³² movement in an outdoor pond." Whittaker (1961) commented as follows on the difficulties he encountered:

(a) Sampling difficulties resulting from the small size and limited biomass of aquaria. (b) The highly mixed character of plankton, attached algae, and mud, which prevents effective distinction of rates and concentrations in different kinds of organisms and living and dead components, and gives most measurements a gross or synthetic character. (c) Adsorption onto surfaces of organisms and particles, and the difficulty of distinguishing this from other uptake. (d) Binding of P³² to aquarium walls and other surfaces by films of microorganisms. (e) Aquarium individuality, the marked differences between aquaria with similar conditions which result from minor, uncontrolled factors and are a major limitation on reproducibility and statistical adequacy of the data. (f) Irregularity or dispersion of P³² content of organisms or other samples from a given aquarium. (g) The inescapable complexity of aquarium processes, the changing character of these as the aquarium ages, and the interrelatedness of almost all that happens in the aquarium. Aquarium communities are small but not simple; they are scarcely simpler to study and interpret than full-scale natural communities.

Other than application of radionuclide techniques to hydrological studies, the only ecosystem study involving introduction of a radiotracer into a natural free-flowing aquatic habitat of some size was that of R.C. Ball, F. F. Hooper, and their associates in the west branch of the Sturgeon River located in the northern part of the lower peninsula of Michigan. These workers were permitted to inject ³²P in this river because apparently no health hazard was involved, since the injection point was in a remote section about 1/2 mile from a road. The study was concerned with transport downstream (Ball and Hooper, 1963) and upstream (Ball *et al.*,1963) of radiophosphorus in this relatively infertile trout stream. The study as described by Ball and Hooper (1963) was basically one of the relationship of phosphorus and stream productivity. The ³²P tracer was introduced into the stream from a 55-gal oil drum containing a polyethylene tube. The drum was placed in the center of the stream on a fallen log, and 23 mCi ³²P, as $H_3{}^{32}PO_4$, diluted by the water of a full drum, was discharged at 1.22×10^{-5} $\mu Ci/ml$. Interestingly, the head required to maintain this rate of flow was attained by lowering the discharge nozzle along a board attached to the barrel. The board was marked off with nails so that the nozzle would be lowered to the next nail every 33 min timed from the initiation of the experiment. Sampling stations were located along the stream (Figure 93a), and personnel at these stations were instructed to take water samples every 5 min following their first sample, which coincided with the appearance of a dye marker that had been released at the inoculation point 5 min prior to release of the tag. When the drum was emptied and washed, another injection of dye was made that marked the upstream movement of the spike. After the main mass of ³²P had passed, the sampling period was extended. It was necessary to enhance the dye marker at three points downstream. Following this collection by personnel, automatic water-samplers were placed in operation at selected stations (8, 11, 14). The sample water was passed through a filter and the filtrate counted, giving an indication of the amount of water-soluble ^{32}P. The filter was washed with 0.1 N HCl that released the adsorbed phosphorus. The activity of the filter was then attributed to the incorporated ^{32}P in some solid. At 2 weeks prior to tagging, a series of Plexiglas plates was suspended on metal stands in the stream at Stations 3, 8, 12, and 14 to allow growth of periphyton on them. These plates were later sampled at various periods, and the periphyton was counted for ^{32}P by scraping the material from the plates and processing it prior to counting. At Stations 3, 8, 12, and 14, routine collections of aquatic plants were made, processed in the laboratory, and counted. At the same stations, aquatic invertebrates were collected periodically and counted. Fish and trees adjacent to the stream were also sampled. Some of the data are presented in Figure 93b,c.

It has been observed that addition of phosphorus to lakes may result in increased productivity. Thus, the cycling of phosphorus is of interest to aquatic ecologists interested in lake dynamics. Hayes and Coffin (1951) discussed their studies of exchange of phosphorus in lakes using ^{32}P. They stated that the first such study using ^{32}P was conducted by Hutchinson and Bowen (1947), who surface-labeled a 14-acre Connecticut lake. Hayes and Coffin (1951) introduced 100 mCi ^{32}P at the surface of an acid bog lake of less than 1 acre. At 2 hr after introduction of the ^{32}P, samples of various organisms were collected periodically. In another experiment, the tracer was introduced into the same bog lake at a depth 3 ft above the bottom in a bottle in which a dynamite cap had been placed. After the material in the bottle reached thermal equilibrium with the lake water, the cap was detonated. Water samples were also collected in this experiment, and primary movement was observed to be horizontal rather than vertical. In another experiment, Hayes and Coffin used an 8-acre lake containing little vegetation and no sphagnum moss. They introduced 1000 mCi ^{32}P onto the lake surface. Some results of the bog-lake study involving introduction of the tracer at the surface are shown in Figure 94a. The distribution of the tracer within an organism was studied by autoradiography as illustrated by the autoradiograph of a frog in Figure 94b.

Hooper and Imes (1973) also used ^{32}P in a study of a bog lake, which was approximately 50 × 40 m in area and slightly over 8 m deep. Their study of the physical and biological dispersion of phosphorus was by injection of ^{32}P into deep strata to isolate vertical transport processes. In a 1969 study, the tracer was applied through ice cover, while a 1970 study involved tagging during open-water conditions. Their procedure was to obtain 50 gal water from the 7-m depth, to which were added rhodamine dye and 176 mCi ^{32}P as orthophosphate, the water and additions then being mixed thoroughly. Labeled orthophosphate is the compound that Hayes and Coffin (1951) stated to be the form most often used

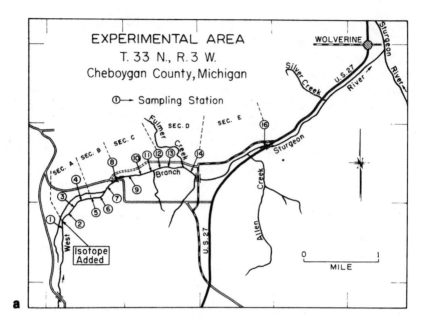

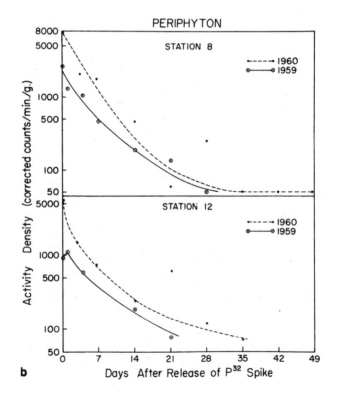

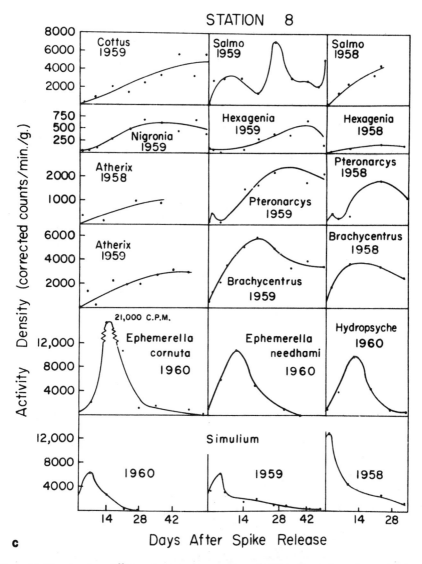

Figure 93. Translocation of ^{32}P in a trout-stream ecosystem. (a) Map of experimental area showing location of sampling stations. (b) Concentration–time curves for periphyton at Stations 8 and 12 in 1959 and 1960. The curves were fitted by eye. Each plotted point is based on a single observation. (c) Concentration–time curves for a selected series of consumer organisms collected at Station 8 in 1958, 1959, and 1960. Each plotted point is based on one observation. From Ball and Hooper (1963).

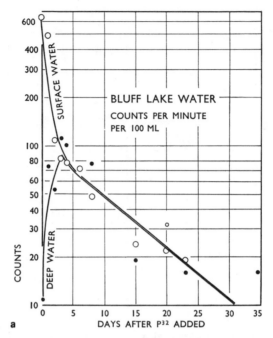

a

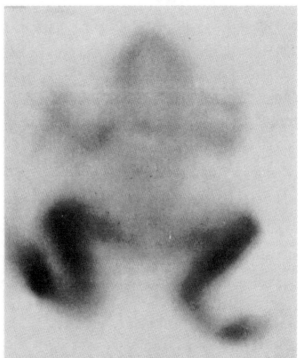

b

in tracer work. This mixture was then injected back into the stratum from which the water had been collected. This was done through an ice cover by drilling 50 holes spaced in a grid in the area of the stratum contour. One gallon of the mixture was injected through each hole at the 7-m stratum via a 2-inch plastic tube fitted with a device that permitted horizontal flowing. The tube was flushed with unlabeled water from the 7-m stratum so that withdrawal of the tube would not result in the label's being released at other depths. During the year when labeling was performed in open water, the same sampling procedure of injection was followed, but from an open boat. In this case, the tube was flushed with surface water rather than water from the stratum being labeled. Since this water was warmer than that at 7 m, the ^{32}P was distributed through a thicker stratum. Dispersion of the radiotracer was determined by measurement of sample activity at various locations. The investigators determined the radioactivity associated with the soluble reactive and nonreactive phosphorus and total phosphorus. The concentration of rhodamine dye was also determined. To determine whether or not radioactivity was transported by organisms other than phantom midges (*Chaoborus*), which were observed at the surface to be radioactive, they collected other invertebrates at various depths. The dye was used to facilitate visual observation of water movement.

Because ^{131}I is an important constituent of fallout from nuclear testing, Kolehmainen *et al.* (1969) studied its distribution in a small Finnish oligotrophic lake (volume 23,000 m^3) by introducing 17 mCi into the lake. From a moving boat that passed around the lake 20 times, carrier-free Na^{131}I was pumped into the lake at depths of 1 and 5 m as it was being diluted in the pump with 20,000 liters of lake surface water. Water samples were collected at three depths from four sampling stations. Sufficient samples for counting were not available for plankton and bottom organisms. Samples of the following plants were taken: yellow water lily (*Nuphar luteum*), a green alga (*Oedogonium* sp.), and sphagnum moss (*Sphagnum recurvum*). In addition, mud, a sponge (*Spongilla lacustris*), and a fish (*Cyprinus carassius*) were collected. A pulse-height analyzer in conjunction with a NaI(Tl) crystal was used to count samples in the "fresh state." Some results are presented in Figure 95. This is, to our knowledge, the second study in an aquatic habitat that involved the addition by investigators of an important fission product to a natural system; the other was in Fern Lake (Chase, 1971), which is discussed below.

$\longleftarrow$

Figure 94. Exchange of lake nutrients studied with ^{32}P. (a) Concentrations of ^{32}P in surface water and deep waters of a lake in which complete mixing occurred. Time is measured from the deposition of ^{32}P at the surface. The ordinate is logarithmic. (b) Autoradiograph of a frog taken from a lake, 40 days after addition of ^{32}P. The concentration of tracer in the skeleton is evident. Exposure 15 days, on dental X-ray plate. From Hayes and Coffin (1951).

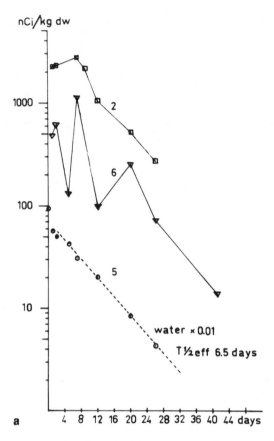

Figure 95. Iodine-131 tracer experiment in an oligotrophic lake. (a) Iodine-131 content (nCi/kg dry wt.) in a green alga *(Oedogonium* sp.) (2) and a moss *(Sphagnum recurvum)* (6) and in the water (10^{-2} nCi/liter) (5). (b) Iodine-131 content (nCi/kg dry wt.) in a sponge *(Spongilla lacustris)* (1),

A pilot study of the cycling of important radioactive waste products was conducted in an experimental pond in Ohio (Brungs, 1967). A 50 × 70 ft pond with a maximum depth of 3 ft was constructed with an 8-mil polyethelene liner installed so as to prevent surface runoff from entering the pond and to prevent seepage water loss (Figure 96). The primary pond was filled with spring water 2 months prior to addition of the radionuclides of interest, namely, ^{60}Co, ^{65}Zn, ^{85}Sr, and ^{137}Cs. After addition of the water, a layer of washed sand was placed on the bottom of the pond. Two wooden tanks lined with polyester resin were constructed with facilities to circulate filtered pond water through them. The tanks were built to hold fish in pond water so that the fish would not have contact

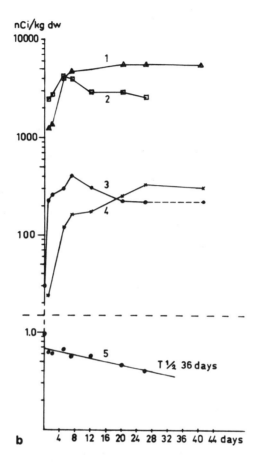

a green alga (*Oedogonium* sp.) (2), a yellow water lily *(Nuphar luteum)* (3), and the crucian carp *(Cyprinus carassius)* (4), and in the water, (nCi/liter) (5), all corrected for decay to the moment of labeling. From Kolehmainen *et al.* (1969).

with food organisms that contained radioactivity. Certain organisms were placed in the pond and later sampled for radioactivity. According to Brungs (1967), the radionuclides used in the study were selected because they are common radioactive waste products and because they or their daughters are gamma emitters, which favored sample preparation and counting. A dose of 4 mCi of each radionuclide was placed in 50 gal of pond water contained in a polyethylene tank; the solution was pumped into the pond on the surface and beneath the surface. While the solution was being pumped, another pump filled the tank with pond water. Finally, the recirculating pump was used to mix the pond water. The final concentrations of the radionuclides were within the safety limits spec-

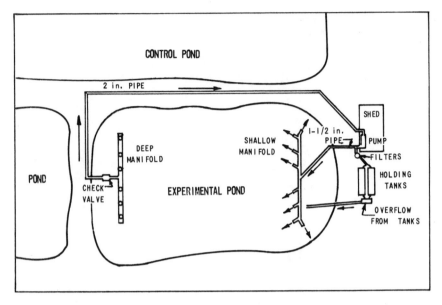

Figure 96. Pond-water recirculation system used in a study of radionuclide distribution in a freshwater pond. From Brungs (1967).

ified for the general human population. The following macrofauna were introduced into the pond: the blue gill (*Lepomis macrochirus*), an omnivore; carp
(*Cyprinus carpio*), a bottom feeder; clams (*Anodonta grandis* and *Lampsilis
radiata siloquoidea*); a snail (*Viviparus malleatus*); bullfrog tadpoles (*Rana ca-
tesbiana*); and "minnows and aquatic insects." The fish were placed in both the
pond and the tanks; in the latter, they were fed dry fish food. As expected, some
organisms that were not stocked invaded the pond: snapping turtles (*Chelydra
serpentina*), crayfish (*Orconectes rusticus*), and a filamentous alga (*Cladophora*
sp.). These were collected and analyzed for radioactivity. The samples were
collected at various times for 80 days after introduction of the radionuclides and
analyzed for radioactivity with a 512-channel analyzer in conjunction with a
NaI(Tl) crystal. Details concerning sampling, sample-processing, and counting
are described by the author. A portable U.S. Army Corps of Engineers water-
treatment unit and a twin-bed de-ionizer were used at the termination of the
study to remove radioactivity from the pond water, which was then returned to
a water course on the area. Brungs (1967) stated:

It should be emphasized that the experimental pond system would be an example prin-
cipally of a situation in which radioactive wastes were discharged to a standing impound-

ment. In a flowing system, any attempt at precise mass balances would be most difficult because of an unknown biomass and other factors. . . . The most striking general conclusion from these calculations from a biological point of view, was that the maximum accumulation in the biota for a single radionuclide, zinc 65, was only slightly above 1 percent. Cobalt 60 and cesium 137 never exceeded 0.25 percent.

Another radionuclide of contemporary importance is ^{65}Zn. In a laboratory investigation of zinc cycling in fresh water, Bachmann (1963) used the tracer ^{65}Zn to study its uptake in suspensions of an alga (*Golenkinia paucispina*), natural lake seston and sediments, and organic detritus. In addition, he studied uptake as related to suspended material by two water fleas (*Daphnia pulex* and *D*. magna). An artificial sediment–water system was developed to study the movement of zinc by mayfly nymphs (*Ephemera simulans*) into sediments. A concentrate of 10 μCi ^{65}Zn/ml was introduced in volumes of 0.05–1.0 ml into 100 ml of the suspended material. It was assumed that specific activity of zinc in the tracer solution was the same as that in the experimental containers. Except for one experiment involving *D. pulex*, a well-type crystal scintillation counting system was used in counting samples.

In 1957, the Fern Lake Mineral Metabolism Program was established as a component of the IBP. The study was interdisciplinary in scope, and the lake watershed was considered a geographical unit. One of the studies associated with this ambitious endeavor, namely, that of mineral cycling in a Douglas fir stand (Riekerk and Gessel, 1965), was discussed in Section 10.3.3.2. Rather than discuss the entire program, which is adequately described in the final report (Chase, 1971), we will restrict our comments to the radiological techniques associated with studies of the lake proper. Fern Lake, located in western Washington on the Puget Sound lowland, is 23.8 acres in area with a maximum depth of 7.3 m and is the drainage outlet for a 3.12-square-mile watershed. Studies of the uptake of minerals by biota were conducted in the lake and laboratory. The location and characteristics of the lake permitted safe introduction of radionuclides into this aquatic system. Since the mineral level in the lake water was low, it was expected that the specific activity and demand by biota would be high. Preliminary investigations of 12 radionuclides were made in the laboratory, and 4 were selected for use in the field, namely, ^{32}P, ^{45}Ca, ^{99}Mo, and ^{131}I. These isotopes were introduced into the lake and monitored for 2 months. The objectives of the studies were stated as follows (Chase, 1971):

The aquarium experiments were designed to show the rate and extent of the radionuclide accumulations by organisms and sediments of the lake and to furnish guidelines for the field applications. The general objectives of the field experiments were (1), to measure the accumulations of the selected nuclides in organisms with access to their usual sources of nutrition and (2), to evaluate the role of the food web in the accumulation by measuring relative assimilation directly from the water in organisms held in containers.

The aquarium experiments were conducted in polyethylene-lined containers (150 liters) with 75 liters of unfiltered Fern Lake water; live boxes were suspended in the containers. Clams, crayfish, amphipods, and steelhead trout (*Salmo gairdneri*) were placed in the live boxes, the alga *Nitella flexilis*, was suspended in the aquaria by a cord, and sediment in jars was placed on the bottom of the aquaria (Figure 97a). Radionuclide concentrations in the aquaria were from 0.32 to 5.5 mCi per tank, for ^{59}Fe and ^{131}I, respectively. On the basis of concentrations observed in the various samples, the investigators concluded that the radionuclides selected for field observation would be detectable at dilutions of up to 10,000 times those used in the laboratory studies. The procedure for dispersing the radionuclides, ^{45}Ca, ^{99}Mo, and ^{131}I, on the lake surface is shown in Figure 97b. Application was conducted over a 2-hr period. It was believed that dispersion would be through the thermocline. In a study of dispersion pattern and rate, ^{32}P was applied in 5 min at the lake inlet. Prior to application, rafts were placed at various sampling stations throughout the lake and from these rafts were suspended live boxes containing organisms for periodic sampling. *Nitella* was suspended at various depths from the rafts and at other sampling points. Long-term data on mineral cycling were to have been obtained from observations on ^{45}Ca, but introduction of fallout from September 1961 Russian nuclear tests obscured the results—another irritation associated with field work. Readers interested in details of the experiment are referred to Chase (1971) as well as to the paper of Short *et al.* (1973).

Radionuclide-tracer studies in natural marine environments obviously must rely on natural radioactivity in the environment or on radionuclides introduced from the activities of man such as fallout from nuclear-weapons testing or release of major amounts of nuclear waste such as from the Hanford Operations via the Columbia River. Some studies of this type have been discussed. We will conclude this section with those that are more closely related to investigations of "complete" ecosystems or subsystems.

The cycling of organic carbon is important to an understanding of the ecology of the marine environment. P.M. Williams and Linick (1975) used fallout ^{14}C as a short- and long-term tracer to investigate such cycling. The major source of the ^{14}C was assumed to be the 1961–1962 nuclear-weapons testing program. Samples of surface, bathypelagic, and benthic marine organisms and surface waters from various areas in the Pacific Ocean and Ross Sea were collected. The ^{14}C content of the organisms, or selected portions, and the amounts in dissolved organic matter in sea water were determined. Details concerning sample-processing and counting were presented by the investigators. Concerning the technique, they commented: "One critical phase in all these techniques is in using nets and gear which are not heavily contaminated with large amounts of

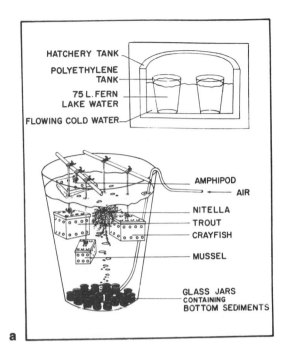

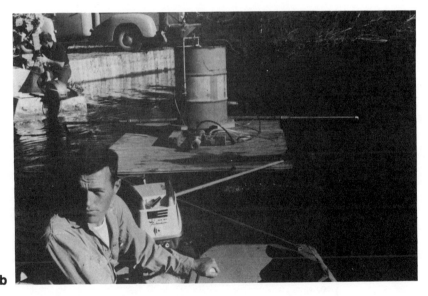

Figure 97. Uptake of radionuclides by biota in an aquarium and a freshwater lake. (a) Diagram of the aquarium experiment. (b) Application of radioactive nuclides to Fern Lake. The tank and distribution pipe were on a raft towed by a boat. From Short *et al.* (1973). (b) courtesy of L. R. Donaldson.

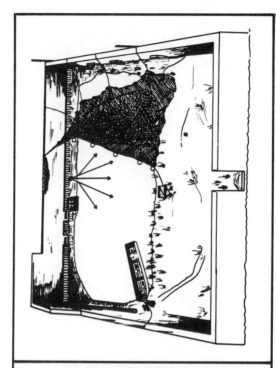

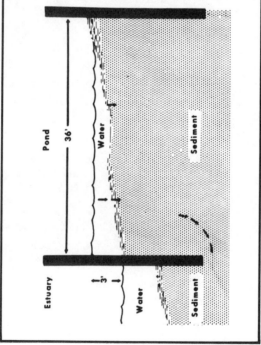

Pond

36'

Water

Sediment

Estuary

3'

Water

Sediment

a

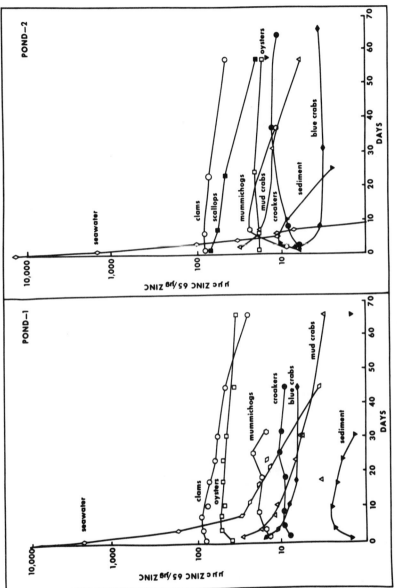

Figure 98. Cycling of ^{65}Zn in an experimental estuarine environment. (a) Diagrammatic sketches of experimental ponds. Arrows in Pond I (*left*) indicate the flow of water, and in Pond II the location of the pipe through which water was exchanged with the adjoining estuary. The position of the sampling net is shown in Pond II. (b) Specific activity of components in experimental ponds. The specific activity of the water at the time ^{65}Zn was introduced into the pond (0 days) was 18,100 $\mu\mu Ci$ $^{65}Zn/\mu g$ zinc in Pond I and 14,200 in Pond II. From T. W. Duke *et al.* (1966).

'dead' carbon (oils, etc.), or with 'hot' carbon (^{14}C) oftentimes in heavy use on biological cruises in connection with photosynthetic rate studies."

T.W. Duke *et al.* (1966) reported on a study of cycling of trace elements in experimental estuarine ponds in which they utilized radiotracers. Two modified concrete ponds adjoining an estuary in North Carolina were utilized in the experiment (Figure 98a). Pond I was filled with 45 m^3 of seawater taken from the estuary. A plastic liner was placed in the pond, and a layer of sediment was laid atop the liner. To balance seepage from the pond, an inflow of seawater from the estuary was used. Since no liner was put in Pond II, there was no consequent disturbance of the bottom as there was in Pond I. Pond II was connected directly to the estuary by a pipe, the end of which was covered with a mesh net to prevent egress or ingress of organisms. At low tide, this pond contained 78 m^3 of water and at high tide, 173 m^3. Organisms of various types, including plants and animals, were collected in the estuary and placed in both ponds. The authors presented considerable detail concerning the species used and related aspects that we will not reiterate. Since the element of interest was zinc, ^{65}Zn was used as a tracer. The investigators were interested in the factors that controlled the distribution of radioactive and stable zinc and in determining whether the distributions were related. A dose of 10 mCi ionic ^{65}Zn in 0.92 N HCl was introduced into each pond by spraying a stream of the solution and pond water onto the pond surface. Sediment, water, and biota samples were collected periodically. At 100 days after initiation of the experiment, a composite sediment sample and three samples of water and of each organism were collected. Animals in Pond II were free-ranging and those in Pond I were restricted, with one exception, to cages. Samples were processed and counted on a single-channel spectrometer and a liquid scintillation detector. Some results are presented in Figure 98b. The investigators commented:

> Organisms in Pond II contained less zinc 65 at each sampling period than those in Pond I even though the same amount of radioisotope was released in each pond. Most of this difference undoubtedly resulted from the greater dilution of the zinc 65 in Pond II. Tidal exchange contributed to this dilution and steadily lowered the concentration of zinc 65 in the water and thus reduced the amount available to the organisms.

Miscellaneous Techniques and Equipment

11.1. Environmental Pollutants

11.1.1. General Comments

Application of radiotracers to studies of environmental pollution source and distribution is rather widespread. This is partly due to encouragement by the International Atomic Energy Agency (IAEA), which through its various symposia, e.g., on radiological techniques in pesticide research (IAEA, 1966a, 1970c) and also on other environmental pollutants (IAEA, 1975a, 1976), has disseminated knowledge on the subject. Perhaps the most extensive use has been in the study of pesticides (Dedek, 1967a,b, 1970, 1975; Casida, 1961; Dahm, 1957; Redemann and Meikle, 1958; Winteringham, 1960; Peterle, 1966; and documented in the bibliographies of Bingelli, 1963, 1965, 1967, 1969). Citing 110 references, DeWitt (1978) summarizes the application of isotopes in investigations of air, soil, and water pollution and concludes:

> Based on established isotope uses, on the projected increase in the pollution problem, and on the apparent social and economic pressure for pollution abatement, a significant demand for enriched isotopes appears to be developing for the assessment and control of air, water, and soil pollutants. Isotopic techniques will be used in combination with conventional methods of detection and measurement, such as gas chromatography, x-ray fluorescence, and atomic absorption. Recent advances in economical isotope separation methods, instrumentation, and methodology promise to place isotopic technology within the reach of most research and industrial institutions. Increased application of isotope techniques appears most likely to occur in areas where data are needed to characterize the movement, behavior, and fate of pollutants in the environment.

Our discussion of radionuclide techniques associated with environmental-pollution studies will be restricted to pesticide studies of an ecological nature. We have decided to emphasize pesticides because their application in the environment has been of significant concern to ecologists for many years. Readers interested in other environmental pollutants are referred to the references cited above.

11.1.2. Applications

Considerable controversy existed in the past as to the effect of DDT on natural populations of animals, particularly the impact on specific bird populations. Research efforts included the use of labeled DDT in laboratory and field experiments.

Harvey (1967) studied the concentration and translocation of this insecticide in the starling *(Sturnus vulgaris)* by means of ^{14}C-labeled DDT. Wild juvenile starlings were maintained in outdoor cages and fed chicken mash and canned peas containing the labeled insecticide. A solution of DDT containing corn oil, the labeled DDT, and a carrier was injected into a pea with a microinjector. Every day for 5 days, a bird was force-fed labeled peas, totaling 4.75 mg DDT. At predetermined intervals, birds were sacrificed, and the fat-soluble pesticide in the brain, liver, and carcass was extracted. Radioactivity in the extract was determined with a scintillation counting system. A portion of the results is presented in Figure 99.

Dr. T. J. Peterle was one of the first ecologists, if not the first, to apply radiotracers in studies of accumulation of insecticides in a natural ecosystem. The studies of Peterle and his students were conducted in Ohio in a marsh, a deciduous forest, and an old-field ecosystem. Meeks (1968) reported on the uptake of ring-labeled [^{36}Cl]-DDT in a freshwater marsh located on the southwestern edge of Lake Erie. The primary objectives of the study were associated with the food-chain aspects of DDT in a freshwater marsh. The study area was a 4-acre diked marsh averaging 1 ft in depth, which was part of a larger marsh of several thousand acres. To prevent some vertebrate movement into and out of the area, a ½-inch-mesh fence was placed on the dike with the lower portion buried 8 inches deep and an electric wire on the top. Since all the ethane-chain chlorides on the DDT molecule may be lost during metabolism, ring-labeled DDT was selected because none of the phenyl-ring chlorides is removed. Thus, ^{36}Cl in a sample implied the presence of an integral part of the molecule or one of the degradation products. Chlorine-36 has a physical half-life of 3.1×10^5 years and decays by emission of a negative beta particle with energy adequate for efficient counting. The investigator commented that the radionuclide, in addition to having these characteristics, did not present an external human health hazard. The labeled DDT was mixed with a granular formulation to facilitate

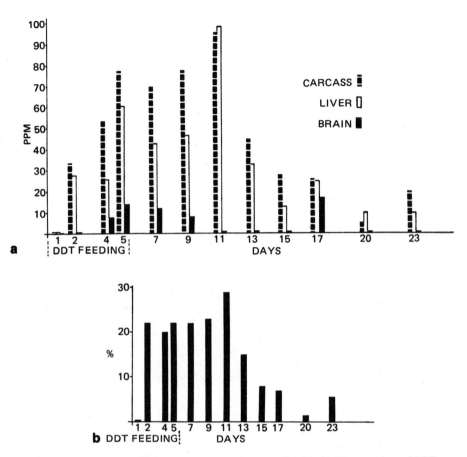

Figure 99. Excretion of [¹⁴C]DDT by starlings *(Sturnus vulgaris)*. (a) Concentrations of DDT or metabolites recovered from carcass, liver, and brain. (b) DDT or metabolites recovered, as percentage of total ingested DDT. From Harvey (1967).

aerial application and prevent drifting. The level of application was similar to standard larvacide levels. It was applied at the rate of 0.2 lb of "technical material" with 100 lb of granules per acre-foot of water, involving 3.9 mCi of the tracer. To extend the time the DDT would remain dispersed in the water, an emulsifier was mixed with the solution. The mixture was applied from a helicopter with the same equipment used in a terrestrial investigation (Bandy and Peterle, 1973) (Figure 100). Personnel safety precautions were taken, and the helicopter landed on a plastic sheet to facilitate cleanup in case a spill occurred. To detect drift if it occurred during application, air was passed through a filter located on the periphery of the treated area. No radioactivity was observed above

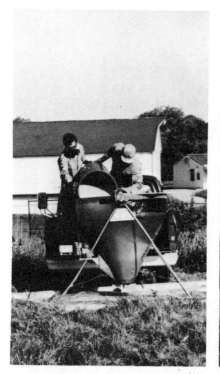 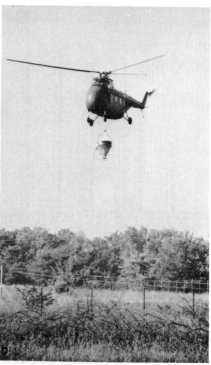

Figure 100. Helicopter application of ^{36}Cl-ring-labeled DDT to a terrestrial study area. (a) Radio-controlled, gasoline-powered rotary applicator used to apply insecticide to study area. (b) DDT granules being applied to an old-field ecosystem. Courtesy of T. J. Peterle.

background on the filter, through which over 4000 ft^3 of air was passed. Samples of water, bottom soil, plants, and animals were collected periodically, some for a period of 15 months. The samples were processed and counted with a Tri-Carb liquid scintillation counting system and corrected for background. Meeks (1968) observed that the majority of the granules settled to the bottom during application and that the DDT was released into the water when the granules dissolved. He noted that very little DDT was in the water at any time. Concerning the use of this radiotracer, Meeks (1968) commented:

> A direct relationship exists between the radioactivity above background and the quantity of radiolabeled material in a sample from the treated marsh. Microquantities of a labeled compound can therefore be detected if the specific activity of the original material is known. This is very useful when the compound in question is difficult or costly to analyze by standard chemical methods, or when unknown products are involved. Although very small amounts of DDT can be detected by standard chromatographic methods, such

techniques are impractical for large-scale environmental studies involving dozens of different biological materials and hundreds of samples.

In a study conducted concurrently with that described above, Dindal (1970) collected wild mallards *(Anas platyrhynchos)* and lesser scaup ducks *(Aythya affinis)*, and the animals, after being marked and pinioned, were introduced intermittently into the marsh enclosure and periodically collected. Every group introduced was tagged with a different-colored streamer bird tag; thus, the period of exposure associated with a particular bird was known, and a bird that had been exposed to the tagged DDT for a specific period could be collected. Background radioactivity was determined for the two species from individuals collected from areas distant from the overall marsh study area. Various tissues and organs from many individuals were analyzed for the tracer.

Using these data, Eberhardt *et al.* (1971) constructed the food-chain model for the DDT kinetics of this aquatic system with equations of first-order kinetics.

Chlorine-36-labeled DDT with carrier was applied to an old-field ecosystem in west-central Ohio and its bioelimination and translocation followed for 1 month (Bandy and Peterle, 1973). The labeled DDT was distributed in a 10-acre plot enclosed by a 2.44-m high cyclone fence with a partially buried sheet-metal barrier and electric stock fence at its base. To prevent drift, the DDT was applied in impregnated clay granules. An emulsifier was also applied to xylene-solubilized DDT to facilitate release from the granules. As the granules were rotated in a concrete mixer drum, the mixture of labeled and carrier DDT in xylene and emulsifier was sprayed on the clay granules. On June 10, the material was distributed over the study area with a specially designed applicator carried beneath a helicopter. Area samplers consisted of the bottom half of petri dishes placed on wooden stands throughout the study area. The distribution pattern of the granules over the area following application was determined from the concentration of granules in the dishes. Plants and animals within the plot were collected at weekly intervals for a month and then monthly until the end of the growing season. A Tri-Carb liquid scintillation spectrometer was used to count samples. It was observed that the release time of the DDT from the clay granules was a function of moisture on the area. Background levels of radiation were determined in samples collected from the study area the year prior to application and also from a control area at each sampling period. In addition to the normal plant and animal populations on the plot, wing-clipped ring-necked pheasants *(Phasianus colchicus)* were released within the study area. An air sampler was used to see whether there was a loss of DDT to the atmosphere. Of the 10.2 mCi ^{36}Cl delivered by the helicopter, 2.07 μCi was lost to the 1.8-m buffer strip around the study area. Following this application in June 1969, Forsyth and Peterle (1973) collected two species of shrews *(Blarina brevicauda* and *Sorex cinereus)* during the period June–November 1970 and in February of 1971 and 1972.

Specimens were also collected away from the study area to be used as controls. Various portions of the animals were processed and counted. In a study of the uptake rate of DDT in *Blarina,* individuals were collected from the area, toe-clipped, and marked with a numbered aluminum leg band for identification. In addition, a 100-μCi piece of ^{182}Ta wire was sealed in a nylon tube that was then placed under the skin in the intrascapular region with a modified hypodermic needle. As contrasted with other uses of this tagging method, it was necessary to anesthetize the shrew prior to injecting the wire. The ^{182}Ta tag was intended to facilitate locating the animals with a Geiger–Müller (GM) field survey meter for periodic collection. The investigators commented that the use of this tag to facilitate recapture was "almost totally unsuccessful," since the animals were apprently too far below the surface to locate with the survey meter.

The deciduous-forest study was conducted on a 41.5-acre tract in east-central Ohio by Giles (1970). The area consisted of two watersheds of which one was treated with the insecticide ^{35}S-labeled malathion. The selection of ^{35}S provided a physical half-life of 88 days, but the relatively weak beta energy (0.167 MeV) can complicate detection and measurement. According to Giles (1970), malathion metabolizes into 10–12 metabolites. Using paper chromatograms, he investigated the association of ^{35}S to the metabolites and concluded that the results suggested that the ^{35}S was distributed with all the metabolites, but not equally. During development of the techniques to be applied on the large study area, Giles hand-applied the labeled insecticide to four plots, each 6.1 × 66.4 m, located 50 m from the boundary of the watershed to be studied. This was accomplished with a back-pack spray apparatus that he developed to simulate aerial application. Numbered stakes were placed in a grid pattern on the control and treated plots. A frosted glass disk was placed at each stake to collect the spray. Cages and faunal sampling devices were placed throughout the plots. In addition, GM survey meter readings were taken of vegetation and the ground following application of the labeled insecticide. On the basis of plot observations, 4.5 mCi per acre was applied to the one watershed. An attempt was made to capture and place wild animals in cages on the treated watershed. This was unsuccessful for a variety of reasons. To assist in aerial application, the area to be sprayed was marked with colored balloons placed above the canopy. The first attempt at aerial application resulted in an airplane crash on the study area, but another airplane completed the spraying on May 25, 1962. The distribution of the insecticide released by the first airplane is shown in Figures 101 and 102. Details and results of measuring the distribution of the labeled insecticide are presented by the investigator. A large number (over 3000 total) of different types of samples were collected. Due to the low concentration of ^{35}S in these samples and the relatively low emission energy of ^{35}S, the samples had to be processed in the laboratory using a low-background automatic sample-changer with a thin-window detector and a cosmic-ray shield. The comprehensive nature of this

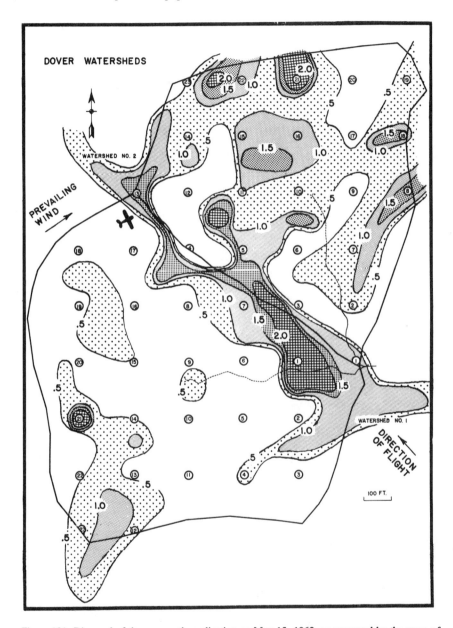

Figure 101. Dispersal of the one-swath application on May 15, 1962, as measured by the mean of two frosted glass disks placed on the ground at all grid intersections less than one hour before spraying and collected six hours later every 30.5 m along the path between intersections, and every 15.2 m along lines running at right angles to the boundaries. The position of the crashed plane between thirteen and seventeen is shown. From Giles (1970).

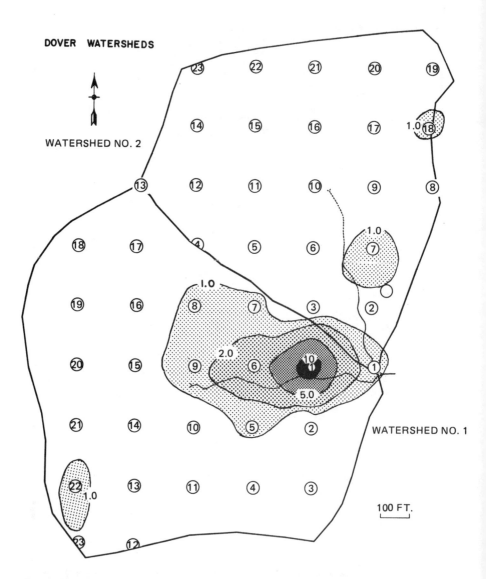

Figure 102. Dispersal of the one-swath application on May 15, 1962, as measured by the mean of two enamel-coated papers placed 15 cm above the ground at all grid intersections, less than one hour before spraying and collected six hours later. From Giles (1970).

study precludes an adequate description of all the collection and processing techniques; therefore, readers interested in performing a similar study are urged to read this monograph in detail. In his discussion of the project, Giles (1970) comments:

> In one sense, malathion tagged with sulfur 35 was a poor choice for study since its total ecological effects were not spectacular. That radionuclide and the insecticide are both short-lived and used in small amounts. The insecticide is relatively specific for insects. The isotope could only be adequately quantified in the laboratory. But in another sense it was an excellent choice because (1) it is replacing the chlorinated hydrocarbons in forest insect control work and information on its effects is needed for practicing control agencies; (2) it has specific effects on insects and was short-lived enough so that it could have provided information on secondary effects on birds and fishes; (3) it has required, and therefore, demonstrated, the great amount of effort needed to study and conclusively interpret the ecological effects of certain insecticides. . . . Sample preparation lagged far behind field work during the study so there was no periodic review and modifications in sampling procedures. The dispersal patterns, if they could have been calculated and plotted in time (if they had ever been suspected), would have suggested alternate sampling intensities and programs. . . . An optimum ecological study using a radioactively labeled insecticide would require a radionuclide having an optimum of "mix" of half-life, type of emission, minimum health hazard, and minimal incompatibility with the major nutrients of the biota of an ecosystem. Then, an insecticide should be sought that was highly toxic to a large segment of the biota and virtually nontoxic to one or more segments and that could be labeled with the selected radionuclide.

Carbon-14-labeled dieldrin has been used in a study of its uptake by fish (Grzenda *et al.*, 1971) and in another of its presence in feathers of birds with surgically removed uropygial glands (Greichus and Greichus, 1974). In the former study, ^{14}C-labeled dieldrin was fed to goldfish *(Carassius auratus)* at regular intervals, and the uptake was determined in various tissues and organs. The experiment was conducted in Plexiglas chambers that were submersed in a constant-temperature bath. The chambers were arranged in three rows of eight chambers each, and a single fish was placed in each chamber. Constant water flow was maintained in each row. Feces were removed during experimentation to minimize readsorption of the pesticide from feces. Two groups of fish were fed diets, each with a different level of [^{14}C]dieldrin. At intervals of 8, 16, 32, 64, 128, and 192 days, fish were sacrificed, and tissues were processed and counted with a low-background gas-flow GM counting system.

Greichus and Greichus (1974) were interested in the source of oils on bird feathers. Since organochlorine insecticides are lipid-soluble and are mobilized along with fat, the investigators reasoned that the residues would be present on the feathers because the oil on feathers is thought to arise from the uropygial gland. They were interested in seeing whether significant amounts of the residue came from within the body of the bird via the gland. In addition to chickens, double-crested cormorants *(Phalacrocorax a. auritus)* and mallard ducks *(Anas platyrhynchos)* were used in the experiment. Birds with and without uropygial glands were given the labeled insecticide; the chickens and mallard ducks received the ^{14}C-labeled dieldrin by injection of a mixture of 6.19 μCi in 80% ethanol deep into the breast. The cormorants were fed a fish that had been injected with 10.36 μCi. Controls were maintained. After a period of time, the birds were sacrificed and feathers collected from various areas on the bird. The feathers were processed, and the dieldrin was eluted through a column containing Florisil and sodium sulfate. These samples and samples of the uropygial glands were counted by liquid scintillation. It was concluded that the mechanism of distribution of dieldrin onto feathers was other than via the uropygial gland.

The pesticide lindane has been widely used in agriculture as a seed dressing. Using ^{14}C-labeled lindane, Saha (1975) studied its biodegradation in plants and animals. He studied the residue distribution over time in chicks and eggs of pheasants fed the labeled pesticide in gelatin capsules. Pheasants were also fed treated wheat seeds. In addition, the occurrence of residue was determined in samples of brain, liver, breast muscle, and fat from five hen pheasants.

In a different use of a radionuclide tracer, Crossley and Witkamp (1964) studied the effects of naphthalene on arthropods and the breakdown of forest litter. They used white oak leaves *(Quercus alba)* that had been tagged with ^{134}Cs by tree-trunk inoculation. The experiment involved placing different amounts of naphthalene flakes on plots of leaf litter. Litter bags containing the tagged leaves were placed on the plots, and the loss of ^{134}Cs and the number of arthropods were determined at weekly intervals. The investigators observed a difference between the control and treated plots in the ^{134}Cs retention in the litter bags. They commented:

> New techniques in such studies—radioisotopes, litter bags, use of insecticides, and other experimental approaches—can provide a fresh insight into the ecological problems confronting biologists and agronomists alike. Such experimentation is best approached from a functional viewpoint; that is, an over-all consideration of the ecosystem as a dynamic unit, and the soil fauna and soil microflora as parts of that unit

Environmental contamination by mercury from various sources has resulted in a large number of investigations. Reports on the subject have been published, for example, by the IAEA (1972b). Nuclear techniques in the study of environmental mercury have assumed importance because the element lends itself to identification and quantification by neutron activation at great sensitivity. In addition, the radioisotopes of mercury have been used directly to study its behavior in the environment and in organisms.

The comparative metabolism of two mercury compounds, ^{203}Hg(NO$_3$)$_2$ and CH$_3$^{203}HgCl, was studied in the freshwater mussel *(Margaritifera margaritifera)* (Mellinger, 1973). Mercury-203 has a physical half-life of 46.57 days and decays by beta emission to the excited state ^{203}Tl, which emits a gamma ray, thus permitting use of a scintillation detector. Daily assays were made of the test solution, and additional radioactive solution was added to maintain a specific concentration of mercury. Mussels in the solution were removed periodically and placed in nonradioactive water to remove nonbound mercury. The mussel was then removed, drained of water, and replaced in the radioactive solution to continue uptake. Retention curves were computed from whole-body levels observed periodically while the mussels were kept in nonradioactive water. During the retention studies, the water was changed daily, thus avoiding readsorption of excreted mercury. Whole-body counts were made prior to removing tissues, which were individually counted. Whole-body accumulation data for the two compounds are presented in Figure 103.

In another laboratory experiment, Fang (1973) added ^{203}Hg-labeled phenylmercuric acetate (PMA), a slimicide used in the paper and pulp industry, to glass aquaria containing single guppies *(Lebistes reticulatus),* snails *(Helisoma campanulata),* and the aquatic plants elodea *(Elodea canadensis)* and coontail *(Ceratophyllum demersum)* in 4–7 liters of water. A scintillation spectrometer was used to measure activity in periodic samples of water and biota. Retention studies were made by transferring the guppies and elodea to fresh water that was changed periodically to minimize reabsorption. Some of the data are displayed in Figures 104 and 105.

The extensive use of herbicides in modern agricultural and other activities has resulted in very great interest in the impact of these chemicals on the natural environment and its components. The number of ecological or ecologically related studies using radionuclide-labeled herbicides is considerably less than that of studies involving labeled insecticides such as described above.

Osborn *et al.* (1954) reported on a study using eight formulations of ^{14}C-labeled 2,4-D to control aquatic weeds. They were interested in the role of the waterline as a barrier in the translocation of the herbicide, the distribution of the herbicide in untreated parts of treated plants, the role of point of application in the distribution in plants, the effects of chemical additives on the distribution pattern within plants, and the effect of different exposure times on the distribution pattern. The ^{14}C was incorporated in the carboxyl group of 2,4-D, and this tracer was used in preference to ^{131}I, since the former is structurally similar to 2,4-D and the latter more similar to 2,4,5-T; the ^{14}C atom is in the most reactive portion of the molecule, while the ^{131}I label is in the benzene ring; lastly, ^{14}C has a considerably longer physical half-life than ^{131}I. Autoradiographic techniques were utilized to attain the study objectives. The following plants were studied: the filamentous green algae, *Cladophora* sp. and *Spirogyra* sp.; a parasitic fungus, *Phoma* sp.; and the vascular plants, American pondweed *(Potamogeton nodosus)* and broad-leaved cattail *(Typha latifolia).* The cattail was treated in

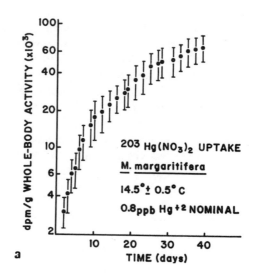

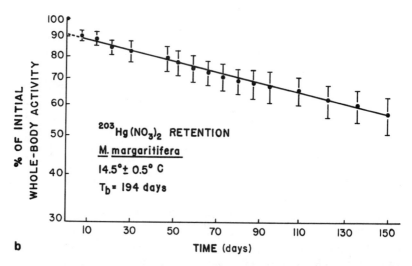

Figure 103. Uptake and retention of two tagged mercury compounds by a freshwater mussel *(Margaritifera margaritifera)*. (a) Uptake of ^{203}Hg(NO$_3$)$_2$ during chronic exposure. (b) Whole-body retention of ^{203}Hg(NO$_3$)$_2$ following chronic exposure. (c) Uptake of CH$_3$^{203}HgCl during chronic exposure. (d) Whole-body retention of CH$_3$^{203}HgCl following chronic exposure. From Mellinger (1973).

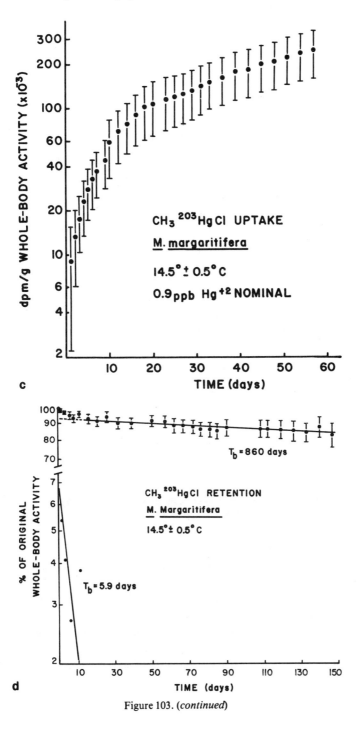

Figure 103. (*continued*)

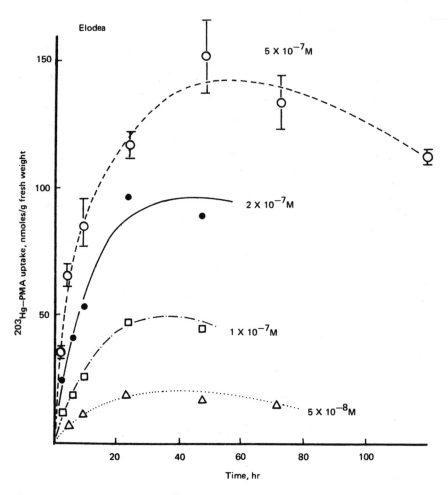

Figure 104. Time-course uptake of [²⁰³Hg]-PMA by elodea *(Elodea canadensis)* from water containing various concentrations of PMA; each point is the mean ± 1 S.E. of results from four or more elodea. From Fang (1973).

a small lake, the pondweed in metal tanks, the fungus on the cattail, and the algae in tanks containing pondweed. The method of application of the labeled herbicide varied with the organism being treated. No special attempt was made to treat the algae and fungus with the herbicide; they came in contact with the herbicide because of their association with the vascular plants that were treated. The herbicide was applied with a micropipette within a small circle of lanolin on the treated leaf of the pondweed. A narrow band of lanolin was applied on both sides of the cattail leaf about 6–7 inches from the tip, and the herbicide was applied above the band in a ½- to ¾-inch strip. The band of lanolin prevented the herbicide from running down the leaf from the area of application. During a period of 8 days, 14 days postapplication, approximately half the plants were harvested. The remaining specimens were harvested 48 days later. Details concerning the selection of a control leaf and the portions of plant from which radioautographs were made were presented by the authors. Regarding the technique, the investigators observed that the high water content of the samples posed problems, since they tended to soften the film emulsion that resulted when the plant samples were applied to the film. Since both plant species dried out rapidly and in the process twisted and became brittle, other difficulties arose in preparing autoradiographs from such specimens. To alleviate these problems,

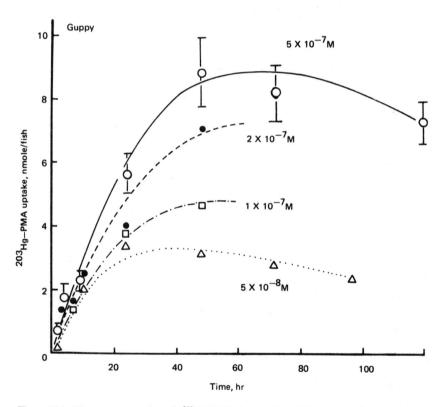

Figure 105. Time–course uptake of [^{203}Hg]-PMA by guppies *(Lebistes reticulatus)* from water containing various concentrations of PMA; each point is the mean ± 1 S.E. of results from four guppies. From Fang (1973).

the specimens were processed the same day as collected after being surface-dried with an absorbent paper towel. To prevent cross-contamination during processing, a new razor blade portion was used for each cut and then discarded. In a study of the possibility that the emulsion might be activated by plant juices and other contaminants, the investigators prepared a series of blanks from cattails collected away from the treatment area. They also applied the labeled herbicide directly to the film and compared the texture of the autoradiographs with that of those associated with the labeled material. It is recommended that the interested reader consult the original paper for details. A large number of interesting autoradiographs also accompany the report.

Sodium arsenite, which is used widely to control aquatic plants, was used in labeled form by Ball and Hooper (1966) in a study of the effects of this herbicide on the ecology of a ⅓-acre natural pond and aquaria ecosystems. Arsenic-74-labeled sodium arsenite was used in the studies. Arsenic-74 has a physical half-life of 17.9 days and decays by beta and gamma emission. The investigators prepared the mixture of labeled sodium arsenite and carrier with distilled water and allowed 12 hr after mixing for the equilibration of the radiolabeled and stable sodium arsenite. The strength of 10 ml of the solution in 1 gal of water was 8 ppm of sodium arsenite, and the activity was 6 dps/ml. A well-type scintillation countering system with a NaI(Tl) crystal was used in counting, and a single-channel spectrum analyzer was used for measuring emissions of the desired energy. The aquarium studies included observations of individual groups of the same species as well as a "complete ecosystem" that contained organisms from more than one trophic level. The individual aquarium studies included three species of plants (*Potamogeton praelongus, Elodea canadenis,* and *Isoetes* sp.); three species of fish, green sunfish *(Lepomis cyanellus),* black bullhead *(Ictalurus melas),* and the golden shiner *(Notemigonus crysoleucas);* crayfish (species not given); snails *(Physa* sp.); and dragonfly naiads *(Gomphus* sp.). The "complete ecosystem" contained individuals of the organisms listed. In addition, slides were placed in aquaria containing only pond water and the labeled sodium arsenite–carrier mixture to study the adsorption of the herbicide to the sides of the aquaria. Background of the different organisms was determined from specimens from the same source as those used in the experiment. Details concerning the composition of the aquarium systems are presented by the authors in a table that contains number of aquaria, substrate, and kinds of plants, animals, and organisms per aquarium for the various experiments. Samples were taken from the aquaria at various intervals; some organisms were sacrificed and counted, while the snails were returned after being counted.

The natural-pond study was conducted in a pond that had been studied for a number of years. The pond had a maximum depth of 2 m; *Chara* and higher aquatic vegetation covered approximately one third of the bottom. A total of 100 pots containing the plant species used in the aquarium experiments were placed on platforms at median depth in the pond. The herbicide mixture was applied and the abundance of various organisms was observed while the water chemistry was studied. The potted plants were used to study the effects of the herbicide. Samples of the same organisms used in the aquarium experiments were collected, and activity was determined in them, the water, and the substrate.

The last study (Radwan, 1967) we will discuss in this section is that of the translocation and metabolism of ^{14}C-labeled tetramine—a compound that is used to control animal damage to plants—in three plant species: Douglas fir (Pseudotsuga menziesii), orchard grass (Dactylis glomerata), and blackberry (Rubus ursinus). Seedlings of Douglas fir and orchard grass were grown from seed in sand, and when the plants were 3–5 inches tall, they were placed in quart Mason jars containing a nutrient solution and covered with aluminum foil. Blackberry plants were obtained from cuttings and were also placed in Mason jars as described. The jars were placed in a growth chamber under controlled temperatures and light at a pH of 5.0. Solutions in the jars were continuously aerated. After 10 days of acclimation, the labeled tetramine was applied to the roots via the solution in the jars. Foliar application was by means of a micropipette. Samples of the three species were taken periodically to relate the distribution and uptake to time (Figure 106a). The metabolism of tetramine was studied by chromatography of extracts and determination of the amount of carbon dioxide evolved. In addition to the counting of radioactivity, observations were made by means of autoradiography. The activity in tissues and Ba^{14}CO$_3$, collected in the metabolism study, was determined with a thin-window gas-flow GM tube and scaler. In addition, the activity on some of the autoradiograph spots was determined by counting the spots directly (Figure 106b).

11.2. Sterile-Male Method of Insect Control

Ionizing radiation can be used in two ways to control insect populations: (1) by killing the insect outright as in its use with stored crops and (2) by sterilization of the males followed by their release into the natural population in such competitive numbers that most matings result in sterile eggs. Although description of either of these procedures plays a minor role in meeting the objectives of this book, a discussion of the first procedure would more appropriately be found in a book on radiation effects, while the second merits at least brief mention here.

The development of a successful sterilization program depends on many factors, the least of which may be the ability to sterilize the male with ionizing

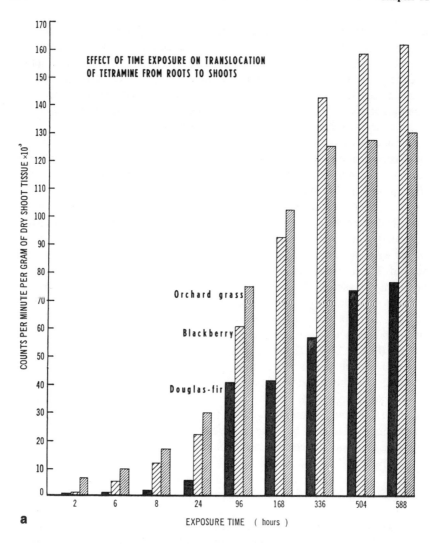

EFFECT OF TIME EXPOSURE ON TRANSLOCATION OF TETRAMINE FROM ROOTS TO SHOOTS

radiation or some chemical sterilant. Consequently, we will only refer the reader to some reference sources. As with other techniques that utilize radionuclides and ionizing radiation, the IAEA has played a primary role in developing and promoting sterile-male techniques. This organization has sponsored proceedings (IAEA, 1968a,b, 1969a,b, 1970a, 1971a,b, 1973d, 1974a) and a technical report (LaBrecque and Keller, 1965) on this subject. Persons interested in reading material on the technique other than proceedings of symposia are referred to Bushland (1960), O'Brien and Wolfe (1964b), and Knipling (1965).

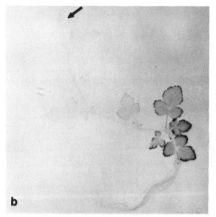
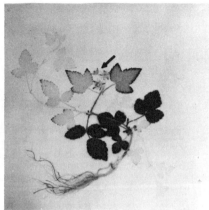

Figure 106. Translocation of ^{14}C-labeled tetramine by some plants. (a) Effect of time of exposure on translocation of tetramine from roots to shoots of orchard grass *(Dactylis glomerata)*, blackberry *(Rubus ursinus)*, and Douglas fir *(Pseudotsuga menziesii)* grown in nutrient solution containing 2.5 ppm of the tracer. (b) Autoradiographs of blackberry plants showing distribution of tetramine in the flowers. Plants were treated for 48 hr before they were transferred to tetramine-free solution. Autoradiographs are from plants treated before and after flowering . (←) Images of the flowers. From Radwan (1967).

11.3. Other Techniques

11.3.1. Terrestrial

11.3.1.1. Plants

Let us first consider the labeling of plants and plant products with radionuclides, whatever the purpose of the study.

The subject was reviewed by Sudia and Linck (1963) in a paper presented in 1961 at the First National Symposium on Radioecology. Since their review of the literature, new techniques have been developed and older ones modified, some of which have been discussed in previous sections. The application methods Sudia and Linck mention are drop, well, spray, leaf-flap, wick, injection, excised root, intact root, and procedures for introducing gases into roots. The names of the methods are, in a general way, descriptive of the procedures, with the exception of the wick method, which involves placing a cotton thread through the midvein of the leaf with one end in the radioactive solution. Some of the methods are illustrated in Figure 107. Olson (1968), in a paper on tracer techniques for study of geochemical cycles, discussed methods of tagging trees, including: (1) boring holes into tree trunks and surrounding the trees with troughs in which the radioactive solution is placed; (2) the Mauget feeder, which consists

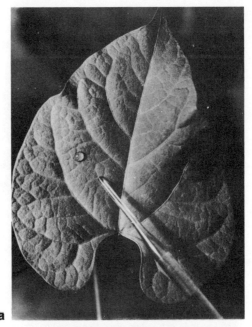

a

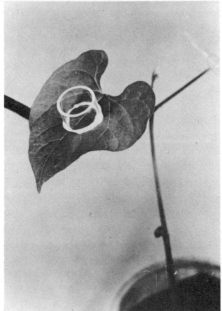

b

Figure 107. Some methods for introducing radionuclides into plants. (a) Drop method. A drop of solution is delivered to a leaf with a micropipette. (b) Well method. A glass well is sealed to the leaf surface. (c) Glass chamber for supplying radionuclides as gases to the leaves of plants. (d) Plastic bottle, mounted on a small farm tractor, for delivering radionuclide solutions to the soil. (e) Glass chamber for introducing $^{14}CO_2$ into the roots of plants. From Suida and Linck (1963).

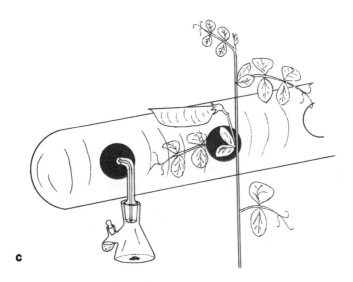

c

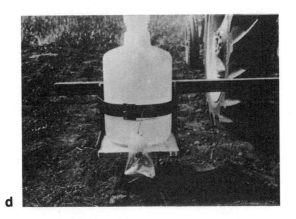

d

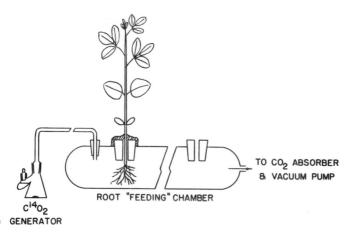

c¹⁴0₂
● GENERATOR

ROOT "FEEDING" CHAMBER

TO CO₂ ABSORBER
& VACUUM PUMP

of a plastic reservoir containing the radionuclide attached to an aluminum tube inserted into a bored hole; (3) the chisel-cut and trough method used in the tulip poplar forest at Oak Ridge National Laboratory [discussed in (Section 10.3.2)]; (4) direct spraying or using gauze saturated in a radioactive solution and wrapped around branches; (5) excised root or cut branches placed in the radioactive solution; and (6) direct application on cut tree stumps.

Tagging of dogwood *(Cornus florida)* at Oak Ridge National Laboratory is illustrated in Figure 84 (Section 10.3.2). A triple tag (^{42}K, ^{45}Ca, and ^{85}Sr) was introduced into the dogwood tree under pressure from a garden spray. The distribution data of gamma activity in an injected tree are presented in Table 14. Figure 70b (Section 10.2.2) is a schematic presentation of the results of injection of ^{134}Cs into white oak *(Quercus alba)* with Mauget feeders.

Monk (1967) proposed a method of tagging plants using seeds that had been soaked in a radioactive solution. In studying food-chain relationships, one must give serious consideration to indirect labeling; therefore, the labeling of individual plants by some of the aforementioned methods may not be satisfactory. Since the hand-labeling of a large number of individual plants may not be practical, Monk (1967) proposed the following method: He soaked seeds of oats *(Avena sativa)* for 24 hr in a solution of approximately 2 mCi/100 cc of ^{45}Ca, ^{59}Fe, and ^{65}Zn. He also soaked corn seeds *(Zea mays)* in the solution of ^{45}Ca for the same period. After the plants had reached a certain height in the greenhouse, the researcher harvested them, processed various portions, and counted

Table 14. Gamma Activity in Dogwood Injected with Mixed Isotopes on May 4[a]

Time and tree part	Distance from source (cm)	^{85}Sr (cpm)	^{42}K (cpm)
At 30 min after tagging			
Lower trunk branches	60	140	33,994
Lower crown branches	130	0[b]	—
Upper crown branches	266	0[b]	—
At 5 hr after tagging	115	0[b]	281
Branches from four forks	110	124	27,558
	140	11,237	430,562
	210	0[b]	2,844
Top of tree	330–480	0[b]	2,697
Selected top branchlet	480	0[b]	18,301
At 22 hr after tagging			
Top of tree	330–480	0[b]	4,193
Selected top branchlet	480	0[b]	—
Total activity in 0.1 N KCl (pH$_5$): ^{45}Ca, 2.18 mCi; ^{85}Sr, 0.79 mCi; ^{42}K, 4.0 mCi.			

[a] From Olson (1968).
[b] No activity detectable above background.

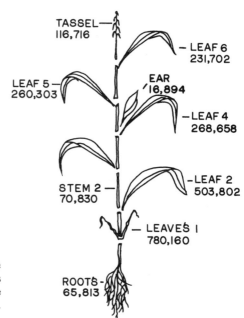

TASSEL—
116,716

– LEAF 6
231,702

LEAF 5—
260,303

EAR
16,894

–LEAF 4
268,658

STEM 2 —
70,830

–LEAF 2
503,802

– LEAVES I
780,160

ROOTS-
65,813

Figure 108. Mean cpm/g dry wt. for nine corn plants *(Zea mays)* grown from seeds soaked for 24 hr in a ^{45}Ca solution. One S.E. is approximately 17% of the mean. From Monk (1967).

them using an ultra-thin-window gas-flow counting system for ^{45}Ca and ^{59}Fe and a NaI(Tl) crystal scintillation counting system to count ^{65}Zn. Calcium-45 distribution in corn plants grown from labeled seeds is shown in Figure 108. Monk (1967) commented:

> Seed tagging offers several major advantages. First, mass inoculation can be more easily accomplished. Second, contamination is lessened, because the seeds are placed below ground, and no solutions are left exposed. Third, the fate of the radionuclide can be followed in all stages of the plant development.
>
> The seed-tag method is not without difficulties. One disadvantage, which is also shared with other inoculation methods, is illustrated by the marked gradient in isotope activity in corn. . . . [see Figure 108]. Herbivores feeding on different portions of such plants would probably ingest different amounts of label. This uneven tagging may be inherent in any radionuclide that is not easily redistributed in plants. Seed size may restrict the seed-tag method. Plants with small seeds may imbibe insufficient quantities of the isotope to obtain a satisfactory tag.

The tagging of native grassland vegetation was accomplished by Dahlman and Kucera (1969) by placing a plastic tent over the vegetation and introducing $^{14}CO_2$ gas. Sand was placed on the ground edge of the plastic, which sealed the plastic tightly to the ground. A solution of $Na_2{}^{14}CO_3$ and 1 M NaOH was placed in an open vial within the tent. By means of adding excess 1 M H_2SO_4 to the vial with a syringe that was inserted through the tent, 1 mCi $^{14}CO_2$ was released. After the syringe was withdrawn from the plastic, the puncture was sealed with tape. The plants were exposed to the labeled CO_2 for 6 hr during which time a small fan powered by a 6V automobile battery was operated to assure mixing. Air temperatures within the tent were higher than ambient, but did not cause any observable damage for the remainder of the growing period. Although liquid scintillation counting is best for this weak beta emitter, it was decided that this procedure was too time-consuming, so another technique was used to measure activity in the plant parts. Uniformly ground plant material was placed on a planchet and counted at saturation thickness with a gas-flow counting system with a Mylar film window. Since this procedure accounted for only a fraction of the total activity, the investigators developed a correction factor that they described in detail. They commented:

> This technique for labeling prairie grasses with radiocarbon was judged satisfactory because appreciable radioactivity was recovered in the plant biomass when the plants were exposed to a single application of 151 μCi/m^2. Estimates of 41–67 μCi/m^2, depending on the physiological condition of the foliage and the respiration loss, imply C^{14} incorporation from 27% to 45% of the total quantity available inside the enclosure in 6 hr. The balance of the available C^{14}O$_2$ escaped as the tents were removed from the areas. Diffusion of CO_2 through the film was negligible during the labeling operation, based on calculations from the manufacturer's specifications. Assimilation of the radioisotope by native vegetation under field conditions resulted in specific activities in the order of 0.01–0.1 μCi/g biomass, and this level of activity proved suitable for subsequent evaluation of C^{14} transfer among other components of the prairie ecosystem. This technique is particularly useful for tagging root systems with an isotope to study in situ turnover and processes of organic transfer.

In another study concerned with prairie vegetation, Mitchell (1972) evaluated the use of beta-attenuation for estimating the standing crop of shortgrass prairie vegetation. The principle involved is that the vegetation absorbs or attenuates beta particles emitted from certain radionuclides, and this is a function of the biomass between the radiation source and the detector. Although other radionuclides are suitable beta emitters, he used 10 μCi ^{90}Sr in liquid form in this investigation. The radionuclide was spread uniformly over the surface of an 8 × 10 inch sheet of grid paper. After the sheet had dried, it was placed inside an "acetate document protector." The detection system included a thin-window GM tube and portable scaler. The sheet containing the radioactive material was attached inside a cardboard box, the upper edge of which contained notches for placing the GM tube, serving as a porthole. The box was placed upside-down over the vegetation to be investigated. Three 1-min counts were made, the box was removed, the vegetation was clipped, and the biomass was determined. The relationship between the biomass and activity readings that were associated with low biomass showed the highest variability. Thus, the investigator concluded that the technique is influenced by microtopography and has doubtful value for use on moderately to heavily grazed shortgrass prairie. He suggested that the technique may be especially useful in double-sampling.

A radionuclide technique for studying root systems in the field was devised by Price (1965). The radionuclide ^{131}I was introduced into ⅜-inch-diameter color-labeled tubes placed at different depths into the ground. The objectives of the experiment determined the number, location, and depth of the tubes. To minimize animal damage, it was found best to use stoppers in the tubes and to have the tubes protrude no more than 1 dm above the ground. The pointed spout cap of a plastic bottle containing the tracer was inserted into the tube. To facilitate draining, a hole was made in the bottom of the bottle before the bottle was filled; the hole was then covered with tape and exposed after the bottle was inserted into the tube. Price noted that it was advantageous to prime the bottle by filling the tube partially before attaching the bottle to the tube. Since small animals were observed to damage bottles, it was found best to remove the bottles when empty. If the flow rate decreased after repeated use, this was alleviated by forcing a wire down the tube and through the compacted soil at the base of the tube. Figure 109 illustrates a portion of the procedure. Price (1965) commented:

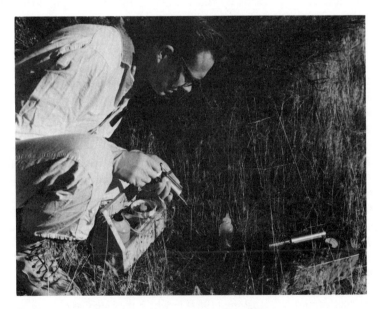

Figure 109. K. R. Price demonstrating soil contamination with ^{131}I in the field. Note the implanted ⅜-inch aluminum tube and the disconnected 120 cm^3 polyethylene bottle with a "spout cap." From Price (1965). Reproduced from *Health Physics* **11**:1521–1525 (1965) by permission of the Health Physics Society.

Due to its rapid decay rate ^{131}I is useful for time sequence studies because the same plants can be sampled following treatment through the same injection tube or tubes. While soil-injected ^{131}I is a valuable aid in studying root systems, there are certain limitations and precautions, and data must be interpreted with care. The method described above is limited to relatively stonefree soils. Furthermore, because iodine is very reactive with organic matter the method is probably less useful for soils with high organic content. An improved method, using ^{32}P to study root sytems of plants growing on deep peat, has been described. . . . the soil moisture content at the time of contamination influences the degree of movement of ^{131}I outward from the bottom of the injection tube.

Price also discussed the interpretation of data obtained with this technique.

Labeling of fungi for ecological studies has been accomplished by Coleman (1968), who labeled fungi with ^{65}Zn by inoculating a tagged old-field soil extract with 1 cm^2 of mycelia in 250-ml flasks. The soil extract was enriched, and 1 mCi ^{65}Zn, as ZnCl$_2$ in 0.5 N HCl, was added per 100 ml of the extract. After the enriched soil extract was incubated for 1 week in a controlled area at 25 $\pm$ 1°C, approximately 130 mg dry wt. per flask was obtained. It was observed that the intensity of labeling increased if the mixture was shaken a few seconds each day. Before the fungi were placed in the field, they were washed. During this washing, it was observed that the zinc was tightly bound.

The destruction of seeds by rodents during forest-reseeding operations is of concern to foresters. In a study of the fate of sown Douglas fir seed (*Pseudotsuga menziesii*), Lawrence and Rediske (1962) labeled the seed by soaking it with ^{46}Sc, which has a physical half-life of 83.80 days and decays to stable titanium with emission of beta particles and hard gamma rays. The latter were used to locate the tagged seeds. The seeds were treated with different biological agents totaling 16 different treatments. A field design was developed, and the tagged and treated seeds were placed in the field. Weekly checks of the seeds were made with a NaI(Tl) crystal scintillator. The detection equipment involved a hand probe, portable battery, and earphones. With the scintillometer used, it was possible to detect seeds at twice background at a distance of approximately 30 inches through air and a depth of 18 inches through dry soil. It was observed that some of the ^{46}Sc leached from the seeds.

Quink *et al.* (1970) used ^{46}Sc-labeled white pine seeds (*Pinus strobus*) to locate successfully the seed caches of small mammals. They used a procedure similar to that of Lawrence and Rediske (1962). Mathies (1972) used ^{60}Co- and ^{137}Cs-labeled pine seeds to study food consumption of pine seeds by small mammals in an oak–hickory forest.

A unique application of ionizing radiation to plant systematics was developed by McCormick and Rushing (1964) in which they studied three cytogenetic races of *Sedum pulchellum*, a succulent spring plant that appears on rock outcrops in the southeastern United States. Seeds were exposed to relatively high levels of radiation, and it was observed that in at least two of three experiments,

". . . there was indicated a direct relationship between chromosome number and radiation resistance." Thus, it was possible to use ionizing radiation as a means of distinguishing seed and seedlings of races that were not morphologically distinguishable.

11.3.1.2. Animals

In this section, we will discuss the use of radionuclide tracers in a metabolic index study. This subject is related to the subjects discussed in our section on cycling (Section 10.2), which included ingestion, biological uptake and retention, and excretion. However, we included in that section references wherein the investigators were interested in a specific radionuclide or its stable isotope. We will consider here cases in which the specific tracer was not of concern, but rather was used as a means to an end.

Since it is impossible to measure respiration rates in free-ranging animals, a search has been made for a substitute measurement in order that ecologists can conduct field studies of energy flow. One such approach has been the study of the elimination rates of radionuclides. Baker and Dunaway (1975) presented a literature review of the subject and discussed their selection of ^{137}Cs and ^{59}Fe for such an investigation. They conducted a study on elimination of ^{137}Cs, as well as that of ^{59}Fe, which is produced by neutron bombardment of enriched ^{58}Fe in a reactor. The study utilized three species of wild rodents, the cotton rat *(Sigmodon hispidus komareki)*, the white-footed deer mouse *(Peromyscus leucopus leucopus)*, and the harvest mouse *(Reithrodontomys humulis humulis)*. The biological half-lives of the two radionuclides were computed for each species for winter and spring under various laboratory conditions (ambient temperature, cold exposure, irradiation, and chemical metabolic inhibition). Experiments were conducted in the field and the laboratory. The investigators were interested in the correlation of elimination and metabolic rates of two nuclides; one, ^{137}Cs, has either little or no relationship to metabolic rates, and the other, ^{59}Fe, is actively involved in metabolism. The radionuclides were injected intraperitoneally in a combined form. Although the investigators realized that injection was not a natural way of introducing the radionuclides into the animals, they selected the method because it was the most practical and convenient for field studies. Whole-body counts were made at weekly intervals by placing a rodent in a paper carton (Figure 110) that was inserted into an Armac liquid scintillation detector connected to an auto-gamma spectrometer (Figure 111). Although the study was concerned with metabolism methodology, it did furnish data on the biological uptake and retention of the fission product, ^{137}Cs. The investigators stated:

> The data suggested that elimination of ^{59}Fe is influenced by metabolic rates of rodents in the field, but laboratory experiments were unable to demonstrate any predictable

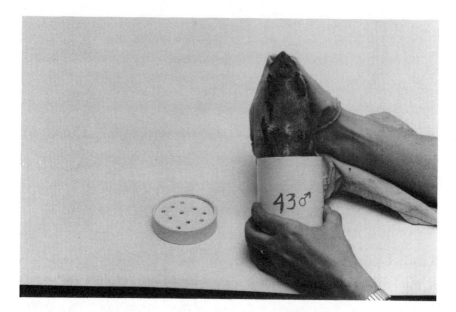

Figure 110. Cotton rat *(Sigmodon hispidus komareki)* being placed into a container prior to whole-body counting. From Baker *et al.* (1968).

relationship. Neither did the rate of final-component ^{137}Cs loss from rodents appear to be influenced by metabolic rate in the laboratory or in the field. However, final-component Y-axis intercept values of ^{137}Cs exhibited a linear correlation with metabolic rates. . . . Prediction of metabolism by the intercept method as reported here is based only on intraperitoneal injection of isotopes. Further investigation will be required to determine whether similar relations exist with other modes of administration.

Although estimates of various parameters were presented, it is unfortunate that measures of variability were not associated with them and that the data points were not plotted on the many figures containing the fitted regression lines. It is essential that the reader have at least one, and preferably both, to evaluate the feasibility of the method in predicting metabolic rates.

In a study involving the rock ptarmigan *(Lagopus mutus)*, Gasaway (1976) used ^{14}C-labeled cellulose in a study of cellulose digestion and metabolism in this bird. The test birds were fed orally 0.5 ml of a solution of uniformly labeled methylcellulose with an activity of 7 µCi. The solution was administered from a syringe into a polyethylene tube that had been placed in the bird's mouth and extended to the esophagus. Prior to administration, the solution had been treated with HCl to release volatile CO_2 and then neutralized with KOH. The bird was placed in an air-tight chamber, and the $^{14}CO_2$ produced was collected as

$Ba(^{14}CO_3)_2$. The activity of the $Ba(^{14}CO_3)_2$ collected was determined with a scintillation counting system. The presence of labeled carbon dioxide implied that the cellulose was digested; however, carbon dioxide could have been released as a result of microbial fermentation or oxidation by bird tissues. In another study with rock ptarmigan, Gasaway *et al.* (1976) used ^{51}Cr-labeled EDTA and ^{144}Ce in a study of the digestion of dry matter (DM) and adsorption of water in the cecum and intestine. The birds that had been maintained on a nonlabeled diet were fed food labeled by spraying the food with a solution containing the radionuclides, and the birds were kept on this diet for 24 hr to allow for equilibrium in the gut. During the experimental period, excreta were collected and separated into cecal and intestinal droppings. The samples were counted with a scintillation counting system. The amount of DM and water entering the cecum was estimated from data on the amount of labeled cecal droppings and total droppings. The authors commented.

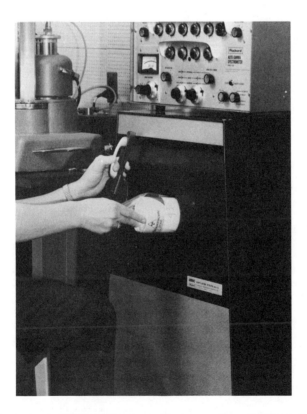

Figure 111. Packard Armac whole-body counter, with cotton rat *(Sigmodon hispidus komareki)* being inserted for assay. From Baker *et al.* (1968).

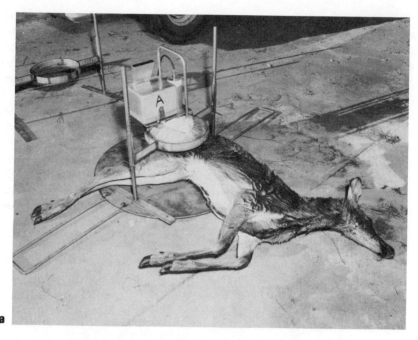

Figure 112. Field measurement of ^{137}Cs in white-tailed deer *(Odocoileus virginianus)*. (a) Modified single-channel analyzer used to obtain measurements in the field. (b) Field estimate vs. laboratory analysis. From McMahan and Wright (1973).

Digestibility estimates of the Purina flight conditioner using ^{51}Cr-EDTA and Ce-144 as nondigestible markers gave good approximation of the total collection method (i.e. 3% under and 2% over, respectively) indicating that both markers were suitable for digestibility studies in ptarmigan.

Since 86% of the ^{51}Cr-EDTA is excreted in only 2 to 4 cecal droppings (i.e. in only 15% of the excreta) per day, it is important to use a sufficiently long sample period to insure a representative sampling of each feces type, otherwise significant errors in digestibility estimates will result. On the other hand, Ce-144 concentration is only slightly higher in cecal than intestinal droppings and hence an incomplete daily recovery of one feces type should have less bias on the final estimate of digestibility. . . .

Estimates of the disappearance of DM based on changes in marker concentrations may be in error if the marker does not bind with DM uniformly. Nonuniform labeling of the DM with Ce-144 was suggested. . . .

This study showed that caution must be used in interpreting cecal digestibility information obtained from water soluble markers. The concentration of ^{51}Cr-EDTA in cecal DM has little relationship to the digestion of DM occurring in the cecum.

Controlled hunting of white-tailed deer *(Odocoileus virginianus)* at the U.S. Department of Energy's Savannah River Plant provided McMahon and Wright

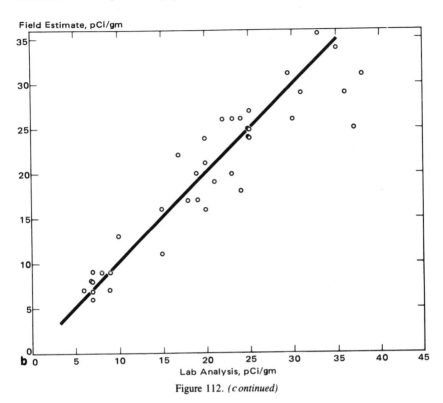

Figure 112. (*c ontinued*)

(1973) with an opportunity to measure the ^{137}Cs content in an animal living on a nuclear-energy site. Further, as a safety precaution, measurements were taken before the hunter was allowed to remove the deer from the site. A single-channel analyzer was modified for field measurements of ^{137}Cs and its performance compared with laboratory analyses (Figure 112).

The effect of ionizing radiation on the hemopoietic system has received considerable investigation. In developing an index to hemopoietic damage, Kitchings *et al.* (1968) developed a tracer technique and tested it on seven species of wild rodents. The procedure was basically that of studying the elimination rate and biological half-life of [59]Fe. Iron-59 was selected because the bulk of iron resides in red-cell hemoglobin and its rate of loss from the body of mammals is very small. Wild-trapped rodents of the seven species were acclimated to the laboratory for 2 weeks and then assigned to a control group or to one of two groups to receive either 0.475 or 0.110 μCi ^{59}Fe injected intraperitoneally. Activity was determined with a whole-body counter at various periods until the animals were irradiated on the 114th day. Animals in each of the two treatment groups were exposed to radiation from a ^{60}Co source with the group injected with the highest level of ^{59}Fe receiving 400 rads and the second group, 125–150 rads. On the 2nd and 5th days following irradiation, whole-body counts were made, and the effect of ionizing radiation on the biological elimination of ^{59}Fe was noted for the various species and treatment groups. An effect of ionizing radiation resulting in a decrease in retention of the radionuclide was observed.

Fox *et al.* (1975) reported on the development of a field procedure using beta-backscatter for measuring eggshell qualities of density, thickness, and structure. They observed that sensitivity of the method was great enough to detect inter- and intraspecific variability in quality. The beta-backscatter device and a diagram of its components are shown in Figure 113. The investigators reported the use of 10 μCi ^{106}Ru and 15 μCi ^{90}Sr as the beta source. Results obtained using the device were correlated with three physicochemical measurements. Concerning their use of equipment, the authors commented:

> The number of beta particles backscattered per unit thickness is affected by the energy of the particles, which is characteristic of the particular isotope, and the atomic number of the reflecting material. The lower the energy of the beta particles, the larger the number backscattered per unit thickness. Hence, it is possible that by choosing an isotope whose beta particles are much less energetic than ^{90}Strontium (2.18 MeV) and ^{106}Ruthenium (3.5 MeV), one may increase the sensitivity of the measurement and eliminate most of the variability introduced by backscatter from the shell membranes and albumen.
>
> It has been suggested that the performance of the present gauge would be improved by substituting a surface-barrier detector for the GM tube. . . .
>
> The BBS technique allows one to make nondestructive, physiologically and ecologically meaningful measurements of shell quality of eggs of any species at the nest site. It is sensitive, highly portable, and relatively inexpensive, and deserves the consideration of ecologists and environmental toxicologists.

Tanner and Tolbert (1975) also used a radiation procedure to measure eggshell thickness. However, rather than using beta-backscatter as a means of measurement, they used a gamma-radiation densitometer that had been used to measure density of small sections of wood cores. The radiation source was ^{55}Fe. They concluded that ". . . radiation absorption methods are only slightly superior to optical methods in measuring this effect. The optical methods are much faster and cheaper." It should be noted that their procedure, as contrasted with that of Fox *et al.* (1975), required destruction of the egg and use of laboratory equipment.

Although it may be questioned whether or not it is appropriate to discuss in this book a technique involving X-ray spectrometry, the uniqueness of the application to an ecological problem and the use of a radiation source justify its inclusion. A problem of interest to waterfowl biologists has been the geographic origin of waterfowl in a hunter's bag. The use of numbered leg bands attached to birds of various age classes from specific areas has obvious limitations, par-

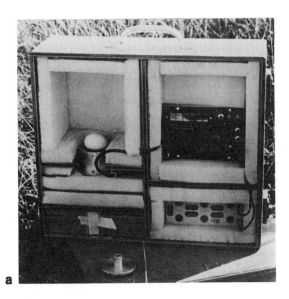

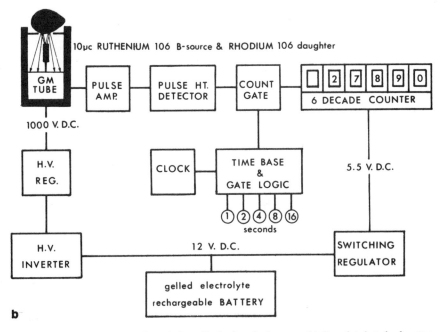

Figure 113. Field assessment of eggshell quality by beta-backscatter. (a) Complete beta-backscatter gauge, as used at the nest site, with an egg in counting position. The aluminum lid that is used as a standard is in the foreground. (b) Block diagram showing components of the portable beta-backscatter eggshell-quality gauge. From Fox *et al.* (1975).

ticularly the problem of labeling a large number of individuals. It was proposed that the chemical content of certain tissues might be an indicator of the area in which the animal was hatched or lived. We have discussed the use of a radiotracer by Hanson and Case (1963) to identify waterfowl on the Columbia River in the vicinity of Hanford (Section 6.3.3) and also the study of Devine and Peterle (1968), in which neutron activation analysis was used in an attempt to identify natal areas of North American waterfowl (Section 3.2.1). Kelsall and Calaprice (1972), in a study using the chemical content of feathers of waterfowl to identify geographic origins, tested the efficacy of X-ray spectrometry as an analytical tool. Three populations of male mallards *(Anas platyrhynchus)* were compared using this procedure. A sample of whole primary feathers was washed, and a central portion of the feather was irradiated with a gamma-ray source of 25 mCi ^{241}Am. Irradiation resulted in a fluorescence pattern that is characteristic of each of the various kinds and concentrations of element present. A lithium-drifted silicon detector and a pulse-height analyzer were used to identify the X-ray fluorescence pattern. Multiple discriminant analysis was used in data interpretation. In regard to the X-ray spectrometric portion of their overall study, the investigators commented:

> We consider that our test of X-ray spectrometric analysis of waterfowl plumage shows promise for the future. The technique is much faster and more convenient than conventional wet chemical methods of analysis, and it has the great advantage of being nondestructive. It could be applied to the plumage of living birds in the field.

11.3.2. Aquatic

Within this category, we have included descriptions of techniques that seem to be of marginal relevance to our other sections. In addition, we will describe some equipment of interest. The subject of X-ray spectrometry in aquatic studies will not be discussed here, but readers interested in this subject are referred to Calaprice and Calaprice (1970) and Calaprice *et al.* (1971).

Using isotopes of carbon and sulfur in studies of lake metabolism, Deevey *et al.* (1964) reported their observations and reviewed other works on the subject. The stable isotope ^{34}S was discussed by them in the sulfur-balance studies. Our comments here will be restricted to the radioactive isotope of carbon, ^{14}C. None of the isotopes used was artificially introduced into the pond or other water bodies studied. The ^{14}C was for the most part naturally occurring ^{14}C, with a small amount resulting from nuclear testing. The basis of this study was the isotopic fractionation of carbon, which can be used to gain an insight into the intensity and nature of geochemical processes. Particular attention was centered on lacustrine metabolism. However, most of the differences in isotopic abundance could be attributed to ordinary processes (e.g., mixing) rather than to metabolism.

In a review of previous observations from a softwater lake, it was commented that there was a fractionation of isotopes between CO_2 and CH_4 with enrichment of CO_2 in mud gases by ^{13}C and that ordinary oxidative metabolism yields CO_2 with less ^{13}C. Consequently, the heavier CO_2 resulting from methane production can be distinguished. However, in Lindsley Pond, a medium-hard-water pond that these investigators studied, the differential relationship was not clear.

Emerson *et al.* (1973) reported on a study of gas exchange in a small lake using a technique involving the determination of radon gas movement from the pond into the atmosphere. The origin of radon was from the disintegration of radium. According to Shilling and Shilling (1964), 1 kg radium generates spontaneously $100mm^3$ of this gas per day. The investigators stated that dissolved radium must be the source of radon in a lake to use the technique. To increase the radon level well above background, they introduced radium into the lake they studied. Although the method was complicated by radium uptake by algae, they were able to establish limits to the rate of gas exchange.

The role that is played in the cycling of radionuclides by the assemblage of organisms attached to surfaces below the water surface known as "periphyton" has been investigated at Hanford and Oak Ridge National Laboratory. Since it is rather difficult to study this process in the field, techniques have been developed for laboratory investigations. Cushing and Porter (1969) reported on a system developed at Hanford that permitted continuous observations of periphyton uptake of radionuclides in a controlled aquatic system. The modified system is shown in Figure 114. A tube labeled in the figure as the "periphyton tube" was placed in the river for several weeks, removed, and placed in an exposure chamber and over a GM detector as indicated, and water was circulated as either a closed or an open system. The closed system was similar to aquarium studies except that a unidirectional flow of water was maintained. Two reservoirs of water were connected to the system, one consisting of uncontaminated water used in retention-time studies. Current flow and light intensity were controlled. Since the ambient level of a tracer could not be maintained during experimentation in the closed system, the investigators designed an open system that maintained constant tracer concentrations by means of a "pipetting machine" that injected the tracer into the system in constant amounts. The reader is referred to the article for additional details. Concerning the equipment, Cushing and Porter (1969) commented:

> The types of experiments theoretically feasible with this system are many and varied. Retention and half-time studies can be accomplished by switching to the uncontaminated water reservoir in the closed system or merely by shutting off the pipetting machine in the open system and continuing the periodic counts. The effects of photoperiod, light intensity, water velocity, temperature, and chemical composition of the water upon nutrient cycling can be investigated. Non-metabolic uptake can be studied by use of inhib-

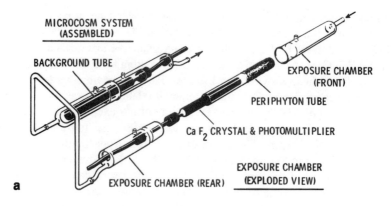

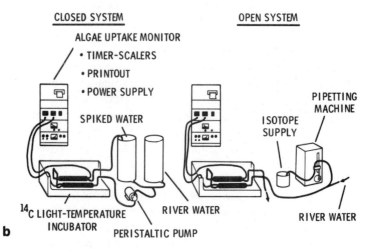

Figure 114. Periphyton radionuclide-cycling microcosm. (a) Exposure chambers and components. (b) Method of operation in closed and open systems. From Cushing and Rose (1970).

itors, killed communities, or chemical alteration of the water. The effects of either multiple spikes or isotope dilution can be investigated with appropriate addition to or dilution of the water.

Concurrent with radionuclide cycling studies, basic algal physiological data can be obtained, such as upstream–downstream (in this case above–below) changes in dissolved O_2 and CO_2. Hopefully, it may be possible to use the system for ^{14}C productivity studies of periphyton communities, although the weak beta energy of this isotope may require a more sensitive detection system or a different arrangement between the algae and detector.

In a study using a technique of introducing ^{32}P into a running stream and observing the uptake of the radionuclide by periphyton on rocks and on emplaced glass slides as well as the ^{32}P remaining in the water, D. J. Nelson *et al.* (1969) estimated the mass of periphyton and stream-bottom area in a portion of White Oak Creek (Oak Ridge National Laboratory) using a material balance procedure.

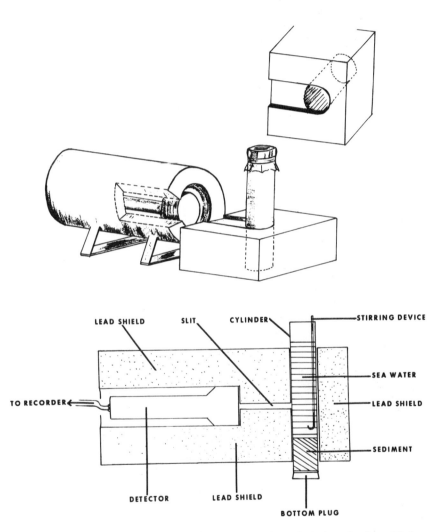

Figure 115. Apparatus for measuring instantaneously and continuously the loss of radionuclide from water to sediment. From T. W. Duke *et al.* (1968).

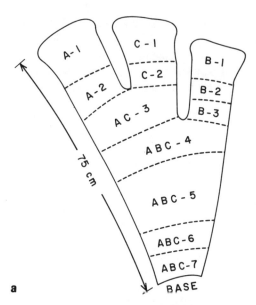

Figure 116. Coral growth rates using ^{228}Ra and ^{210}Pb. (a) Longitudinal sectional view of the coral (*Stephanocoenia* sp.) collected from Discovery Bay, Jamaica. Branching at about 25 cm from the top is clearly evident. Samples analyzed are designated with a letter and number. (b) Plot of activity of ^{228}Ra/^{226}Ra in the Jamaica coral head and the North Carolina coral *(Solenastrea hyades)* head vs. distance from outer surface. The estimated growth rates based on decay of excess ^{228}Ra activity are 0.5 and 0.15 cm/yr, respectively. From Moore and Krishnaswami (1972).

Briefly, the study was of material balance of ^{32}P after a 30-min release of a known amount of the radionuclide into the stream. The mass and bottom area were determined from data on substrate concentration per unit area and concentration per unit weight of periphyton on the substrate and the total amount of ^{32}P retained within the study area. The latter was determined by measuring water flow rate and activity of water leaving the area.

Elwood and Nelson (1972) described another study of periphyton, utilizing the same field methods as in the previous study, in which periphyton production and grazing rates were measured. Their concluding statement was:

> This material balance method would appear to have wide application for studying process rates in natural streams regardless of their location since less than maximum permissible concentrations of ^{32}P were used while radionuclide levels in periphyton and water were sufficient to monitor for at least six weeks following the release. . . . Since ^{32}P has a short physical half-life (14.3 days), there is no danger of high residual concentrations in a stream ecosystem following the release because of radioactive decay. Thus, repeated releases may be made to the same stream to determine changes in biomass, primary production rate, and primary consumption rate on a seasonal basis.

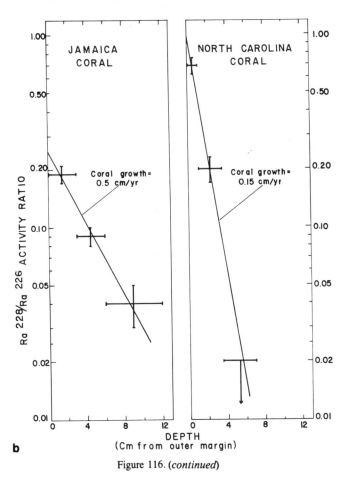

b

Figure 116. (*continued*)

An interesting procedure for studying the exchange of trace elements between water and estuarine sediments was devised by T. W. Duke *et al.* (1968).
They described a field device used to collect cores and overlying water. After
the cylinder containing the sediment and water was returned to the laboratory,
the cylinder was placed in a 30-gal container of water collected at the sampling
site and allowed to come to equilibrium with the trace element in the water in
the container. It was advised that caution be exercised not to disturb the sediment
in this step as well as in the following steps, which included removing and
filtering water overlying the sediment in the cylinder. The inside of the exposed
portion of the cylinder was wiped clean, and an aliquot sample of the filtered
water was returned to the cylinder. The cylinder containing the sediment and
filtered water was placed in a special apparatus in which the activity of the tracer
of interest could be determined for various water segments (Figure 115). The

carrier-free tracer was introduced into the water column below the surface of the water with a pipette. It should be noted that when the cylinder was in position, radioactivity in the sediment could not be detected and only the tracer in the water was measured. A blank containing only filtered water and tracer was used to correct for processes other than exchange with the sediment that affected concentration of the tracer. Application of the technique was used with ^{65}Zn and cores collected from a North Carolina estuary. The investigators stated: "This technique is applicable to studies of any other element with a convenient gamma-emitting isotope, as long as no isotopic effects occur."

Moore and Krishnaswami (1972) studied the growth rate of head corals (*Stephanocoenia* sp. and *Solenastrea hyades*) by two radiometric methods. Assuming an initial incorporation of ^{228}Ra (or ^{210}Pb) to ^{226}Ra, which has a long half-life (1600 years) as contrasted to ^{228}Ra and ^{210}Pb, they used the decay of the latter in the coral as an index of growth rate. Since ^{228}Ra has a shorter half-life (5.77 years) than ^{210}Pb (21 years), the presence of ^{228}Ra would approach zero in the older areas of the coral, and if no additional material was incorporated into the coral, it would be measurable for about 30 years. The ^{210}Pb would reach equilibrium with its parent, ^{226}Ra, in older sections of the coral head. Figure 116 shows the procedure for sampling a coral head and the graphic results of the ^{228}Ra/^{226}Ra ratio method.

The previously discussed investigation of Hanson and Case (1963) used the measurement of ^{32}P and ^{65}Zn in waterfowl as an indicator of waterfowl use of the Columbia River in the vicinity of Hanford. Romberg and Renfro (1973) used the same radionuclides in a study of juvenile-salmon movement and feeding habits in the Columbia River. Of interest is the use of 200,000 hatchery fish that were marked by cold-branding and released into the Columbia River about 25 miles downstream from the reactors. Samples of the fish were collected down-

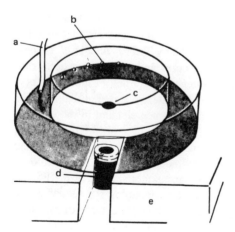

Figure 117. Ring-shaped testing container used in investigations of periodicity of freshwater invertebrates with radionuclides. Locomotor activity was measured in the container. (a) Water supply; (b,c) water discharge; (d) scintillation counter; (e) lead shielding. From Lehmann (1965).

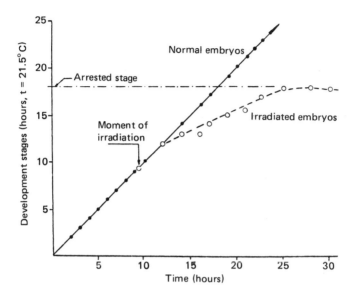

Figure 118. Method of determination of the maximal developmental stage reached (arrested stage). Irradiation with 20/kR at the 9½-hr stage. Development is arrested at the 18-hr stage. From Neyfakh (1959).

stream at two dams. In addition, samples of unmarked fish were collected from the river in a study to see whether the sample consisted of distinguishable groups of fish. The fish were returned to the laboratory, and the levels of ^{32}P and ^{65}Zn were measured. A graphic model of the data was developed. Commenting on the model, the authors stated:

> The best application of the graphical model may be to identify, within a population of seemingly identical fish, groups which apparently have had quite different recent histories. Boundaries for the graphical model are variable, being highly dependent on season, reactor operation, species of fish, and location along the river.

Lehmann (1965) utilized radionuclides to study periodicity of larvae of the invertebrate, *Anabolia nervosa*. Locomotor activity was observed in a special test container (Figure 117) that when in use was placed in a light-tight box. Marked animals passing over a detector were recorded, and this record for a single animal provided a means of studying locomotor activity. The animals were tagged externally with a mixture containing ^{137}Cs by pasting the substance on the animal. The detector was a NaI(Tl) crystal. The activity of the tag was 0.1–0.01 μCi/animal.

The effects of exposing early stages of egg development to ionizing radiation have been studied extensively. In a study of the function of nuclei in the early development of fishes, Neyfakh (1959) inactivated the nuclei of fish embryos with X-rays. The procedure requires the use of a level of radiation that inactivates the nuclei and has little effect on the cytoplasm. Neyfakh irradiated embryos of the loach *(Misgurnus fossilis)* in closely packed groups in a small volume of water at doses of 20–60 kR. The doses used had the desired effect, and the investigator concluded that the inactivation of nuclei by X-ray was a satisfactory means to investigate the role of the nuclei in developing embryos. Figure 118 illustrates the determination of the maximal developmental stage reached.

Appendix

Physical Characteristics of Radionuclides Discussed in This Volume

The primary source of physical half-life data was Heath (1971), with supplementary information from Lederer *et al.* (1967). The latter publication was the principal source of the tabulated "major radiations."

Atomic number	Radionuclide	Physical half-life	Major radiations
1	Hydrogen-3 (^{3}H)	12.26 years	β^-
6	Carbon-14 (^{14}C)	5730 years	β^-
11	Sodium-22 (^{22}Na)	2.602 years	β^+, γ
	Sodium-24 (^{24}Na)	15.0 hours	β^-, γ
14	Silicon-32 (^{32}Si)	650 years	β^-
15	Phosphorus-32 (^{32}P)	14.3 days	β^-
	Phosphorus-33 (^{33}P)	25 days	β^-
16	Sulfur-35 (^{35}S)	88 days	β^-
17	Chlorine-36 (^{36}Cl)	3.1×10^5 years	β^-, γ
	Chlorine-38 (^{38}Cl)	37.3 minutes	β^-, γ
19	Potassium-40 (^{40}K)	1.28×10^9 years	β^-, β^+, γ
	Potassium-42 (^{42}K)	12.4 hours	β^-, γ
20	Calcium-45 (^{45}Ca)	165 days	β^-
	Calcium-47 (^{47}Ca)	4.53 days	β^-, γ
21	Scandium-46 (^{46}Sc)	83.80 days	β^-, γ
24	Chromium-51 (^{51}Cr)	27.8 days	γ, e^-
25	Manganese-54 (^{54}Mn)	303 days	γ, e^-
26	Iron-55 (^{55}Fe)	2.6 years	γ
	Iron-59 (^{59}Fe)	45.1 days	β^-, γ

Atomic number	Radionuclide	Physical half-life	Major radiations
27	Cobalt-58 (^{58}Co)	71.3 days	β^+, γ
	Cobalt-60 (^{60}Co)	5.26 years	β^-, γ
29	Copper-64 (^{64}Cu)	12.9 hours	β^-, β^+, e^-, γ
30	Zinc-65 (^{65}Zn)	243.6 days	β^+, e^-, γ
33	Arsenic-74 (^{74}As)	17.9 days	β^-, β^+, γ
34	Selenium-75 (^{75}Se)	120.4 days	γ, e^-
35	Bromine-82 (^{82}Br)	35.5 hours	β^-, γ
37	Rubidium-86 (^{86}Rb)	18.66 days	β^-, γ
38	Strontium-85 (^{85}Sr)	64 days	γ, e^-
	Strontium-89 (^{89}Sr)	52 days	β^-, γ
	Strontium-90 (^{90}Sr)	28.1 years	β^-
40	Zirconium-95 (^{95}Zr)	65 days	β^-, γ
42	Molybdenum-99 (^{99}Mo)	66.69 hours	β^-, γ
44	Ruthenium-103 (^{103}Ru)	39.6 days	β^-, γ
	Ruthenium-106 (^{106}Ru)	367 years	β^-
47	Silver-110m (^{110m}Ag)	253 days	β^-, e^-, γ
51	Antimony-124 (^{124}Sb)	60.3 days	β^-, γ
53	Iodine-125 (^{125}I)	60 days	γ
	Iodine-126 (^{126}I)	13 days	β^-, β^+, γ
	Iodine-131 (^{131}I)	8.070 days	β^-, e^-, γ
54	Xenon-133 (^{133}Xe)	5.27 days	β^-, γ
55	Cesium-134 (^{134}Cs)	2.05 years	β^-, γ
	Cesium-137 (^{137}Cs)	30.23 years	β^-, e^-, γ
56	Barium-133 (^{133}Ba)	7.2 years	β^+, γ
	Barium-140 (^{140}Ba)	12.8 days	β^-, e^-, γ
57	Lanthanum-140 (^{140}La)	40.22 hours	β^-, γ
58	Cerium-144 (^{144}Ce)	284.9 days	β^-, e^-, γ
69	Thulium-170 (^{170}Tm)	128.6 days	β^-, e^-, γ
73	Tantalum-182 (^{182}Ta)	115 days	β^-, e^-, γ
74	Tungsten-181 (^{181}W)	140 days	γ, e^-
77	Iridium-190 (^{190}Ir)	11 days	γ, e^-
	Iridium-192 (^{192}Ir)	74 days	β^-, e^-, γ
79	Gold-198 (^{198}Au)	2.693 days	β^-, e^-, γ
80	Mercury-203 (^{203}Hg)	46.57 days	β^-, e^-, γ
82	Lead-210 (^{210}Pb)	21 years	β^-, e^-, γ, α
88	Radium-226 (^{226}Ra)	1600 years	α, γ, e^-
	Radium-228 (^{228}Ra)	5.77 years	β^-, e^-
90	Thorium-230 (^{230}Th)	8×10^4 years	α, γ
91	Protactinium-230 (^{230}Pa)	17.7 days	β^-, e^-, γ, α
	Protactinium-231 (^{231}Pa)	3.25×10^4 years	α, γ, e^-
92	Uranium-238 (^{238}U)	4.51×10^9 years	α, γ, e^-
95	Americium-241 (^{241}Am)	458 years	α, γ

Literature Cited

Aitken, M. J. 1974. *Physics and Archaeology*, 2nd ed. Oxford University Press, London. viii + 291 pp.

Alldredge, A. W., J. F. Lipscomb, and F. W. Whicker. 1974. Forage intake rates of mule deer estimated with fallout cesium-137. *J. Wildl. Manage.* **38**(3):508–516.

Amiard, J.-C. 1974a. Utilization of radioactive tracers in biological oceanography. *Union Oceanogr. Fr.* **6**(2):35–40 (in French).

Amiard, J.-C. 1974b. Utilization of radioactive tracers in biological oceanography: Bibliography. *Union Oceanogr. Fr.* **6**(3):21–25 (in French).

Arena, V. 1971. *Ionizing Radiation and Life.* C. V. Mosby, Saint Louis. xi + 543 pp.

Arnold, D. E. 1966. Marking fish with dyes and other chemicals. Tech. Pap. No. 10. U.S. Fish and Wildlife Service, Washington, D.C. 44 pp.

Attix, F. H. (ed.). 1967. *Luminescence Dosimetry.* U.S. AEC Symp. Ser. No. 8. 532 pp.

Auerbach, S. I., J. S. Olson, and H. D. Waller. 1964. Landscape investigations using caesium-137. *Nature (London)* **201**(4921):761–764.

Bachmann, R. W. 1963. Zinc-65 in studies of the freshwater zinc cycle. pp. 485–496. In: *Radioecology* (V. Schultz and A. W. Klement, Jr., eds.). Reinhold, New York.

Bailey, G. N. A., I. J. Linn, and P. J. Walker. 1973. Radioactive marking of small mammals. *Mammal Rev.* **3**(1):11–23.

Bailey, R. E. 1953. Radiosurgery and uptake of radioactive iodine by the thyroid of the Oregon junco. *Auk* **70**(2):196–199.

Baker, C. E., and P. B. Dunaway. 1975. Elimination of ^{137}Cs and ^{59}Fe and its relationship to metabolic rates of wild small rodents. *J. Exp. Zool.* **192**(2):223–236.

Baker, C. E., P. B. Dunaway, and S. I. Auerbach. 1968. Measurement of metabolism in cotton rats by retention of cesium-134. U.S. AEC, Oak Ridge National Lab. Rep. ORNL-TM-2069. v + 46 pp.

Baldwin, W. F., J. R. Allen, and N. S. Slater. 1966. A practical field method for the recovery of blackflies labelled with phosphorus-32. *Nature (London)* **212**(5065):959–960.

Ball, R. C., and F. F. Hooper. 1963. Translocation of phosphorus in a trout stream ecosystem. pp. 217–228. In: *Radioecology* (V. Schultz and A. W. Klement, Jr., eds.). Reinhold, New York.

Ball, R. C., and F. F. Hooper. 1966. Use of ^{74}As-tagged sodium arsenite in a study of effects of a herbicide on pond ecology. pp. 149–161. In: *Isotopes in Weed Research.* International Atomic Energy Agency, Vienna. Publ. No. STI/PUB/113.

Ball, R. C., T. A. Wojtalik, and F. F. Hooper. 1963. Upstream dispersion of radiophosphorus in a Michigan trout stream. *Pap. Mich. Acad. Sci. Arts Lett.* **48**:57–64.

261

Bandy, L. W., and T. J. Peterle. 1973. Transfer of chlorine-36-DDT in a meadow. pp. 232–239. In: *Radionuclides in Ecosystems* (D. J. Nelson, ed.). U.S. AEC Rep. CONF-710501-P1.

Baptist, J. P., and C. W. Lewis, 1969. Transfer of ^{65}Zn and ^{51}Cr through an estuarine food chain. pp. 420–430. In: *Symposium on Radioecology* (D. J. Nelson and F. C. Evans, eds.). U.S. AEC Rep. CONF-670503.

Barbour, R. W., and M. J. Harvey. 1968. The effect of radioactive tags on the activity of rodents. *Am. Midl. Nat.* **79**(2):519–522.

Baserga, R. and D. Malamud. 1969. *Autoradiography: Techniques and Application.* Harper and Row, New York, xii + 281 pp.

Bate, L. C., W. S. Lyon, and E. H. Wollerman. 1974. Gold tagging of elm bark beetles and identification by neutron activation analysis. *Radiochem. Radioanal. Lett.* **17**(1):77–85.

Baxter, M. S., and A. Walton. 1971. Fluctuations of atmospheric carbon-14 concentrations during the past century. *Proc. R. Soc. London Ser. A* **321**(1544):105–127.

Bergner, P.-E. E. 1966. Tracer theory: A review. *Isot. Radiat. Technol.* **3**(3):245–262.

Berlin, M., and R. Rylander. 1963. Autoradiographic detection of radioactive bacteria introduced into sea water and sewage. *J. Hyg.* **61**:307–315.

Beyers, R. J., and B. J. Beyers. 1974. Partial bibliography of interest to those measuring the primary productivity of aquatic ecosystems (revision). Savannah River Ecology Lab., U.S. AEC Rep. SRO-819-2. 137 pp. (Available from National Technical Information Service, Springfield, Virginia.)

Bilinski, E., and R. E. E. Jonas. 1973. Effects of cadmium and copper on the oxidation of lactate by rainbow trout *(Salmo gairdneri)* gills. *J. Fish. Res. Board Can.* **30**(10):1553–1558.

Binggeli, M. 1963, 1965, 1967, 1969. Radioisotopes and ionizing radiation in entomology. *IAEA Bibl. Ser.,* 1963, No. 9, 414 pp. (STI/PUB/21/9); 1965, No. 15, viii + 564 pp. (STI/PUB/21/15); 1967, No. 24, xx + 454 pp. (STI/PUB/21/24); 1969, No. 36, xvi + 805 pp. (STI/PUB/21/36).

Blaylock, B. G. 1966. Cytogenetic study of a natural population of *Chironomus* inhabiting an area contaminated by radioactive waste. pp. 835–845. In: *Disposal of Radioactive Wastes into Seas, Oceans and Surface Waters.* International Atomic Energy Agency, Vienna. Publ. No. STI/PUB/126.

Blaylock, B. G., and J. P. Witherspoon, Jr. 1965. Environmental factors affecting glass rod dosimetry. *Health Phys.* **11**(6):549–552.

Bonham, K. 1965. Growth rate of giant clam *Tridacna gigas* at Bikini Atoll as revealed by radioautography. *Science* **149**(3681):300–302.

Breckenridge, W. J., and J. R. Tester. 1961. Growth, local movements and hibernation of the Manitoba toad, *Bufo hemiophrys. Ecology* **42**(4):636–646.

Broecker, W. 1963. Radioisotopes and large-scale oceanic mixing. pp. 88–108. In: *The Sea,* Vol. 2 (M. N. Hill, ed.). Interscience, New York.

Broecker, W. S., R. D. Gerard, M. Ewing, and B. C. Heezen. 1961. Geochemistry and physics of ocean circulation. pp. 301–322. In: *Oceanography* (M. Sears, ed.). American Association for the Advancement of Science, Washington, D.C.

Brown, J. H., Jr., and F. W. Woods. 1968. Root extension of trees in surface soils of the North Carolina piedmont. *Bot. Gaz.* **129**(2):126–132.

Brungs, W. A., Jr. 1967. Distribution of cobalt 60, zinc 65, strontium 85, and cesium 137 in a freshwater pond. U.S. Public Health Service, Environmental Health Series, Publ. No. 999-RH-25. vi + 52 pp.

Brunn, P. 1962. Tracing of material movement on seashores. *Shore Beach* **1962**(April):10–15.

Bryan, G. W. 1968. Concentrations of zinc and copper in the tissues of decapod crustaceans. *J. Mar. Biol. Assoc. U.K.* **48**(2):303–321.

Bullard, R. W. 1964. Changes in regional blood flow and blood volume, during arousal from hibernation. *Ann. Acad. Sci. Fenn. Ser. A4* **71**:65–74.

Bushland, R. C. 1960. Male sterilization for the control of insects. *Adv. Pest Control Res.* **3**:1–25.

Byrne, A. R., M. Dermelj, and L. Kosta. 1971. A neutron activation study of environmental contamination and distribution of mercury in animals and fish. pp. 415–426. In: *Nuclear Techniques in Environmental Pollution.* International Atomic Energy Agency, Vienna. Publ. No. STI/PUB/268.

Calaprice, J. R., and F. P. Calaprice. 1970. Marking animals with micro-tags of chemical elements for identification by X-ray spectroscopy. *J. Fish. Res. Board Can.* **27**(2):317–330.

Calaprice, J. R., H. M. McSheffrey, and L. A. Lapi. 1971. Radioisotope X-ray fluorescence spectrometry in aquatic biology: A review. *J. Fish. Res. Board Can.* **28**(10):1583–1594.

Calow, P., and C. R. Fletcher. 1972. A new radiotracer technique involving ^{14}C and ^{51}Cr for estimating the assimilation efficiencies of aquatic, primary consumers. *Oecologia* **9**(2):155–170.

Cameron, R. D., R. G. White, and J. R. Luick. 1976. Accuracy of the tritium water dilution method for determining water flux in reindeer *(Rangifer tarandus). Can. J. Zool.* **54**(6):857–862.

Casida, J. E. 1961. Use of radioisotopes in insecticide studies. pp. 427–438. In: *Applications of Radioisotopes and Radiation in the Life Sciences.* Joint Committee on Atomic Energy, Congress of the United States. Hearings before the Sub-committee on Research, Development and Radiation, March 27–30, 1961.

Chapuis, A. M., M. Chartier, H. Francois, G. Soudain, A. Grauby, and M. Fabries. 1973. Radiophotoluminescent glasses as dosimeters in radioecological studies. pp. 59–66. In: *Dosimetry in Agriculture, Industry, Biology, and Medicine.* International Atomic Energy Agency, Vienna. Publ. No. STI/PUB-311 (in French).

Chase, G. D., and J. L. Rabinowitz. 1962. *Principles of Radioisotope Methodology,* 2nd ed. Burgess, Minneapolis. viii + 374 pp. + plus atomic chart.

Chase, G. D., S. Rituper, and J. W. Sulcoski. 1964. *Experiments in Nuclear Science.* Burgess, Minneapolis. xii + 167 pp.

Chase, G. D., S. Rituper, and J. W. Sulcoski. 1971. *Teacher's Guide to Experiments in Nuclear Science,* 2nd ed. Burgess, Minneapolis. 90 pp.

Chase, M. L. (ed.). 1971. The Fern Lake studies. *Univ. Wash. Coll. Fish. Contrib.* No. 352. iv + 75 pp. (Also: U.S. AEC Rep. RLO-2225-T7-6.)

Chipman, W. A. 1959. The use of radioisotopes in studies of the foods and feeding activities of marine animals. *Pubbl. Stn. Zool. Napoli* **31**((suppl.):154–175.*

Coleman, D. C. 1968. A method for intensity labelling of fungi for ecological studies. *Mycologia* **60**(4):960–961.

Coleman, D. C., and J. T. McGinnis. 1970. Quantification of fungus–small arthropod food chains in the soil. *Oikos* **21**(1):134–137.

Conover, R. J.,and V. Francis. 1973. The use of radioactive isotopes to measure the transfer of materials in aquatic food chains. *Mar. Biol.* **18**(4):272–283.

Coons, L. B., and F. E. Guthrie. 1972. High resolution radioautography of ^{3}H-DDT-treated insects. *J. Econ. Entomol.* **65**(4):1004–1007.

Cope, J. B., E. Churchwell, and K. Koontz. 1961. A method of tagging bats with radioactive gold-198 in homing experiments. *Proc. Indiana Acad. Sci.* **70**:267–269.

Cosgrove, G. E., P. B. Dunaway, and J. D. Story. 1969. Malignant tumors associated with subcutaneously implanted ^{60}Co radioactive wires in *Peromyscus maniculatus. Bull. Wildl. Dis. Assoc.* **5**(3):311–314.

Coulson, C. L., and A. J. Peel. 1971. The effect of temperature on respiration of ^{14}C-labelled sugars in stems of willow. *Ann. Bot. (London)* **35**(139):9–15.

Cowan, J. J., and R. B. Platt. 1963. Radiation dosages in the vicinity of an unshielded nuclear reactor. pp. 311–318. In: *Radioecology* (V. Schultz and A. W. Klement, Jr., eds.). Reinhold, New York.

Cowan, R. L., E. W. Hartsook, and J. B. Whelan. 1968. Calcium–strontium metabolism in whitetailed deer as related to age and antler growth. *Proc. Soc. Exp. Biol. Med.* **129**(3):733–737.

Cross, F. A., S. W. Fowler, J. M. Dean, L. F. Small, and C. L. Osterberg. 1968. Distribution of ^{65}Zn in tissues of two marine crustaceans determined by autoradiography. *J. Fish. Res. Board Can.* **25**(11):2461–2466.

Cross, F. A., W. C. Renfro, and E. Gilat. 1975. A review of methodology for studying the transfer of radionuclides in marine foodchains. pp. 185–210. In: *Design of Radiotracer Experiments in Marine Biological Systems.* International Atomic Energy Agency, Vienna. Tech. Rep. Ser. No. 167.

Crossley, D. A., Jr. 1963. Use of radioactive tracers in the study of insect–plant relationships. pp. 43–53. In: *Radiation and Radioisotopes Applied to Insects of Agricultural Importance.* International Atomic Energy Agency, Vienna. Publ. No. STI/PUB/74.

Crossley, D. A., Jr. 1969. Comparative movement of ^{106}Ru, ^{60}Co, and ^{137}Cs in arthropod food chains. pp. 687–695. In: *Symposium on Radioecology* (D. J. Nelson and F. C. Evans, eds.). U.S. AEC Rep. CONF-670503.

Crossley, D. A., Jr., and C. S. Gist. 1973. Use of radioisotopes in modeling soil microcommunities. pp. 258–278. In: *Proceedings of the First Soil Microcommunities Conference,* Syracuse, New York, October 18–20, 1971 (D. L. Dindal, ed.). U.S. AEC Rep. CONF-711076.

Crossley, D. A., Jr., and D. E. Reichle. 1969. Analysis of transient behavior of radioisotopes in insect food chains. *BioScience* **19**(4):341–343.

Crossley, D. A., Jr., and M. Witkamp. 1964. Effects of pesticide on biota and breakdown of forest litter. *Trans. 8th Int. Congr. Soil Sci.* **3**:887–892.

Curnow, R. D., F. A. Glover, and F. W. Whicker, 1967. Uptake, excretion, and distribution of zinc-65 by the mallard. Tech. Pap. No. 10, Colorado Coop. Wildlife Research Unit, Colorado State University, Ft. Collins. 7 pp.

Cushing, C. E., and N. S. Porter. 1969. Radionuclide cycling by periphyton: An apparatus for continuous *in situ* measurements and initial data on zinc-65 cycling. pp. 285–290. In: *Symposium on Radioecology* (D. J. Nelson and F. C. Evans, eds.). U.S. AEC Rep. CONF-670503.

Cushing, C. E., and F. L. Rose. 1970. Cycling of zinc-65 by Columbia River periphyton in a closed lotic microcosm. *Limnol. Oceanogr.* **15**(5):762–767.

Dahlman, R. C., and C. L. Kucera. 1969. Tagging native grassland vegetation with carbon-14. *Ecology* **49**(6):1199–1203.

Dahm, P. A. 1957. Uses of radioisotopes in pesticide research. *Adv. Pest Control Res.* **1**:81–146.

Dalrymple, G. V., and M. A. Lanphere. 1969. *Potassium–Argon Dating: Principles, Techniques and Applications to Geochronology.* W. H. Freeman, San Francisco. xiv + 258 pp.

Davis, W. H., R. W. Barbour, and M. D. Hassell. 1968. Colonial behaviour of *Eptesicus fuscus. J. Mammal.* **49**(1):44–50.

Dean, J. M. 1969. The metabolism of tissues of thermally acclimated trout *(Salmo gairdneri). Comp. Biochem. Physiol.* **29**(1):185–196.

Dean, J. M., and J. D. Berlin. 1969. Alterations in hepatocyte function of thermally acclimated rainbow trout *(Salmo gairdneri). Comp. Biochem. Physiol.* **29**(1):307–312.

Dedek, V. W. 1967a. Radioisotopes in the chemistry of pesticides. II. *Atompraxis* **13**(3):126–129 (in German).

Dedek, V. W. 1967b. Radioisotopes in the chemistry of pesticides. III. *Atompraxis* **13**(4/5):202–206, 208 (in German).

Dedek, V. W. 1970. Radioisotopes in pesticide research. Parts IV and V. *Isotopenpraxis* **6**(7):204–214 (in German).

Dedek, V. W. 1975. Radioisotopes in pesticide research. Part VI. Review papers, general methods of analysis, insecticides. *Isotopenpraxis* **11**(11):378–385 (in German).

Deevey, E. S., Jr., M. Stuiver, and N. Nakai. 1964. Isotopes of carbon and sulfur as tracers of lake metabolism. *Verh. Int. Ver. Limnol.* **15**(1):284–288.

Devine, T., and T. J. Peterle. 1968. Possible differentiation of natal areas of North American waterfowl by neutron activation analysis. *J. Wildl. Manage.* **32**(2):274–279.

DeWitt, R. 1978. Isotope applications in the environmental field. U.S. Department of Energy, Monsanto Research Corp., Rep. MLM-2487. 32 pp.

Dindal, D. L. 1970. Accumulation and excretion of $Cl^{36}DDT$ in mallard and lesser scaup ducks. *J. Wildl. Manage.* **34**(1):74–92.

Dobson, R. M. 1962. Marketing techniques and their application to the study of small terrestrial animals. pp. 228–239. In: *Progress in Soil Zoology*. Papers from a Colloquium on Research Methods Organized by the Soil Zoology Committee of the International Society of Soil Science, Rothamsted Experimental Station, Hertfordshire, July 10–14, 1958 (P. W. Murphy, ed.). Butterworths, London.

Dohrn, R. (ed.). 1959. Marine biological applications of radioisotope research techniques. *Pubbl. Stn. Zool. Napoli* **31**(Suppl.):189 pp. + 7 plates.

Duke, G. E., G. A. Petrides, and R. K. Ringer. 1968. Chromium-51 in food metabolizability and passage rate studies with the ring-necked pheasant. *Poultry Sci.* **47**(4):1356–1364.

Duke, T. W., and T. R. Rice. 1966. Cycling of nutrients in estuaries. *Proc. Gulf Carribean Fish. Inst.* **19**:59–67.

Duke, T. W., J. N. Willis, and T. J. Price. 1966. Cycling of trace elements in the estuarine environment. I. Movement and distribution of zinc-65 and stable zinc in experimental ponds. *Chesapeake Sci.* **7**(1):1–10.

Duke, T. W., J. N. Willis, and D. A. Wolfe. 1968. A technique for studying the exchange of trace elements between estuarine sediments and water. *Limnol. Oceanogr.* **13**(3):541–545.

Dunson, W. A. 1969. Concentration of sodium by freshwater turtles. pp. 191–197. In: *Symposium on Radioecology* (D. J. Nelson and F. C. Evans, eds.). U.S. AEC Rep. CONF-670503.

Duursma, E. K. 1972. Geochemical aspects and applications of radionuclides in the sea. *Oceanogr. Mar. Biol. Annu. Rev.* **10**:137–223.

Eberhardt, L. L., R. L. Meeks, and T. J. Peterle. 1971. Food chain model for DDT kinetics in a freshwater marsh. *Nature (London)* **230**(5288):60–62.

Edmondson, W. T., and G. G. Winberg. 1971. *A Manual on Methods for the Assessment of Secondary Productivity in Fresh Waters*. IBP Handbook No. 17. Blackwell, Oxford, England. xxiv + 358 pp.

Ellis, W. R. 1967. A review of radioisotope methods of stream gaging: Review Paper. *J. Hydrol.* **5**(3):233–257.

Elwood, J. W., and D. J. Nelson. 1972. Periphyton production and grazing rates in a stream measured with a ^{32}P material balance method. *Oikos* **23**(3):295–303.

Emerson, S., W. Broecker, and D. W. Schindler. 1973. Gas-exchange rates in a small lake as determined by the radon method. *J. Fish. Res. Board Can.* **30**(10):1475–1484.

Erickson, J. M. 1972. Mark–recapture techniques for population estimates of *Pogonomyrmex* ant colonies: An evaluation of the ^{32}P technique. *Ann. Entomol. Soc. Am.* **65**(1):57–61.

Fabries, M., A. Grauby, and J. L. Trochain. 1972. Study of a Mediterranean type phytocenose subjected to chronic gamma radiation. *Radiat. Bot.* **12**(3):125–136.

Faires, R. A., and B. H. Parks. 1973. *Radioisotope Laboratory Techniques*, 3rd ed. Halsted Press, New York. 312 pp.

Fang, S. C. 1973. Uptake and biotransformation of phenylmercuric acetate by aquatic organisms. *Arch. Environ. Contam. Toxicol.* **1**(1):18–26.

Filby, R. H., and K. R. Shah. 1974. Activation analysis and applications to environmental research. *Toxicol. Environ. Chem. Rev.* **2**(1):1–44.

Forster, W. O. 1968. Fallout radionuclides (Fe^{55} and Mn^{54}) as indicators of salmon migration in the Northeast Pacific relative to neutron activated radionuclide (Zn^{65}). *Bull. Ecol. Soc. Am.* **49**(2):72.

Forsyth, D. J., and T. J. Peterle. 1973. Accumulation of chlorine-36 ring-labeled DDT residues in various tissues of two species of shrew. *Arch. Environ. Contam. Toxicol.* **1**(1):1–17.

Foster, R. F. 1959. Radioactive tracing of the movement of an essential element through an aquatic community with specific reference to radiophosphorus. *Pubbl. Stn. Zool. Napoli* 31(Suppl.):34–62.

Fourcy, A., A. Fer, C. Poret, M. Neuburger, and J.-P. Garrec. 1967. Application of radioactivation analysis to radioecological studies. *Bull. Inform. Sci. Tech. (Paris)* 119:39–48 (English translation: AEC-tr-7041).

Fox, G. A., F. W. Anderka, V. Lewin, and W. C. MacKay. 1975. Field assessment of eggshell quality by beta-backscatter. *J. Wildl. Manage.* 39(3):528–534.

Fraley, L., Jr., and F. W. Whicker. 1973a. Response of short-grass plains vegetation to gamma radiation. I. Chronic irradiation. *Radiat. Bot.* 13(6):331–341.

Fraley, L., Jr., and F. W. Whicker. 1973b. Response of a native shortgrass plant stand to ionizing radiation. pp. 999–1006. In: *Radionuclides in Ecosystems* (D. J. Nelson, ed.). U.S. AEC Rep. CONF-710501-P2.

Fraser, D. A., and E. E. Gaertner. 1970. Utilization of radioisotopes in forestry research. *Proc. 6th World Forestry Congr. (Madrid)* 2:2264–2274.

French, N. R. 1964. Description of a study of ecological effects on a desert area from chronic exposure to low level ionizing radiation. University of California at Los Angeles, U.S. AEC Rep. UCLA 12–532. 27 pp., 15 figs.

Frigerio, N. A., and W. J. Eisler, Jr. 1968. Low cost, automatic, nest and burrow monitor using radioactive tagging. *Ecology* 49(4):788–791.

Fuhs, G. W., and E. Canelli. 1970. Phosphorus-33 autoradiography used to measure phosphate uptake by individual algae. *Limnol. Oceanogr.* 15(6):962–967.

Gangwere, S. K., W. Chavin, and F. C. Evans. 1964. Methods of marking insects, with especial reference to Orthoptera (Sens. Lat.). *Ann. Entomol. Soc. Am.* 57(6):662–669.

Gasaway, W. C. 1976. Cellulose digestion and metabolism by captive rock ptarmigan. *Comp. Biochem. Physiol. A* 54(2):179–182.

Gasaway, W. C., D. F. Holleman, and R. G. White. 1975. Flow of digesta in the intestine and cecum of the rock ptarmigan. *Condor* 77(4):467–474.

Gasaway, W. C., R. G. White, and D. F. Holleman. 1976. Digestion of dry matter and absorption of water in the intestine and cecum of rock ptarmigan. *Condor* 78(1):77–84.

Gentry, J. B., M. H. Smith, and R. J. Beyers. 1971. Use of radioactively tagged bait to study movement patterns in small mammal populations. *Ann. Zool. Fenn.* 8(1):17–21.

Gerrard, M. 1969. Tagging of small animals with radioisotopes for tracking purposes: A literature review. *Int. J. Appl. Radiat. Isot.* 20(9):671–676.

Gifford, C. E., and D. R. Griffin. 1960. Notes on homing and migratory behavior of bats. *Ecology* 41(2):378–381.

Gifford, D. R. 1967. An attempt to use ^{14}C as a tracer in a Scots pine (*Pinus silvestris* L.) litter decomposition study. pp. 687–693. In: *Secondary Productivity of Terrestrial Ecosystems*, Vol. 2 (K. Petrusewicz, ed.). Institute of Ecology, Polish Academy of Sciences, Warsaw.

Giles, R. H., Jr. 1970. The ecology of a small forested watershed treated with the insecticide malathion-S^{35}. *Wildl. Monogr.*, no. 24. 81 pp.

Glover, F. A., F. W. Whicker, R. J. Buller, and R. D. Curnow. 1967. Distribution of mallards from the Columbia Basin region as indicated by the presence of zinc-65 in birds shot by hunters in the Pacific and Central Flyways. Final Progress Report. Colorado State University Research Foundation, U.S. AEC Rep. COO-1514-3. vi + 36 pp.

Godfrey, G. K. 1953. A technique for finding *Microtus* nests. *J. Mammal.* 34(4):503–505.

Goldman, C. R. (ed.). 1966. *Primary Productivity in Aquatic Environments*. University of California Press, Berkeley. 464 pp.

Golley, F. B. 1967. Methods of measuring secondary productivity in terrestrial vertebrate populations. pp. 99–124. In: *Secondary Productivity of Terrestrial Ecosystems*, Vol. 1 (K. Petrusewicz, ed.). Institute of Ecology, Polish Academy of Sciences, Warsaw.

Golley, F. B., and J. B. McCormick. 1966. Development of a 137-cesium facility for ecological research. U.S. AEC Rep. TID-22499. 24 pp.

Grace, J., and H. W. Woolhouse. 1973. A physiological and mathematical study of the growth and productivity of a *Calluna–Sphagnum* community. III. Distribution of photosynthate in *Calluna vulgaris* L. Hull. *J. Appl. Ecol.* **10**(1):77–91.

Graham, W. J., and H. W. Ambrose, III. 1967. A technique for continuously locating small mammals in field enclosures. *J. Mammal.* **48**(4):639–642.

Greichus, Y. A., and A. Greichus. 1974. Dieldrin-^{14}C residues on feathers of birds with surgically removed uropygial glands. *Bull. Environ. Contam. Toxicol.* **12**(4):413–416.

Griffin, D. R. 1952. Radioactive tagging of animals under natural conditions. *Ecology* **33**(3):329–335.

Grossbard, E. 1973a. Autoradiographic techniques in studies on the decomposition of plant residues labelled with carbon-14. *Bull. Ecol. Res. Comm. (Stockholm)* **17**:279–280.

Grossbard, E. 1973b. An autoradiographic technique to observe uptake and utilization by micro-organisms of carbon-14 derived from labelled herbicides in soil. *Bull. Ecol. Res. Comm. (Stockholm)* **17**:275–276.

Grzenda, A. R., W. J. Taylor, and D. F. Paris. 1971. The uptake and distribution of chlorinated residues by goldfish *(Carassius auratus)* fed a ^{14}C-dieldrin contaminated diet. *Trans. Am. Fish. Soc.* **100**(2):215–221.

Gude, W. D. 1968. *Autoradiographic Techniques: Localization of Radioisotopes in Biological Material.* Prentice-Hall, Englewood Cliffs, New Jersey. xiii + 113 pp.

Guthrie, J. E., and A. G. Scott. 1969. Measurement of radiation dose distribution in a pond habitat by lithium fluoride dosimetry. *Can. J. Zool.* **47**(1):17–20.

Gyllander, C. 1966. Water exchange and diffusion processes in Tvären, a Baltic Bay. pp. 207–219. In: *Disposal of Radioactive Wastes into Seas, Oceans and Surface Waters.* International Atomic Energy, Vienna. Publ. No. STI/PUB/126.

Haber, A. H. 1968. Ionizing radiations as research tools. *Annu. Rev. Plant Physiol.* **19**:463–489.

Hakonson, T. E., and F. W. Whicker. 1969. Uptake and elimination of ^{134}Cs by mule deer. pp. 616–622. In: *Symposium on Radioecology* (D. J. Nelson and F. C. Evans, eds.). U.S. AEC Rep. CONF-670503.

Hakonson, T. E., A. F. Gallegos, and F. W. Whicker. 1973. Use of cesium-133 and activation analysis for measurement of cesium kinetics in a montane lake. pp. 344–348. In: *Radionuclides in Ecosystems* (D. J. Nelson, ed.). U.S. AEC Rep. CONF-710501-P1.

Hall, R. M., Jr. 1970. Thermoluminescent dosimetry. pp. C-37–C-40. In: *A Tropical Rain Forest: A Study of Irradiation and Ecology at El Verde, Puerto Rico* (H. T. Odum and R. F. Pigeon, eds.). U.S. AEC Rep. TID-24270.

Hamilton, E. I., and R. M. Farquhar (eds.). 1968. *Radiometric Dating for Geologists.* Interscience, New York. vii + 506 pp.

Hanson, W. C., and A. C. Case, 1963. A method of measuring waterfowl dispersion utilizing phosphorus-32 and zinc-65. pp 451–453. In: *Radioecology* (V. Schultz and A. W. Klement, Jr., eds.). Reinhold, New York.

Hanson, W. C., F. W. Whicker, and J. F. Lipscomb. 1975. Lichen forage ingestion rates of free-roaming caribou estimated with fallout cesium-137. pp. 71–79. In: *Proc. First Int. Reindeer and Caribou Symp. Biol. Pap. Univ. Alaska, Spec. Rep. No. 1* (J. R. Luick, P. C. Lent, D. R. Klein, and R. G. White, eds.).

Hargrave, B. T. 1970. The utilization of benthic microflora by *Hyalella azteca* (Amphipoda). *J. Anim. Ecol.* **39**(2):427–437.

Harvey, J. M. 1967. Excretion of DDT by migratory birds. *Can. J. Zool.* **45**(5):629–633.

Hawthorn, J., and R. B. Duckworth. 1958. Fall-out radioactivity in a deer's antlers. *Nature (London)* **182**(4645):1294.

Hayes, F. R., and C. C. Coffin. 1951. Radioactive phosphorus and exchange of lake nutrients. *Endeavor* **10**(38):78–81.

Heath, R. L. 1971. Table of isotopes. pp. B245–B541. In: *Handbook of Chemistry and Physics*, 52nd ed. (R. C. Weast, ed.). Chemical Rubber Co., Cleveland.

Hendee, W. R. 1973a. *Radioactive Isotopes in Biological Research*. John Wiley, New York. xvi + 356 pp.

Hendee, W. R. 1973b. Chapt. 17. Activation analysis. pp. 229–236. In: *Radioactive Isotopes in Biological Research*. John Wiley, New York.

Hirth, H. F., R. C. Pendleton, A. C. King, and T. R. Downard. 1969. Dispersal of snakes from a hibernaculum in northwestern Utah. *Ecology* **50**(2):332–339.

Hooper, F. F., and D. G. Imes, 1973. Physical and biological dispersion of the hypolimnetic phosphorus of a bog lake system. pp. 401–409. In: *Radionuclides in Ecosystems* (D. J. Nelson, ed.). U.S. AEC Rep. CONF-710501-P1.

Hooper, F. F., H. A. Podoliak, and S. F. Snieszko. 1961. Use of radioisotopes in hydrobiology and fish culture. *Trans. Am. Fish. Soc.* **90**(1):49–57.

Hoss, D. E. 1967. Marking post-larval paralichthid flounders with radioactive elements. *Trans. Am. Fish. Soc.* **96**(2):151–156.

Hsiao, S. C., and H. Boroughs. 1958. The uptake of radioactive calcium by sea urchin eggs. I. Entrance of Ca^{45} into unfertilized egg cytoplasm. *Biol. Bull.* **114**(2):196–204.

Hubbell, S. P., A. Sikora, and O. H. Paris. 1965. Radiotracer, gravimetric and calorimetric studies of ingestion and assimilation rates of an isopod. *Health Phys.* **11**(12):1485–1501.

Hudson, J. W., and L. C.-H. Wang. 1969. Thyroid function in desert ground squirrels. pp. 17–33. In: *Physiological Systems in Semiarid Environments* (C. C. Hoff and M. L. Riedesel, eds.). University of New Mexico Press, Albuquerque.

Hunn, J. B., and P. O. Fromm. 1964. Uptake, turnover and excretion of I-131 by rainbow trout *(Salmo gairdneri). Biol. Bull.* **126**(2):282–290.

Hutchinson, G. E., and V. T. Bowen. 1947. A direct demonstration of the phosphorus cycle in a small lake. *Proc. Natl. Acad. Sci. U.S.A.* **33**(5):148–153.

Ichikawa, T. 1973. Utilization of X-rays and radioactive isotopes in ichthyology and fishery science. pp. 352–378. In: *Radioactivity and Fishes: Contamination, Injuries, and Utilization* (N. Egami, ed.). Koseiska Kosei Kaku, Tokyo (in Japanese).

International Atomic Energy Agency. 1960. *Large Radiation Sources in Industry*. Proceedings of a conference, Warsaw, September 1959. IAEA, Vienna. Publ. No. STI/PUB/12. Vol. 1, 438 pp.; Vol. II, 456 pp.

International Atomic Energy Agency. 1962a. *Radioisotopes in Soil–Plant Nutrition Studies*. Proceedings of a symposium, Bombay, February 26–March 2, 1962. IAEA, Vienna. Publ. No. STI/PUB/55. 457 pp.

International Atomic Energy Agency. 1962b. *Radioisotopes and Radiation in Entomology*. Proceedings of a symposium, Bombay, December 5–9, 1960. IAEA, Vienna. Publ. No. STI/PUB/38. 307 pp.

International Atomic Energy Agency. 1963a. *Radioisotopes in Hydrology*. Proceedings of a symposium, Tokyo, March 5–9, 1963. IAEA, Vienna. Publ. No. STI/PUB/71. 459 pp.

International Atomic Energy Agency. 1963b. *Radiation and Radioisotopes Applied to Insects of Agricultural Importance*. Proceedings of a symposium, Athens, Greece, April 22–26, 1963. IAEA, Vienna. Publ. No. STI/PUB/74. 508 pp.

International Atomic Energy Agency. 1964. *Laboratory Training Manual on the Use of Isotopes and Radiation in Soil–Plant Relations Research, IAEA, Vienna. Tech. Rep. Ser. No. 29. Publ. No. 165 pp. STI/DOC/10/29.*

International Atomic Energy Agency. 1965. *Isotopes and Radiation in Soil-Plant Nutrition Studies*. Proceedings of a symposium, Ankara, June 28–July 2, 1965. IAEA, Vienna. Publ. No. STI/PUB/108. 624 pp.

International Atomic Energy Agency. 1966a. *Radioisotopes in the Detection of Pesticide Residues.* Proceedings of a panel, Vienna, April 12–15, 1965. IAEA, Vienna, Panel Proceedings Series. Publ. No. STI/PUB/123. 118 pp.

International Atomic Energy Agency. 1966b. *Isotopes in Weed Research.* Proceedings of a symposium, Vienna, October 25–29, 1965. IAEA, Vienna. Publ. No. STI/PUB/113. 246 pp.

International Atomic Energy Agency. 1966c. *Guide to the Safe Handling of Radioisotopes in Hydrology.* IAEA, Vienna, Safety Ser. No. 20. Publ. No. STI/PUB/131. 38 pp.

International Atomic Energy Agency. 1967. *Isotopes in Hydrology.* Proceedings of a symposium, Vienna, November 14–18, 1966. IAEA, Vienna. Publ. No. STI/PUB/141. 740 pp.

International Atomic Energy Agency. 1968a. *Control of Livestock Insect Pests by the Sterile-Male Technique.* Proceedings of a panel, Vienna, January 23–27, 1967. IAEA, Vienna. Publ. No. STI/PUB/184. 108 pp.

International Atomic Energy Agency. 1968b. *Radiation, Radioisotopes, and Rearing Methods in the Control of Insect Pests.* Proceedings of a panel, Tel Aviv, October 17–21, 1966. IAEA, Vienna. Publ. No. STI/PUB/185. 153 pp.

International Atomic Energy Agency, 1968c. *Isotopes and Radiation in Soil Organic-Matter Studies.* Proceedings of a symposium, Vienna, July 15–19, 1968. IAEA, Vienna. Publ. No. STI/PUB/190. 593 pp.

International Atomic Energy Agency. 1968d. *Guidebook on Nuclear Techniques in Hydrology.* IAEA, Vienna, Tech. Rep. Ser. No. 91. Publ. No. STI/DOC/10/91. 214 pp.

International Atomic Energy Agency. 1968e. *Isotope Techniques in Hydrology,* Vol. I (1957–1965). IAEA, Vienna, Bibl. Ser. No. 32. Publ. No. STI/PUB/21/32. 228 pp.

International Atomic Energy Agency, 1969a. *Insect Ecology and the Sterile-Male Technique.* Proceedings of a panel, Vienna, August 7–11, 1967. IAEA, Vienna. Publ. No. STI/PUB/223. 102 pp.

International Atomic Energy Agency. 1969b. *Sterile-Male Technique for Eradication or Control of Harmful Insects. Proceedings of a panel, Vienna, May 27–31, 1968. IAEA, Vienna. Publ. No. STI/PUB/224. 151 pp.*

International Atomic Energy Agency. 1970a. *Sterile-Male Technique for Control of Fruit Flies.* Proceedings of a Panel on the Application of the Sterile-Male Technique for Control of Insects with Special Reference to Fruit Flies, Vienna, September 1–5, 1969. IAEA, Vienna. Publ. No. STI/PUB/276. 185 pp.

International Atomic Energy Agency. 1970b. *Reference Methods for Marine Radioactivity Studies.* IAEA, Vienna, Tech. Rep. Ser. No. 118. Publ. No. STI/DOC/10/118. 284 pp.

International Atomic Energy Agency. 1970c. *Nuclear Techniques for Studying Pesticide Residue Problems.* Proceedings of a panel, Vienna, December 16–20, 1968. IAEA, Vienna. Publ. No. STI/PUB/252. 84 pp.

International Atomic Energy Agency. 1970d. *Isotope Hydrology 1970.* Proceedings of a symposium on the Use of Isotopes in Hydrology, Vienna, March 9–13, 1970. IAEA, Vienna. Publ. No. STI/PUB/255. 918 pp.

International Atomic Energy Agency, 1971a. *Application of Induced Sterility for Control of Lepidopterous Populations.* Proceedings of a panel, Vienna, June 1–5, 1970. IAEA, Vienna. Publ. No. STI/PUB/281. 176 pp.

International Atomic Energy Agency. 1971b. *Sterility Principle for Insect Control or Eradication.* Proceedings of a symposium, Athens, Greece, September 14–18, 1970. IAEA, Vienna. Publ. No. STI/PUB/265. 542 pp.

International Atomic Energy Agency. 1971c. *Rapid Methods for Measuring Radioactivity in the Environment.* Proceedings of a symposium, Neuherberg, Germany, July 5–9, 1971. IAEA, Vienna. Publ. No. STI/PUB/289. 967 pp.

International Atomic Energy Agency. 1971d. *Nuclear Techniques in Environmental Pollution.* Pro-

ceedings of a symposium, Salzburg, October 26–30, 1970. IAEA, Vienna. Publ. No. STI/
PUB/268. 824 pp.

International Atomic Energy Agency. 1972a. *Radiotracer Studies of Chemical Residues in Food and Agriculture*. Proceedings of a combined panel and research coordination meeting, Vienna, October 25–29, 1971. IAEA, Vienna. Publ. No. STI/PUB/332. 172 pp.

International Atomic Energy Agency. 1972b. *Mercury Contamination in Man and His Environment*. IAEA, Vienna, Tech. Rep. Ser. No. 137, Publ. No. STI/DOC/10/137. 181 pp.

International Atomic Energy Agency. 1972c. *Isotopes and Radiation in Soil–Plant Relationships including Forestry*. Proceedings of a symposium, Vienna, December 13–17, 1971. IAEA, Vienna, Publ. No. STI/PUB/292. 684 pp.

International Atomic Energy Agency. 1973a. *Tracer Techniques in Sediment Transport*. Panel meeting, Saclay, France, June 21–25, 1971. IAEA, Vienna, Rep. Ser. No. 145. Publ. No. STI/DOC-10/145. 240 pp.

International Atomic Energy Agency. 1973b. *Soil-Moisture and Irrigation Studies*, Vol. II. Proceedings of a panel, Vienna, November 2–6, 1970. IAEA, Vienna. Publ. No. STI/PUB-327. 194 pp.

International Atomic Energy Agency. 1973c. *Dosimetry in Agriculture, Industry, Biology and Medicine*. Proceedings of a symposium, Vienna, April 17–21, 1972. IAEA, Vienna. Publ. No. STI/PUB/311. 685 pp.

International Atomic Energy Agency. 1973d. *Computer Models and Application of the Sterile-Male Technique*. Proceedings of a panel, December 13–17, 1971. IAEA, Vienna. Publ. No. STI/PUB/340. 195 pp.

International Atomic Energy Agency. 1973e. *Isotope Techniques in Hydrology*, Vol. II (1966–1971). IAEA, Vienna, Bibl. Ser. No. 41. Publ. No. STI/PUB/21/41. 233 pp.

International Atomic Energy Agency. 1974a. *The Sterile-Insect Technique and its Field Applications*. Proceedings of a panel, Vienna, November 13–17, 1972. IAEA, Vienna. Publ. No. STI/PUB/364. 137 pp.

International Atomic Energy Agency. 1974b. *Isotope and Radiation Techniques in Soil Physics and Irrigation Studies 1973*. Proceedings of a symposium, Vienna, October 1–5, 1973. IAEA, Vienna. Publ. No. STI/PUB-349. 525 pp.

International Atomic Energy Agency. 1974c. *Comparative Studies of Food and Environmental Contamination*. Proceedings of a symposium, Otaniemi, Finland, August 27–31, 1973. IAEA, Vienna. Publ. No. STI/PUB-348. 633 pp.

International Atomic Energy Agency. 1975a. *Origin and Fate of Chemical Residues in Food, Agriculture and Fisheries*. IAEA, Vienna, Panel Proceedings Series. Publ. No. STI/PUB/399. 189 pp.

International Atomic Energy Agency. 1975b. *Isotope Ratios as Pollutant Source and Behaviour Indicators*. Proceedings of a symposium, Vienna, November 18–22, 1974. IAEA, Vienna. Publ. No. STI/PUB/382. 491 pp.

International Atomic Energy Agency. 1975c. *Design of Radiotracer Experiments in Marine Biological Systems*. IAEA, Vienna, Tech. Rep. Ser. No. 167. Publ. No. STI/DOC/10/167. 289 pp.

International Atomic Energy Agency. 1976. *Measurement, Detection and Control of Environmental Pollutants*. Proceedings of a symposium, Vienna, March 15–19, 1976. IAEA, Vienna. Publ. No. STI/PUB/432, 643 pp.

International Atomic Energy Agency. 1977. *Laboratory Training Manual on the Use of Isotopes and Radiation in Entomology*, 2nd ed. IAEA, Vienna, Tech. Rep. Ser. No. 61. Publ. No. STI/DOC/10/61/2. 274 pp.

Jenkins, D. W. 1957. Radioisotopes in entomology. pp. 195–229. In: *Atomic Energy and Agriculture* (C. L. Comar, ed.). American Association for the Advancement of Science, Washington, D.C., Publ. No. 49.

Jenkins, D. W. 1962a. Radioisotopes in ecological and biological studies of agricultural insects. pp. 3–20. In: *Radioisotopes and Radiation in Entomology*. International Atomic Energy Agency, Vienna. Publ. No. STI/PUB/38.

Jenkins, D. W. 1962b. Radioisotopes in entomological studies of endemic and tropical diseases. pp. 235–262. In: *Radioisotopes in Tropical Medicine*. International Atomic Energy Agency, Vienna. Publ. No. STI/PUB/31.

Jenkins, D. W. 1963. Use of radionuclides in ecological studies of insects. pp. 431–440. In: *Radioecology* (V. Schultz and A. W. Klement, Jr., eds.). Reinhold, New York.

Johanningsmeier, A. G., and C. J. Goodnight. 1962. Use of iodine-131 to measure movements of small animals. *Science* **138**(3537):147–148.

Jorgensen, C. D., and P. V. Wells. 1964. Pleistocene wood rat middens and climatic change in Mohave Desert: A record of juniper woodlands. *Science* **143**(3611):1171–1174.

Karlstrom, E. L. 1957. The use of Co^{60} as a tag for recovering amphibians in the field. *Ecology* **38**(2):187–195.

Karzinkin, G. S. 1962. *The Use of Radioactive Isotopes in the Fishing Industry (Ispol'zovaniye Radioaktivnykh Izotopov v Rybnom Khozyaystve)*. Pishichepromizdat, Moscow. 73 pp. (English translation: Joint Publication Research Service, New York, JPRS 21109; U.S. National Technical Information Service, OTS-63-31775.

Kaye, S. V. 1960. Gold-198 wire used to study movements of small mammals. *Science* **131**(3403):824.

Kaye, S. V. 1961. Movements of harvest mice tagged with gold-198. *J. Mammal.* **42**(3):323–337.

Kaye, S. V. 1965. Use of miniature glass rod dosimeters in radiation ecology. *Ecology* **46**(1/2):201–206.

Keller, G. H. 1969. Radioisotopes and oceanography. *Isot. Radiat. Technol.* **6**(4):376–381.

Kelsall, J. P., and J. R. Calaprice. 1972. Chemical content of waterfowl plumage as a potential diagnostic tool. *J. Wildl. Manage.* **36**(4):1088–1097.

Kenagy, G. J., and C. B. Smith. 1970. Depth and activity measurements of a heteromyid rodent community using radioisotopes. School of Engineering and Applied Science, University of California at Los Angeles, Rep. UCLA-ENG-7075. xi + 51 pp.

Kenagy, G. J., and C. B. Smith. 1973. Radioisotopic measurement of depth and determination of temperatures in burrows of heteromyid rodents. pp. 265–273. In: *Radionuclides in Ecosystems* (D. J. Nelson, ed.). U.S. AEC Rep. CONF-710501-P1.

Kennington, G. S., and C. F. T. Ching. 1966. Activation analysis of ungulate hair. *Science* **151**(3714):1085–1086.

Kerstetter, T. H., L. B. Kirschner, and D. D. Rafuse. 1970. On the mechanisms of sodium ion transport by the irrigated gills of rainbow trout *(Salmo gairdneri)*. *J. Gen. Physiol.* **56**(3):342–359.

Kevern, N. R. 1966. Feeding rate of carp established by a radioisotopic method. *Trans. Am. Fish. Soc.* **95**(4):363–371.

Kitchings, J. T., III, P. B. Dunaway, J. D. Story, and L. E. Tucker. 1968. Use of radioiron (^{59}Fe) as an index to hemopoietic damage caused by ionizing radiation. *J. Tenn. Acad. Sci.* **43**(3):85–87.

Kkmeleva, N. N. 1959. An experiment with radioactive phosphorus (^{32}P) in the study of inorganic fertilization of ponds. pp. 41–48. In: *Transactions of the 6th Conference on the Biology of Inland Waters*, June 10–19, 1957 (*Trudy VI Soveschchaniya po Problemam Biologii Vnutrennykh Vod*, 10–19 Iyunya 1957g.) (B. S. Kuzin and S. I. Kuznetsov, eds.). Publishing House of the USSR, Academy of Sciences, Moscow and Leningrad. [English translation: AEC-tr-6880 (1969).]

Klement, A. W., Jr., and V. Schultz. 1980. *Freshwater and Terrestrial Radioecology: A Selected Bibliography*. Dowden, Hutchinson and Ross, Stroudsburg, Pennsylvania. viii + 587 pp.

Kline, J. R., M. L. Stewart, and C. F. Jordan. 1972. Estimation of biomass and transpiration in coniferous forests using tritiated water. pp. 159–166. In: *Proceedings—Research on Coniferous*

Forest Ecosystems—A Symposium (J. F. Franklin, L. J. Dempster, and R. H. Waring, eds.). Pacific Northwest Forest and Range Experiment Station, U.S. Forest Service, Portland, Oregon.

Knipling, E. F. 1965. The sterility method of pest population control. pp 233–249. In: *Research in Pesticides* (C. O. Chichester, ed.). Academic Press, New York.

Knox, K. L., J. G. Nagy, and R. D. Brown. 1969. Water turnover in mule deer. *J. Wildl. Manage.* 33(2):389–393.

Knutson, D. W., R. W. Buddemeier, and S. V. Smith. 1972. Coral chronometers: Seasonal growth bands in reef corals. *Science* 177(4045):270–272.

Kodrich, W. R., and C. A. Tryon. 1973. Effect of season on thyroid release of iodine-131 in free-ranging eastern chipmunks *(Tamias striatus)*. pp. 260–264. In: *Radionuclides in Ecosystems* (D. J. Nelson, ed.) U.S. AEC Rep. CONF-710501-P1.

Kolehmainen, S. E. 1974. Daily feeding rates of bluegill *(Lepomis macrochirus)* determined by a refined radioisotope method. *J. Fish. Res. Board Can.* 31(1):67–74.

Kolehmainen, S., S. Takatalo, and J. K. Miettinen. 1969. A tracer experiment with I-131 in an oligotrophic lake. pp. 278–284. In: *Symposium on Radioecology* (D. J. Nelson and F. C. Evans, eds.) U.S. AEC Rep. CONF-670503.

Kowal, N. E., and D. A. Crossley, Jr. 1971. The ingestion rates of microarthropods in pine mor, estimated with radioactive calcium. *Ecology* 52(3):444–452.

Kuenzler, E. J. 1969. Elimination of iodine, cobalt, iron, and zinc by marine zooplankton. pp 462–473. In: *Symposium on Radioecology* (D. J. Nelson and F. C. Evans, eds.). U.S. AEC Rep. CONF-670503.

Kuzin, A. M. 1960. The application of radioisotopes in biology. International Atomic Energy Agency, Vienna, Rev. Ser. No. 7. Publ. No. STI/PUB/15/7. 63 pp.

LaBrecque, G. C., and J. C. Keller (eds.). 1965 *Advances in Insect Population Control by the Sterile-Male Technique*. International Atomic Energy Agency, Vienna, Tech. Rep. Ser. No. 44. Publ. No. STI/DOC/10/44. 79pp.

Lappenbusch, W. L., D. G. Watson, and W. L. Templeton. 1971. *In situ* measurement of radiation dose in the Columbia River. *Health Phys.* 21(2):247–251.

Lawrence, W. H., and J. H. Rediske. 1962. Fate of sown Douglas-fir seed. *For. Sci.* 8(3):210–218.

Leddicotte, G. W. 1969. Specific activation analysis techniques and methods for the assay of trace substances in aquatic and terrestrial environments. pp. 76–80. In: *Modern Trends in Activation Analysis*, Vol. 1 (J. R. DeVoe, ed.). National Bureau of Standards Rep. NBS-Spec. Publ. 312.

Lederer, C. M., J. M. Hollander, and I. Perlman. 1967. *Table of Isotopes*, 6th ed. John Wiley, New York. 594 pp.

Lee, J. J., M. McEnery, S. Pierce, H. D. Freudenthal, and W. A. Muller. 1966. Tracer experiments in feeding littoral foraminifera. *J. Protozool.* 13(4):659–670.

Lehmann, U. 1965. Investigations of periodicity of freshwater invertebrates by radioactive isotopes. pp. 318–320. In: *Circadian Clocks* (J. Aschoff, ed.). North-Holland, Amsterdam.

Lewis, C. T., and N. Waloff. 1964. The use of radioactive tracers in the study of dispersion of *Orthotylus virescens* (Douglas & Scott) (Miridae, Heteroptera). *Entomologia Exp. Appl.* 7:15–24.

Likens, G. E., and A. D. Hasler. 1962. Movements of radiosodium (Na^{24}) within an ice-covered lake. *Limnol. Oceanogr.* 7(1):48–56.

Linn, I., and J. Shillito. 1960. Rings for marking very small mammals. *Proc. Zool. Soc. London* 134(3):489–495.

Loeffel, R. E., and W. O. Forster. 1970. Determination of movement and identity of stocks of coho salmon in the ocean using the radionuclide zinc-65. *Res. Rep. Fish Comm. Oreg.* 2(1):15–27.

Longhurst, W. M., N. F. Baker, G. E. Connolly, and R. A. Fisk. 1970. Total body water and water turnover in sheep and deer. *Am. J. Vet. Res.* 31(4):673–677.

Lucas, A. C., and N. R. French. 1967. A miniature thermoluminescent dosimeter and its application in radioecology. pp. 402–411. In: *Luminescence Dosimetry* (F. H. Attix, ed.) U.S. AEC Symp. Ser. No. 8.

Lucas, H. F., Jr., D. N. Edgington, and P. J. Colby. 1970. Concentrations of trace elements in Great Lakes fishes. *J. Fish. Res. Board Can.* **27**(4):677–684.

Lutz, G. J. (ed.). 1970a. *Oceanography: A bibliography of Selected Activation Analysis Literature.* U.S. National Bureau of Standards Rep. NBS-TN-534. 36 pp.

Lutz, G. J. (ed.). 1970b. *Pollution Analysis: A Bibliography of the Literature of Activation Analysis.* U.S. National Bureau of Standards Rep. NBS-TN-532. 32 pp.

Lutz, G. J., R. J. Boreni, R. S. Maddock, and J. Wing (eds.). 1972. *Activation Analysis: A Bibliography through 1971.* U.S. National Bureau of Standards Rep. NBS-TN-467. 892 pp.

Lynn, W. G., and J. N. Dent. 1961. A comparison of the responses of *Triturus* and *Desmognathus* to thyroid-stimulating hormone administration. *Biol. Bull.* **120**(1):54–61.

Madison, D. M., and C. R. Shoop. 1970. Homing behavior, orientation, and home range of salamanders tagged with tantalum-182. *Science* **168**(3939):1484–1487.

Maguire, B., Jr., and W. E. Neill. 1971. Species and individual productivity in phytoplankton communities. *Ecology* **52**(5):903–907.

Malone, C. R., and D. J. Nelson. 1969. Feeding rates of freshwater snails *(Goniobasis clavaeformis)* determined with cobalt[60]. *Ecology* **50**(4):728–730.

Mason, W. H., and E. P. Odum. 1969. The effect of coprophagy on retention and bioelimination of radionuclides by detritus-feeding animals. pp 721–724. In: *Symposium on Radioecology* (D. J. Nelson and F. C. Evans, eds.). U.S. AEC Rep. CONF-670503.

Mathies, J. B. 1972. Annual consumption of cesium-137 and cobalt-60 labeled pine seeds by small mammals in an oak–hickory forest. Dissertation, Michigan State University. xviii + 213 pp. (Also: Mathies, J. B., P. B. Dunaway, G. Schneider, and S. I. Auerbach, Oak Ridge National Laboratory Rep. ORNL-TM-3912).

Mautz, W. W. 1971. Comparison of the ^{51}CrCl$_3$ ratio and total collection techniques in digestibility studies with a wild ruminant, the white-tailed deer. *J. Anim. Sci.* **32**(5):999–1002.

Mautz, W. W., and G. A. Petrides. 1967. The usefulness of chromium-51 in digestive studies of the white-tailed deer. *Trans. North Am. Wildl. and Nat. Resour. Conf.* **32**:420–429.

McBrayer, J. F., and D. E. Reichle. 1971. Trophic structure and feeding rates of forest soil invertebrate populations. *Oikos* **22**(3):381–388.

McCabe, R. A., and G. A. LePage. 1958. Identifying progeny from pheasant hens given radioactive calcium (Ca^{45}). *J. Wildl. Manage.* **22**(2):134–141.

McCormick, J. F. 1970. Patterns of radiation exposure in the tropical rain forest. pp. C-41–C-47. In: *A Tropical Rain Forest: A Study of Irradiation and Ecology at El Verde, Puerto Rico* (H. T. Odum and R. F. Pigeon, eds.). U.S. AEC Rep. TID-24270.

McCormick, J. F., and F. B. Golley. 1966. Irradiation of natural vegetation: An experimental facility, procedures and dosimetry. *Health Phys.* **12**(10):1467–1474.

McCormick, J. F., and R. B. Platt. 1962. Effects of ionizing radiation on a natural plant community. *Radiat. Bot.* **2**(3/4):161–188.

McCormick, J. F., and W. N. Rushing. 1964. Differential radiation sensitivities of races of *Sedum pulchellum* Michx.: A useful method of plant identification. *Radiat. Bot.* **4**(3):247–251.

McEnery, M., and J. J. Lee. 1970. Tracer studies on calcium and strontium mineralization and mineral cycling in two species of foraminifera, *Rosalina leei* and *Spiroloculina hyalina. Limnol. Oceanogr.* **15**(2):173–182.

McHenry, J. R. 1969. Use of tracer technique in soil erosion research. *Isot. Radiat. Technol.* **6**(3):280–287.

McMahan, J. W., and C. N. Wright. 1973. Field measurement of cesium-137 in deer. U.S. AEC, E. I. du Pont de Nemours, Rep. DPSPU-73-30-8. 4 pp.

Meeks, R. L. 1968. The accumulation of ^{36}Cl ring-labeled DDT in a freshwater marsh. *J. Wildl. Manage.* **32**(2):376–398.

Mellinger, P. J. 1973. The comparative metabolism of two mercury compounds as environmental contaminants in the freshwater mussel, *Margaritifera margaritifera.* pp 173–180. In: *Trace Substances in Environmental Health*–VI (D. D. Hemphill, ed.) University of Missouri, Columbia.

Mellinger, P. J., and V. Schultz. 1975. Ionizing radiation and wild birds: A review. *CRC Crit. Rev. Environ. Control* **5**(3):397–421.

Meslow, F. C., and L. B. Keith. 1968. Demographic parameters of a snowshoe hare population. *J. Wildl. Manage.* **32**(4):812–834.

Metcalf, R. L. 1972. A model ecosystem for the evaluation of pesticide biodegradability and ecological magnification. *Outlook Agric.* **7**(2):55–59.

Michael, H. N., and E. K. Ralph (eds.). 1971. *Dating Techniques for the Archaeologist.* MIT Press, Cambridge. xii + 227 pp.

Michels, J. W. 1973. *Dating Methods in Archaeology.* Seminar Press, New York. xiv + 230 pp.

Miller, L. S. 1957. Tracing vole movements by radioactive excretory products. *Ecology* **38**(1):132–136.

Mitchell, J. E. 1972. An analysis of the beta-attenuation technique for estimating standing crop of prairie range. *J. Range Manage.* **25**(4):300–304.

Moghissi, A. A., and M. W. Carter. 1977. Chapt. 14. Radionuclides in environmental studies. pp. 659–687. In: *Radiotracer Techniques and Applications,* Vol. 1 (E. A. Evans and M. Muramatsu, eds.). Marcel Dekker, New York.

Monk, C. D. 1967. Radioisotope tagging through seed soaking. *Bull. Ga. Acad. Sci.* **25**(1):13–17.

Monk, C. D. 1971. Leaf decomposition and loss of ^{45}Ca from deciduous and evergreen trees. *Am. Midl. Nat.* **86**(2):379–384.

Moore, W. S., and S. Krishnaswami. 1972. Coral growth rates using ^{228}Ra and ^{210}Pb. *Earth Planet. Sci. Lett.* **15**(2):187–190.

Myllymäki, A., A. Paasikallio, and U. Häkkinen. 1971. Analysis of a 'standard trapping' of *Microtus agrestis* (L.) with triple isotope marking outside the quadrat. *Ann. Zool. Fenn.* **8**(1):22–34.

Nellis, D. W., J. H. Jenkins, and A. D. Marshall. 1967. Radioactive zinc as a feces tag in rabbits, foxes, and bobcats. *Proc. Conf. Southeastern Association of Game and Fish Commissioners.* **21**:205–207.

Nelson, D. J., N. R. Kevern, J. L. Wilhm, and N. A. Griffith. 1969. Estimates of periphyton mass and stream bottom area using phosphorus-32. *Water Res.* **3**(5):367–373.

Nelson, D. M., P. F. Gustafson and J. Sedlet. 1970. Fallout radionuclides as tracers of lake mixing. *Proc. Conf. on Great Lakes Research* **13**(1): 490–494.

Nelson, J. L., R. W. Perkins, and W. L. Haushild. 1966. Determination of Columbia River flow times downstream from Pasco, Washington, using radioactive tracers introduced by the Hanford reactors. *Water Resour. Res.* **2**(1):31–39.

Nelson, V. A., and A. H. Seymour. 1972. Oyster research with radionuclides: A review of selected literature. *Proc. Natl. Shellfish. Assoc.* **62**:89–94.

Neyfakh, A. A. 1959. X-ray inactivation of nuclei as a method for studying their function in the early development of fishes. *J. Embryol. Exp. Morphol.* **7**(2):173–192.

Nishimura, M., N. Urakawa, and M. Ikeda. 1971. An autoradiographic study on the distribution of mercury and its transfer to the egg in the laying quail. *Jpn. J. Pharmacol.* **21**(5):651–659.

O'Brien, R. D., and L. S. Wolfe. 1964a. Chapt. 3. Tagging. pp. 55–69. In: *Radiation, Radioactivity, and Insects.* Academic Press, New York.

O'Brien, R. D., and L. S. Wolfe. 1964b. *Radiation, Radioactivity, and Insects. (Monograph Series on Radiation Biology.)* Academic Press, New York. xv + 211 pp.

Odum, E. P., and F. B. Golley. 1963. Radioactive tracers as an aid to the measurement of energy flow at the population level in nature. pp. 403–410. In: *Radioecology* (V. Schultz and A. W. Klement, Jr., eds.). Reinhold, New York.

Odum, E. P., and E. J. Kuenzler. 1963. Experimental isolation of food chains in an old-field ecosystem with the use of phosphorus-32. pp.113–120. In: *Radioecology* (V. Schultz and A. W. Klement, Jr., eds.) Reinhold, New York.

Odum, E. P., and A. J. Pontin. 1961. Population density of the underground ant, *Lasius flavus*, as determined by tagging with P^{32}. *Ecology* **42**(1):186–188.

Odum, H. T., and G. Drewry. 1970. The cesium source at El Verde. pp. C-23–C-36. In: *A Tropical Rain Forest: A Study of Irradiation and Ecology at El Verde, Puerto Rico* (H. T. Odum and R. F. Pigeon, eds.) U.S. AEC Rep. TID-24270.

O'Farrell, T. P., and P. B. Dunaway. 1967. Incorporation and tissue distribution of a thymidine analog in the cotton rat *Sigmodon hispidus*. *Comp. Biochem. Physiol.* **22**(2):435–450.

Olson, J. S. 1968. Use of tracer techniques for the study of biogeochemical cycles. pp. 271–288. In: *Functioning of Terrestrial Ecosystems at the Primary Production Level* (F. E. Eckardt, ed.) UNESCO, Paris.

Olson, J. S., and D. A. Crossley, Jr. 1963. Tracer studies of the breakdown of forest litter. pp. 411–416. In: *Radioecology* (V. Schultz and A. W. Klement, Jr., eds.). Reinhold, New York.

Olsson, I. U. 1968. Modern aspects of radiocarbon datings. *Earth-Sci. Rev.* **4**(3):203–218.

Osborn, E. T., E. T. Lyons, and L. O. Timblin, Jr. 1954. Studies of herbicidal action on aquatic weeds using radioactive 2,4-D-1-C^{14}. Engineering Laboratories, Bureau of Reclamation, Denver, Laboratory Rep. SI-4. 17pp., 16 figs.

Osterberg, C., N. Cutshall, and J. Cronin. 1965. Chromium-51 as a radioactive tracer of Columbia River water at sea. *Science* **150**(3703):1585–1587.

Paris, O. H. 1965. Vagility of P^{32}-labelled isopods in grassland. *Ecology* **46**(5):635–648.

Paris, O. H., and A. Sikora. 1965. Radiotracer demonstration of isopod herbivory. *Ecology* **46**(5):729–734.

Pendleton, R. C. 1956. Labeling animals with radioisotopes. *Ecology* **37**(4):686–689.

Pendleton, R. C., and A. W. Grundmann. 1954. Use of ^{32}P in tracing some insect–plant relationships of the thistle, *Cirsium undulatum*. *Ecology* **35**(2):187–191.

Pendleton, R. C., and E. W. Smart. 1954. A study of the food relations of the least chub, *Iotichthys phlegethontis* (Cope), using radioactive phosphorus. *J. Wildl. Manage.* **18**(2):226–228.

Pennington, W., R. S. Cambray, and E. M. Fisher. 1973. Observations on lake sediments using fallout ^{137}Cs as a tracer. *Nature (London)* **242**(5396):324–326.

Peterle, T. J. 1966. The use of isotopes to study pesticide translocation in natural environments. *J. Appl. Ecol.* **3**(Suppl.):181–191.

Peters, D. S., and D. E. Hoss. 1974. A radioisotopic method of measuring food evacuation time in fish. *Trans. Am. Fish. Soc.* **103**(3):626–629.

Petrides, G. A. 1968. The use of 51-chromium in the determination of energy-flow and other digestive characteristics in animals. pp. 25–31. In: *Proc. Symp. Recent Adv. Trop. Ecol.*, Vol. 1 (Misra, R. M., and B. Gopal, eds.) International Society for Tropical Ecology, Banares Hindu University, Varanasi, India.

Pillay, K. K. S., and C. C. Thomas, Jr. 1971. Determination of the trace element levels in atmospheric pollutants by neutron activation analysis. *J. Radional. Chem.* **7**(1):107–118.

Piper, D. S., and G. G. Goles. 1969. Determination of trace elements in seawater by neutron activation analysis. *Anal. Chim. Acta* **47**(3):560–563.

Platt, R. B. 1963. Ecological effects of ionizing radiation on organisms, communities and ecosystems. pp. 243–255. In: *Radioecology* (V. Schultz and A. W. Klement, Jr., eds.). Reinhold, New York.

Platt, R. B., and J. A. Mohrbacher. 1959. Studies in radiation ecology. I. The program of study. *Bull. Ga. Acad. Sci.* **17**:1–50.

Platt, R. B., J. T. McGinnis, and J. J. Cowan. 1964. An automatically controlled outdoor gamma irradiation facility at Emory University. *Bull. Ga. Acad. Sci.* **22**(3/4):75–80.

Plummer, G. L., and J. B. Kethley. 1964. Foliar absorption of amino acids, peptides, and other nutrients by the pitcher plant, *Sarracenia flava. Bot. Gaz.* **125**(4):245–260.

Polikarpov, G. G., and V. P. Parchevskiy (eds.). 1972. *Metody Opredeleniya Radioaktivnosii (Methods of Determination of Radioactivity).* "Naukova Dumka" Kiev. 196 pp. (in Russian).

Polikarpov, G. G., and A. V. Tokareva. 1970. On the cellular cycle of dinoflagellatae *Peridinium trochoideum* (Stein.) and *Goniaulax polyedra* (Stein.). *Gidrobiol. Zh.* **6**(5):66–69 (Russian with English summary).

Price, K. R. 1965. A field method for studying root systems. *Health Phys.* **11**(12):1521–1525.

Punt, A., and P. J. van Nieuwenhoven. 1957. The use of radioactive bands in tracing hibernating bats. *Experientia* **13**(1):51–54.

Quink, T. F., H. G. Abbott, and W. J. Mellen. 1970. Locating tree seed caches of small mammals with a radioisotope. *For. Sci.* **16**(2):147–148.

Raaen, H. P. 1972. Environments and isotopes. Oak Ridge National Laboratory, U.S. AEC Rep. ORNL-11C-39. vii + 118 pp.

Radwan, M. A. 1967. Translocation and metabolismm of C^{14}-labeled tetramine by Douglas-fir, orchard grass, and blackberry. *For. Sci.* **13**(3):265–273.

Redemann, C. T., and R. W. Meikle. 1958. Isotope dilution techniques for the determination of pesticide residues. *Adv. Pest Control Res.* **2**:183–206.

Reed, J. R., and B. A. Martinedes. 1973. Uptake and retention of tungsten-181 by crayfish (*Cambarus longulus longerostris* Ort.) pp. 390–393. In: *Radionuclides in Ecosystems* (D. J. Nelson, ed.) U.S. AEC Rep. CONF-710501-P1.

Reichle, D. E. 1967. Radioisotope turnover and energy flow in terrestrial isopod populations. *Ecology* **48**(3):351–366.

Reichle, D. E. 1969. Measurement of elemental assimilation by animals from radioisotope retention patterns. *Ecology* **50**(6):1102–1104.

Reichle, D. E., and D. A. Crossley, Jr. 1967. Investigation on heterotrophic productivity in forest insect communities. pp. 563–587. In: *Secondary Productivity of Terrestrial Ecosystems,* Vol. 2 (K. Petrusewicz, ed.). Institute of Ecology, Polish Academy of Sciences, Warsaw.

Reichle, D. E., and D. A. Crossley, Jr. 1969. Trophic level concentrations of cesium-137, sodium, and potassium in forest arthropods. pp. 678–686. In: *Symposium on Radioecology* (D. J. Nelson and F. C. Evans, eds.). U.S. AEC Rep. CONF-670503.

Renfro, W. C., and S. W. Fowler. 1973. General recommendation for designing marine radioecological experiments. *Health Phys.* **24**(5):572–573.

Rerabek, J., and A. Bubenik. 1963. The metabolism of phosphorus and iodine in deer. Unpublished Czech report. (English translation: AEC-tr-5631. v + 51 pp.)

Rice, T. R. 1965. Radioisotope techniques in fishery research. *Trans. North Am. Wildl. Conf.* **30**:66–75.

Rice, T. R., and R. J. Smith. 1958. Filtering rates of the hard clam *(Venus mercenaria)* determined with radioactive phytoplankton. *U.S. Fish Wildl. Serv. Fish. Bull.***58**(129):73–82.

Riekerk, H., and S. P. Gessel. 1965. Mineral cycling in a Douglas fir forest stand. *Health Phys.* **11**(12):1363–1369.

Rigler, F. H. 1961. The uptake and release of inorganic phosphorus by *Daphnia magna* Straus. *Limnol. Oceanogr.* **6**(2):165–174.

Roberts, E. F., and D. P. Snyder. 1973. Use of iodine-125 for identifying mother–offspring relationships in the eastern chipmunk, *Tamias striatus.* pp. 274–281. In: *Radionuclides in Ecosystems* (D. J. Nelson, ed.). U.S. AEC Rep. CONF-710501-P1.

Rogers, A. W. 1973. *Techniques of Autoradiography*. Elsevier, New York. xi + 372 pp.

Romberg, G. P., and W. C. Renfro. 1973. Radioactivity in juvenile Columbia River salmon: A model to distinguish differences in movement and feeding habits. *Trans. Am. Fish. Soc.* **102**(2):317–322.

Rongstad, O. J. 1965. Calcium-45 labeling of mammals for use in population studies. *Health Phys.* **11**(12):1543–1556.

Rose, F. L., and C. E. Cushing. 1970. Periphyton: Autoradiography of zinc-65 adsorption. *Science* **168**(3931):576–577.

Rosenthal, H. L. 1957. The metabolism of strontium-90 and calcium-45 by *Lebistes*. *Biol. Bull.* **113**(3):442–450.

Rudolph, T. D. (ed.), 1974. *The Enterprise, Wisconsin, Radiation Forest: Preirradiation Ecological Studies*. U.S. AEC Rep. TID-26113. v + 150 pp.

Saha, J. G. 1975. Metabolism of (^{14}C)-lindane in plants and animals. pp. 149–156. In: *Origin and Fate of Chemical Residues in Food, Agriculture and Fisheries*. International Atomic Energy Agency, Vienna Panel Proceedings Series. Publ. No. STI/PUB/399.

Salmonson, B. J., R. W. Blank, and R. L. Nelson. 1974. Description of experimental plot design of site L and the control area. pp. 17–31. In: *The Enterprise, Wisconsin, Radiation Forest: Preirradiation Ecological Studies* (T. D. Rudolph, ed.). U.S. AEC Rep. TID-26113.

Schreck, C. B. 1973. Uptake of ^{3}H-testosterone and influence of an antiandrogen in tissues of rainbow trout *(Salmo gairdneri)*. *Gen. Comp. Endocrinol.* **21**(1):60–68.

Schultz, S. L., and V. Schultz. 1975. *Nuclear Technology in Archaeology: Partial Bibliography*. U.S. ERDA Rep. TID-3920. i + 50 pp.

Schultz, V. 1969. *Ecological Techniques Utilizing Radionuclides and Ionizing Radiation: A selected Bibliography*. U.S. AEC Rep. RLO-2213-1. iv + 252 pp.

Schultz, V. 1972. *Ecological Techniques Utilizing Radionuclides and Ionizing Radiation: A Selected Bibliography*. U.S. AEC Rep. RLO-2213-1 (Suppl. 1). i + 129 pp.

Schultz, V. 1974. *Ionizing Radiation and Wild Birds: A Selected Bibliography*. U.S. ERDA Rep. TID-3919. i + 21 pp.

Schultz, V. 1975. *Ecological Techniques Utilizing Radionuclides and Ionizing Radiation: A Selected Bibliography*. U.S. ERDA Rep. RLO-2213 (Suppl. 2). i + 67 pp.

Schultz, V., and F. W. Whicker. 1972. *Ecological Aspects of the Nuclear Age: Selected Readings in Radiation Ecology*. U.S. AEC Rep. TID-25978. 588 pp.

Schulze, W. 1969. Activation analysis: Some basic principles. pp. 1–36. In: *Advances in Activation Analysis*, Vol. 1 (J. M. A. Lenihan and S. J. Thomson, eds.). Academic Press, New York.

Schwoerbel, J. 1970. *Methods of Hydrobiology*. Pergamon Press, New York. ix + 200 pp.

Scott, D. P. 1961. Radioactive iron as a fish mark. *J. Fish. Res. Board Can.* **18**(3):383–391.

Sedell, J. F. 1973. Feeding rates and food utilization of stream caddisfly larvae of the genus *Neophylax* (Trichoptera: Limnephilidae) using cobalt-60 and carbon-14. pp 486–491. In: *Radionuclides in Ecosystems* (D. J. Nelson, ed.). U.S. AEC Rep. CONF-710501-P1.

Selby, J. M., C. A. Willis, B. M. Bowen, and J. H. Edgerton. 1961. Radiation effects of a 10-MW reactor on environs of the Georgia Nuclear Laboratories. *Health Phys.* **6**(3/4):126–135.

Seymour, A. H. 1958. The use of radioisotopes as a tag for fish. *Proc. Gulf Caribbean Fish. Inst.* **10**:118–125.

Seymour, A. H. 1964. Contributions of radionuclides to our understanding of aquatic ecosystems. *Verh. Int. Ver. Limnol.* **15**(1):227–236.

Shilling, C. W., and M. T. Shilling. 1964. *Atomic Energy Encyclopedia in the Life Sciences*. W. B. Saunders, Philadelphia. xxvi + 474 pp.

Shoop, C. R. 1971. A method for short-term marking of amphibians with 24-sodium. *Copeia* **1971**(2):371.

Shoop, C. R., and T. L. Doty. 1972. Migratory orientation by marbled salamanders *(Ambystoma opacum)* near a breeding area. *Behav. Biol.* **7**(1):131–136.

Short, Z. F., P. R. Olson, R. F. Palumbo, J. R. Donaldson, and F. G. Lowman. 1973. Uptake of molybdenum, marked with ⁹⁹Mo, by the biota of Fern Lake, Washington, in a laboratory and a field experiment. pp 474–485. In: *Radionuclides in Ecosystems* (D. J. Nelson, ed.). U.S. AEC Rep. CONF-710501-P1.

Smigel, B. W., W. Jester, J. Blomgren, K. W. Prasad, and M. L. Rosenzweig. 1974. Dietary analysis in granivores through the use of neutron activation. *Ecology* **55**(2):340–349.

Sonenshine, D. E. 1968. Radioisotopes in studies on the ecology of tick vectors of disease. pp. 31–51. In: *Isotopes and Radiation in Entomology*. International Atomic Energy Agency, Vienna. Publ. No. STI/PUB/166.

Sonenshine, D. E., and G. M. Clark, 1968. Field trials on radioisotope tagging of ticks. *J. Med. Entomol.* **5**(2):229–235.

Sonenshine, D. E., and C. E. Yunker. 1968. Radiolabeling of tick progeny by inoculation of procreant females. *J. Econ. Entomol.* **61**(6):*1612–1617.*

Sorokin, Ya. I. 1968. The use of ¹⁴C in the study of nutrition of aquatic animals. *Int. Assoc. Theor. Appl. Limnol., Commun.* No. 16. 41 pp.

Southwood, T. R. E. 1966. Chapt. 3. Absolute population estimates using marking techniques. Methods of marking animals. pp 57–75. In: *Ecological Methods*. Methuen, London.

Sparrow, A. H. 1960. Use of large sources of ionizing radiation in botanical research and some possible practical applications. pp. 195–218. In: *Large Radiation Sources in Industry*, Vol. 2. International Atomic Energy Agency, Vienna. Publ. No. STI/PUB/12.

Sparrow, A. H., and G. M. Woodwell. 1963. Prediction of the sensitivity of plants to chronic gamma irradiation. pp. 257–270. In: *Radioecology* (V. Schultz and A. W. Klement, Jr., eds.). Reinhold, New York.

Spurny, Z., and J. Sulcova. 1973. Bibliography of thermoluminescent dosimetry (1968–1972). *Health Phys.* **24**(5):573–587.

Stark, N. 1973. Radiotracer studies of nutrient cycling pathways. pp. 225–231. In: *Radionuclides in Ecosystems* (D. J. Nelson, ed.). U.S. AEC Rep. CONF-710501-P1.

Steemann Nielsen, E. 1963. Productivity, definition and measurement. pp. 129–164. In: *The Sea*, Vol. 2 (M. N. Hill, ed.). Interscience, New York.

Stephens, G. C. 1962. Uptake of organic material by aquatic invertebrates. I. Uptake of glucose by the solitary coral, *Fungia scutaria. Biol. Bull* **123**(3):648–659.

Stoddart, D. M. 1970. Individual range, dispersion and dispersal in a population of water voles *(Arvicola terrestris* L.). *J. Anim. Ecol.* **39**(2):403–425.

Storteir, S., and A. Palmgren. 1971. 'Long-term' recording of incubating rhythm and feeding frequency with the aid of radioactive tagging. *Ornis Fenn.* **48**(1):33–35 (in Swedish with English summary).

Stout, G. E. (ed.). 1967. *Isotope Techniques in the Hydrologic Cycle*. American Geophysical Union, Washington, D.C., Geophys. Monogr. Ser. No. 11. 199 pp.

Strickland, J. D. H. 1960. *Measuring the Production of Marine Phytoplankton*. Fisheries Research Board of Canada, Ottawa, Bulletin No. 122. viii + 172 pp.

Sudia, T. W., and A. J. Linck. 1963. Methods for introducing radionuclides into plants. pp 417–425. In: *Radioecology* (V. Schultz and A. W. Klement, Jr., eds.). Reinhold, New York.

Suess, H. E. 1973. Natural radiocarbon. *Endeavour* **32**(115):34–38.

Tanner, J. T., and W. W. Tolbert. 1975. Optical and gamma radiation measurements of the effects of chlorinated hydrocarbons on egg shells of red-winged blackbirds. *Wilson Bull.* **87**(3):426–427.

Tester, J. R. 1963. Techniques for studying movements of vertebrates in the field. pp. 445–450. In: *Radioecology* (V. Schultz and A. W. Klement, Jr., eds.). Reinhold, New York.

Thatcher, L. L., and J. O. Johnson. 1973. Determination of trace elements in water and aquatic biota by neutron activation analysis. pp. 277–298. In: *Bioassay Techniques and Environmental Chemistry* (G. E. Glass, ed.). Ann Arbor Science Publishers, Ann Arbor.

Thomas, W. A. 1968. Calcium distribution in leaves: Autoradiography versus chemical analysis. *Int. J. Appl. Radiat. Isot.* **19**(6):544–545.

Thomas, W. A. 1970. Retention of calcium-45 by dogwood trees. *Plant Physiol.* **45**(4):510–511.

Tite, M. S. 1972. *Methods of Physical Examination in Archaeology*. Seminar Press, New York. xxx + 389 pp.

Tiwari, P. N. 1974. *Fundamentals of Nuclear Science: With Applications in Agriculture and Biology*. John Wiley, New York. xi + 167 pp.

Turner, F. B., and J. R. Lannom, Jr. 1968. Radiation doses sustained by lizards in a continuously irradiated natural enclosure. *Ecology* **49**(3):548–551.

Twigg, G. I., and H. Miller. 1963. The use of calcium^{45} as an agent for labeling rat populations. *J. Mammal.* **44**(3):335–337.

Verkhovskaya, I. N. (ed.). 1971. *Metody Radioekologicheskikh Issledovanii (Methods of Radioecological Investigation)*. Atom Press, Moscow. 258 pp. (in Russian).

Vollenweider, R. A. (ed.). 1969. *A Manual on Methods for Measuring Primary Production in Aquatic Environments*. IBP Handbook No. 12. Blackwell, Oxford, England. xvi + 213 pp.

Waid, J. S., K. J. Preston, and P. J. Harris. 1973. Autoradiographic techniques to detect active microbial-cells in natural habitats. *Bull. Ecol. Res. Comm. (Stockholm)* **17**:317–322.

Wang, C. H., and D. L. Willis. 1965. *Radiotracer Methodology in Biological Science*. Prentice-Hall, Englewood Cliffs, New Jersey. xvii + 382 pp.

Ward, P. R. B. 1967. Continuous recording of bird nesting visits using radioactive tagging. *Nature (London)* **216**(5115):592–593.

Ward, P. R. B. 1968. Radioactive labeling of bird nests. *Umsch. Wiss. Tech.* **68**(7):217 (in German).

Watson, D. G., and W. L. Templeton. 1973. Thermoluminescent dosimetry of aquatic organisms. pp. 1125–1130. In: *Radionuclides in Ecosystems* (D. J. Nelson, ed.). U.S. AEC Rep. CONF-710501-P2.

Webster, E. J. 1967. An autoradiographic study of invertebrate uptake of DDT-C1^{36}. *Ohio J. Sci.* **67**(5):300–307.

Wetzel, R. G. 1966. Techniques and problems of primary productivity measurements in higher aquatic plants and periphyton. pp. 249–267. In: *Primary Productivity in Aquatic Environments* (C. R. Goldman, ed.). University of California Press, Berkeley.

Whittaker, R. H. 1961. Experiments with radiophosphorus tracer in aquarium microcosms. *Ecol. Monogr.* **31**(2):157–188.

Wiegert, R. G., and E. P. Odum. 1969. Radionuclide tracer measurement of food web diversity in nature. pp 709–710. In: *Symposium on Radioecology* (D. J. Nelson and F. C. Evans, eds.). U.S. AEC Rep. CONF-670503.

Wiegert, R. G., E. P. Odum, and J. H. Schnell. 1967. Forb–arthropod food chains in a one-year experimental field. *Ecology* **48**(1):75–83.

Wiegert, R. G., D. C. Coleman, and E. P. Odum. 1970. Energetics of the litter-soil subsystem. pp 93–98. In: *Methods of Study in Soil Ecology*. UNESCO, Paris.

Wilkinson, D. H. 1950. Flight records, a technique for the study of bird navigation. *J. Exp. Biol.* **27**(2):192–197.

Williams, E. C., Jr., and D. E. Reichle. 1968. Radioactive tracers in the study of energy turnover by a grazing insect (*Chrysochus auratus* Fab., Coleoptera Chrysomelidae). *Oikos* **19**(1):10–18.

Williams, P. M., and T. W. Linick. 1975. Cycling of organic carbon in the ocean: Use of naturally occurring radiocarbon as a long and short term tracer. pp. 153–166. In: *Isotope Ratios as Pollutant Source and Behavior Indicators*. International Atomic Energy Agency, Vienna. Publ. No. STI/PUB/382.

Winteringham, F. P. W. 1960. The labeled pool technique with particular reference to pesticide research. *Adv. Pest Control Res.* **3**:75–127.

Witherspoon, J. P., Jr. 1963. Cycling of cesium-134 in white oak trees on sites of contrasting soil type and moisture. I. 1960 growing season. pp. 127–132. In: *Radioecology* (V. Schultz and A. W. Klement, Jr., eds.). Reinhold, New York.

Witherspoon, J. P., Jr. 1964. Cycling of cesium-134 in white oak trees. *Ecol. Monogr.* **34**(4):403–420.

Witherspoon, J. P., Jr., S. I. Auerbach, and J. S. Olson. 1962. *Cycling of Cesium-134 in White Oak Trees on Sites of Contrasting Soil Type and Moisture.* U.S. AEC, Oak Ridge National Laboratory, Rep. ORNL-3328. xv + 139 pp.

Wolfe, G. 1964. *Isotopes in Biology.* Academic Press, New York. x + 173 pp.

Woods, F. W., and K. Brock. 1964. Interspecific transfer of Ca-45 and P-32 by root systems. *Ecology* **45**(4):886–889.

Woods, F. W., and D. O'Neal. 1965. Tritiated water as a tool for ecological field studies. *Science* **147**(3654):148–149.

Woodwell, G. M. 1963. Design of the Brookhaven experiment on the effects of ionizing radiation on a terrestrial ecosystem. *Radiat. Bot.* **3**(2):125–133.

Woodwell, G. M., and E. C. Hammond. 1962. *A Descriptive Technique for Study of the Effects of Chronic Ionizing Radiation on a Forest Ecological System.* U.S. AEC, Brookhaven National Laboratory, Rep. BNL-751(T-251). 13 pp.

Woodwell, G. M., and E. V. Pecan (eds.). 1973. *Carbon and the Biosphere.* Proceedings of the 24th Brookhaven Symposium in Biology, Upton, New York, May 16–18, 1972. U.S. AEC Symp. Ser. No. 30. vii + 392 pp.

York, D., and R. M. Farquhar. 1972. *The Earth's Age and Geochronology.* Pergamon Press, New York. viii + 178 pp.

Yousef, M. K., H. D. Johnson, W. G. Bradley, and S. M. Seif. 1974. Tritiated water-turnover rate in rodents: Desert and mountain. *Physiol. Zool.* **47** (3):153–162.

Additional Readings

Allan, J. D. 1973. Competition and the relative abundances of two cladocerans. *Ecology* **54**(3):484–498. [^{14}C]

Alldredge, A. W., and F. W. Whicker. 1972. A method for measuring soil erosion and deposition with beta particle attenuation. *J. Range Manage.* **25**(5):393–398.

Anonymous. 1968. *International Symposium on the Application of Neutron Activation Analysis in Oceanography*, Brussels, June 17–22, 1968. Institut Royal des Sciences Naturelles de Belgique, Bruxelles. 218 pp. [*Nucl. Sci. Abstr.* **25**(8):15535.]

Anonymous. 1975. *Tracer Techniques (1974–1977): Commonwealth Bureau of Soils Annotated Bibliography*. Commonwealth Agricultural Bureaux, Slough, England. 43 pp. [*Nucl. Sci. Abstr.* **32**(5):11869.]

Ashby, W. C., J. N. Beggs, J. Kastner, B. G. Oltman, and H. Moses. 1967. Ecological dosimetry: Radiation levels influenced by plant growth. *Science* **155**(3768):1430–1432.

Attix, F. H., and W. C. Roesch (eds.). 1966. *Radiation Dosimetry*. Vol. II. *Instrumentation*. Academic Press, New York. xviii + 462 pp.

Attix, F. H., and W. C. Roesch (eds.). 1968. *Radiation Dosimetry*, 2nd ed. Vol. 1. *Fundamentals*. Academic Press, New York. xviii + 405 pp.

Attix, F. H., and E. Tochilin (eds.). 1969. *Radiation Dosimetry*, 2nd ed. Vol. III. *Sources, Fields, Measurements, and Applications*. Academic Press, New York. xix + 943 pp.

Avarguès, M., L. Foulquier, A. Vilquin, A. Lambrechts, and G. Moisan. 1973. Comparative study of the experimental contamination in marine and freshwater lamellibranch molluscs by cesium 137. *Radioprotection* **8**(1):19–32 (in French with English abstract).

Barber, S. A., and P. G. Ozanne. 1970. Autoradiographic evidence for the differential effect of four plant species in altering the calcium content of the rhizosphere soil. *Proc. Soil Sci. Soc. Am.* **34**(4):635.

Barbour, R. W. 1963. *Microtus:* A simple method of recording time spent in the nest. *Science* **141**(3582):41. [^{60}Co]

Barker, H. 1970. Critical assessment of radiocarbon dating. *Philos. Trans. R. Soc. London Ser. A* **269**:37–45.

Barrington, E. J. W., and B. B. Rawdon. 1967. Influence of thyroxine upon the uptake of S^{35}-labelled sulphate into the branchial arch skeleton of the rainbow trout (*Salmo gairdneri*). *Gen. Comp. Endocrinol.* **9**(1):116–128.

Beck, J. S., and T. R. Manney. 1962. Neutron activation analysis for phosphorus in a study of development in a beetle wing. *Science* **137**(3533):865–866.

Begemann, F., and W. F. Libby. 1957. Continental water balance, ground-water inventory and storage times, surface ocean mixing rates and world-wide water circulation patterns from cosmic-ray and bomb tritium. *Geochim. Cosmochim. Acta* **12**(4):277–296.

Berthet, P. L. 1964. Field study of the mobility of Oribatei (Acari), using radioactive tagging. *J. Anim. Ecol.* **33**(3):443–449.

Bevelander, G. 1952. Calcification in molluscs. III. Intake and deposition of Ca^{45} and P^{32} in relation to shell formation. *Biol. Bull.* **102**(1):9–15.

Bierly, E. W. 1967. The application of isotopes to some problems in atmospheric sciences. pp. 37–46. In: *Isotope Techniques in the Hydrologic Cycle* (G. E. Stout, ed.). American Geophysical Union, Washington, D. C., Geophys. Monogr. Ser. No. 11.

Blintz, G. L. 1969. Sodium-22 retention as a function of water intake by *Citellus lateralis*. pp. 45–52. In: *Physiological Systems in Semiarid Environments* (C. C. Hoff and M. L. Riedesel, eds.). University of New Mexico Press, Albuquerque.

Bochvar, I. A., I. B. Keirim-Markos, and A. A. Moiseyev. 1971. Using thermoluminescent alumophosphatic glass dosimeters in experimental investigations. pp. 223–230. In: *Methods of Radioecological Investigations* (I. N. Verkhovskaya, ed.). Atom Press, Moscow (in Russian).

Boggie, R., R. F. Hunter, and A. H. Knight. 1958. Studies of the root development of plants in the field using radioactive tracers. *J. Ecol.* **46**(3):621–639.

Bogoyavlenskaya, M. P., I. F. Vel'tishcheva, and G. S. Karzinkin. 1972. Characteristic features of metabolism and the incorporation of C^{14} into organic compounds in sturgeons reared from large and small eggs. *J. Ichthyol.* **12**(1):130–134.

Bonfanti, G., and C. Triulzi. 1974. *Beta and Gamma Detection Efficiencies for Some Typical Radionuclides in Sources of Different Matrix and Geometry*. CISE, Documentation Service, Milan, Italy, Publ. No. CISE-N-169. 15 pp., 19 figs.

Bormann, F. H. 1966. The structure, function, and ecological significance of root grafts in *Pinus strobus* L. *Ecol. Monogr.* **36**(1):1–26. [^{32}P]

Breymeyer, A., and E. P. Odum. 1969. Transfer and bioelimination of tracer ^{65}Zn during predation by spiders on labeled flies. pp. 715–720. In: *Symposium on Radioecology* (D. J. Nelson and F. C. Evans, eds.). U.S. AEC Rep. CONF-670503.

Broecker, W. S., J. Cromwell, and Y. H. Li. 1968. Rates of vertical eddy diffusion near the ocean floor based on measurements of the distribution of excess ^{222}Rn. *Earth Planet. Sci. Lett.* **5**(2):101–105.

Bryan, G. W., and E. Ward. 1965. The absorption and loss of radioactive and non-radioactive manganese by the lobster *Homarus vulgaris*. *J. Mar. Biol. Assoc. U.K.* **45**(1):65–69.

Bul'on, V. V. 1972. Use of Sorokin's apparatus to determine the rate of gas exchange in aquatic animals by the radiocarbon method. *Gidrobiol. Zh.* **8**(4):91–97. [English translation. *Hydrobiol. J.* **8**(4):75–81 (1972).]

Burnett, A. M., W. H. Mason, and S. T. Rhodes. 1969. Reingestion of feces and excretion rates of Zn^{65} in *Popilius disjunctus* versus *Cryptocerus punctulatus*. *Ecology* **50**(6):1094–1096.

Burrage, R. H., and J. G. Saha. 1972. Insecticide residues in pheasants after being fed on wheat seed treated with heptachlor and (^{14}C)-lindane. *J. Econ. Entomol.* **65**(4):1013–1017.

Burrows, W. D., and P. A. Krenkel. 1973. Studies on uptake and loss of methylmercury-203 by bluegills (*Lepomis macrochirus* Raf.). *Environ. Sci. Technol.* **7**(13):1127–1130.

Cammen, L. M. 1977. On the use of liquid scintillation counting of ^{51}Cr and ^{14}C in the twin tracer method of measuring assimilation efficiency. *Oecologia* **30**:249–251.

Carlson, C. A., and M. H. Shealy, Jr. 1972. Marking larval largemouth bass with radiostrontium. *J. Fish. Res. Board Can.* **29**(4):455–458.

Carlsson, S., K. Linden, R. Bertil, and R. Persson. 1971. Use of radionuclides for tracing the origin of marine oil pollution. pp. 361–369. In: *Nuclear Techniques in Environmental Pollution*. International Atomic Energy Agency, Vienna. Publ. No. STI/PUB/268.

Carrick, R. 1956. Radioiodine as an indicator of free feeding of the rabbit, *Oryctolagus cuniculus* (L.). *CSIRO Wildl. Res. (Aust.)* **1**:106–113.

Channell, J. K., and P. Kruger. 1969. Post-sampling activation analysis of stable nuclides for estuary water tracing. pp. 81–86. In: *Modern Trends in Activation Analysis*, Vol. 1 (J. R. DeVoe and P. D. LaFleur, eds.). U.S. National Bureau of Standards Rep. NBS-Spec. Publ.-312.

Chant, G. D., and W. F. Baldwin. 1972. Dispersal and longevity of mosquitoes tagged with ^{32}P. *Can. Entomol.* **104**(6):941–944.

Chew, R. M., and J. G. Hemington. 1973. Turnover of zinc-65 as an index of energy metabolism of *Perognathus longimembris*, the little pocket mouse. pp. 247–252. In: *Radionuclides in Ecosystems* (D. J. Nelson, ed.). U.S. AEC Rep. CONF-710501-P1.

Clayton, C. G., and D. B. Smith. 1963. A comparison of radioisotope methods for river flow measurement. pp. 1–24. In: *Radioisotopes in Hydrology*. International Atomic Energy Agency, Vienna. Publ. STI/PUB/71.

Coffin, C. C., F. R. Hayes, L. H. Jodrey, and S. G. Whiteway. 1949. Exchange of materials in a lake as studied by the addition of radioactive phosphorus. *Can. J. Res. Sect. D* **27**:207–222.

Coleman, D. C. 1970. Food webs of small arthropods of a broomsedge field studied with radio-isotope labelled fungi. pp. 203–207. In: *Methods of Study in Soil Ecology*. UNESCO, Paris.

Constantine, D. G., J. A. Jensen, and E. S. Tierkel. 1959. The use of radiolabeling in determining prey–predator relationships. *J. Mammal.* **40**(2):240–242.

Corey, J. C., A. R. Boulogne, and J. H. Horton. 1970. Determination of soil density and water content by fast neutrons and gamma rays. *Water Resour. Res.* **6**(1):223–229.

Courtois, G. 1967. Radioisotopes in sedimentology. pp. 117–164. In: *Isotopes in Hydrology*. International Atomic Energy Agency, Vienna. Publ. No. STI/PUB/141.

Craig, H. 1957. Isotopic tracer techniques for measurement of physical and chemical processes in the sea and the atmosphere. pp. 103–120. In: *The Effects of Atomic Radiation on Oceanography and Fisheries*. National Academy of Sciences–National Research Council, Washington, D.C. Publ. No. 551.

Crossley, D. A., Jr. 1966. Radioisotope measurement of food consumption by a leaf beetle species, *Chrysomela knabi* Brown. *Ecology* **47**(1):1–8.

Crossley, D. A., Jr., and V. A. Merchant. 1971. Feeding by caeculid mites on fungus demonstrated with radioactive tracers. *Ann. Entomol. Soc. Am.* **64**(4):760–762.

Crossley, D. A., Jr., and R. I. Van Hook, Jr. 1970. Energy assimilation by the house cricket, *Acheta domesticus*, measured with radioactive chromium-51. *Ann. Entomol. Soc. Am.* **63**(2):512–515.

Crozaz, G. 1967. Dating of glaciers by lead-210. pp. 385–393. In: *Radioactive Dating and Methods of Low-Level Counting*. International Atomic Energy Agency, Vienna. Publ. No. STI/PUB/152 (in French with English abstract).

Dansgaard, W., H. B. Clausen, and A. Aarkrog. 1966. The ^{32}Si fallout in Scandinavia: A new method for ice dating. *Tellus* **18**(2/3):187–191.

de la Cruz, A. A., and R. G. Wiegert. 1967. 32-Phosphorus tracer studies of a horseweed–aphid–ant food chain. *Am. Midl. Nat.* **77**(2):501–509.

Denny, M. J. S., and T. J. Dawson. 1973. A field technique for studying water metabolism of large marsupials. *J. Wildl. Manage.* **37**(4):574–578. [^{3}H]

Dent, J. N., and J. S. Kirby-Smith. 1963. Metamorphic physiology and morphology of the cave salamander *Gyrinophilus palleucus*. *Copeia* **1963**(1):119–130. [^{131}I]

DeVoe, J. R., and P. D. LaFleur (eds.). 1969. *Modern Trends in Activation Analysis*, Vol. I and II. Proceedings of the 1968 International Conference, National Bureau of Standards, Gaithersburg, Maryland, October 7–11, 1968. U.S. National Bureau of Standards Rep. NBS-Spec. Publ.-312. Vol. I: xvii + 671 pp.; Vol. II: xv + 673 pp.

Dobrokhotov. B. O., and V. Yu. Litvin. 1971. Radioactivity of pellets of *Falco tuninculus* L. after feeding on mice containing P^{32}. *Zool. Zh.* **50**(10):1591–1592 (in Russian with English summary).

Doty, M. S., and M. Oguri. 1959. The carbon-fourteen technique for determining primary plankton productivity. In: *Marine Biological Applications of Radioisotope Research Techniques. Pubbl. Stn. Zool. Napoli* **31**(Suppl.):70–94.

Draskovic, R., T. Tasovac, and R. Radosavljevic. 1971. Neutron activation analysis of the aquatic environment in the Danube. pp. 329–333. In: *Nuclear Techniques in Environmental Pollution*. International Atomic Energy Agency, Vienna. Publ. No. STI/PUB/268.

Drury, D. E., and J. G. Eales. 1968. The influence of temperature on histological and radiochemical measurements of thyroid activity in the eastern brook trout, *Salvelinus fontinalis* Mitchell. *Can. J. Zool.* **46**(1):1–9. [^{125}I]

Duggus, J. E., and A. H. Gold. 1967. Relationship of tracer-measured aphid feeding to acquisition of beet western yellows virus and to feeding inhibitors in plant extracts. *Phytopathology* **57**(11):1237–1241.

Dustan, G. G. 1966. Effects of tagging amounts of radioactive phosphorus on adults of the oriental fruit moth, *Grapholitha molesta* (Busck) (Lepidoptera: Tortricidae). *Can. Entomol.* **98**(3):305–311.

Duursma, E. K. 1976. Radioactive tracers in estuarine chemical studies. pp. 159–183. In: *Estuarine Chemistry* (J. D. Burton and P. G. Liss, eds.). Academic Press, London.

Dymond, J. 1969. Age determinations of deep-sea sediments: A comparison of three methods. *Earth Planet. Sci. Lett.* **6**(1):9–14.

Eales, J. G. 1969. *In vivo* uptake of radiothyroxine by the tissues of Atlantic salmon (*Salmo salar* L.) parr, presmolt, and smolt. *Can. J. Zool.* **47**(1):9–16.

Eyman, L. D., J. R. Trabalka, and F. N. Case. 1976. Plutonium-237 and -246: Their production and use as gamma tracers in research on plutonium kinetics in an aquatic consumer. pp. 193–203. In: *Environmental Toxicity of Aquatic Radionuclides: Models and Mechanisms* (M. W. Miller and J. N. Stannard, eds.). Ann Arbor Science Publishers, Ann Arbor.

Freely, H. W., A. Walton, C. R. Barnett, and F. Bazan. 1961. *The Potential Applications of Radioisotope Techniques to Water Resource Investigations and Utilization*. Isotopes, Inc., Westwood, New Jersey, U.S. AEC Rep. NYO-9040. xii + 340 pp.

Fink, B. A. 1957. Radioiodine: A method for measuring thyroid activity. *Auk* **74**(4):487–493.

Fleischer, R. L., J. R. M. Viertl, P. B. Price, and F. Aumento. 1971. A chronological test of ocean-bottom spreading in the North Atlantic. *Radiat. Effects* **11**(3–4):193–194. [Fission-track and K–Ar dating of basaltic glass]

Folsom, T. R., and A. C. Vine. 1957. On the tagging of water masses for the study of physical processes in the oceans. pp. 121–132. In: *The Effects of Atomic Radiation on Oceanography and Fisheries*. National Academy of Sciences–National Research Council, Washington, D.C. Publ. No. 551.

Folsom, T. R., R. Grismore, and D. R. Young. 1970. Long-lived γ-ray emitting nuclide silver-108m found in Pacific marine organisms and used for dating. *Nature (London)* **227**(5261):941–943.

Fowler, S. A., J. La Rosa, M. Heyraud, and W. C. Renfro. 1975. Effect of different radiotracer labelling techniques on radionuclide excretion from marine organisms. *Mar. Biol.* **30**(4):297–304.

French, N. R., B. G. Maza, and A. P. Aschwanden. 1966. Periodicity of desert rodent activity. *Science* **154**(3753):1194–1195. [Microthermoluminescent dosimeter]

French, R. L. 1964. A comparative study of radioactive source arrangements for simulating fallout gamma radiation fields. Radiation Research Associates, Inc., Fort Worth, Rep. AFRRI-CR-65-2. 111 pp. [*Nucl. Sci. Abstr.* **20**(13):23345]

Fritzsche, A., and C. Jupiter. 1975. *Development of Snow Water Equivalent Survey Methods Using Airborne Gamma Measurements: Research Progress for January 1975 through September 1975 and Suggested Directions for Future Work.* EG & G, Las Vegas. Publ. No. EGG-1183-1677. iv + 23 pp.

Gakstatter, J. H., and C. M. Weiss. 1967. The elimination of DDT-C^{14}, dieldrin-C^{14}, and lindane-C^{14} from fish following a single sublethal exposure in aquaria. *Trans. Am. Fish. Soc.* **96**(3):301–307.

Gist, C. A., and F. W. Whicker. 1971. Radioiodine uptake and retention by the mule deer thyroid. *J. Wildl. Manage.* **35**(3):461–468.

Gladney, E. S., D. B. Curtis, D. R. Perrin, J. W. Owens, and W. E. Goode. 1980. *Nuclear Techniques for the Chemical Analysis of Environmental Materials.* Los Alamos Scientific Laboratory, Los Alamos. Publ. No. LA-8192-MS. vi + 89 pp.

Godfrey, G. K. 1954. Use of radioactive isotopes in small-mammal ecology. *Nature (London)* **174**(4438):951–952.

Godfrey, G. K. 1955. A field study of the activity of the mole (*Talpa europaea*). *Ecology* **36**(4):678–685. [^{60}Co]

Gold, K. 1964. Aspects of marine dinoflagellate nutrition measured by C^{14} assimilation. *J. Protozool.* **11**(1):85–89.

Goldman, C. R. 1968. The use of absolute activity for eliminating serious errors in the measurement of primary productivity with C^{14}. *J. Cons. Int. Explor. Mer.* **32**(2):172–179.

Golley, F. B., R. G. Wiegert, and R. W. Walter. 1965. Excretion of orally administered zinc-65 by wild small mammals. *Health Phys.* **11**(8):719–722.

Gona, A. G. 1968. Radioiodine studies on prolactin action in tadpoles. *Gen. Comp. Endocrinol.* **11**(2):278–283.

Gösswald, K., and W. Kloft. 1963. Tracer experiments on food exchange in ants and termites. pp. 25–40. In: *Radiation and Radioisotopes Applied to Insects of Agricultural Importance.* International Atomic Energy Agency, Vienna. Publ. No. STI/PUB/74.

Graham, B. F., Jr. 1954. A technique for introducing radioactive isotopes into tree stems. *Ecology* **35**(3):415.

Graham, B. F., Jr. 1957. Labelling pollen of woody plants with radioactive isotopes. *Ecology* **38**(1):156–158.

Grauby, A., and A. Saas. 1974. Reclamation of saline, waterlogged and bog soils. The changes in the soils under the impact of reclamation. pp. 92–102. In: *Tenth International Congress of Soil Science,* Vol. X, Commission VI. Science Press, Moscow (in French with Russian, German, and English summaries).

Green, B. 1978. Estimation of food consumption in the dingo, *Canis familiaris dingo,* by means of ^{22}Na turnover. *Ecology* **59**(2):207–210.

Grigal, D. F. 1973. Calcium cycling: Diffusion into a forest soil. pp. 218–224. In: *Radionuclides in Ecosystems* (D. J. Nelson, ed.). U.S. AEC Rep. CONF-710501-P1. [^{45}Ca]

Grzenda, A. R., D. F. Paris, and W. J. Taylor. 1970. The uptake, metabolism, and elimination of chlorinated residues by goldfish (*Carassius auratus*) fed a ^{14}C-DDT contaminated diet. *Trans. Am. Fish. Soc.* **99**(2):385–396.

Guinn, V. P., and S. C. Bellanca. 1969. Neutron activation analysis identification of the source of oil pollution of waterways. pp. 93–97. In: *Modern Trends in Activation Analysis,* Vol. I (J. R. DeVoe and P. D. LaFleur, eds.). U.S. National Bureau of Standards Rep. NBS-Spec. Publ.-312.

Hakkinen, A., A. Myllymäki, and A. Paassikallio. 1970. Radiation risks and avoidance of hazards in connection with mass marking of small rodents with radio-isotopes. pp. 237–248. In: EPPO Publication Ser. A, No. 58, Helsinki, Finland.

Hakonson, T. E., A. F. Gallegos, and F. W. Whicker. 1975. Cesium kinetics data for estimating food consumption rates of trout. *Health Phys.* **29**(2):301–306. [Neutron activation]

Harris, E. 1957. Radiophosphorus metabolism in zooplankton and microorganisms. *Can. J. Zool.* **35**(6):769–782.

Hickman, C. P., Jr. 1972. Determination of the extracellular fluid volume of a euryhaline flounder by kinetic and net retention methods using tritium-labeled inulin. *Can. J. Zool.* **50**(12):1663–1671.

Higgs, D. A., and J. G. Eales. 1971. Iodide and thyroxine metabolism in the brook trout, *Salvelinus fontinalis* (Mitchill), during sustained exercise. *Can. J. Zool.* **49**(9):1255–1269. [^{125}I]

Hobson, L. A., W. J. Morris, and K. T. Pirquet. 1976. Theoretical and experimental analysis of the ^{14}C technique and its use in studies of primary production. *J. Fish. Res. Board Can.* **33**(8):1715–1721.

Holden, A. V. 1962. A study of the absorption of ^{14}C-labelled DDT from water by fish. *Ann. Appl. Biol.* **50**(3):467–477.

Holleman, D. F., and R. A. Dieterich. 1973. Body water content and turnover in several species of rodents as evaluated by the tritiated water method. *J. Mammal.* **54**(2):456–465.

Holleman, D. F., and J. R. Luick. 1978. Using radioecological data to determine prey selection by the Alaska wolf. pp. 673–681. In: *Environmental Chemistry and Cycling Processes* (D. C. Adriano and I. L. Brisbin, Jr., eds.). U.S. DOE Symp. Ser. 45, Rep. CONF-760429.

Hollibaugh, J. T., J. A. Fuhrman, and F. Azam. 1980. Radioactive labeling of natural assemblages of bacterioplankton for use in trophic studies. *Limnol. Oceanogr.* **25**(1):172–181.

Holm, N. W., and R. J. Berry (eds.). 1970. *Manual on Radiation Dosimetry.* Marcel Dekker, New York. xvi + 450 pp.

Holstein, B. 1971. Metabolism of intraperitoneally injected ^{14}C-histamine in the yellow eel (*Anguilla anguilla*). *Comp. Biochem. Physiol. A* **38**(2):435–441.

Hooper, F. F., and R. C. Ball. 1966. Bacterial transport of phosphorus in a stream ecosystem. pp. 535–549. In: *Disposal of Radioactive Wastes into Seas, Oceans and Surface Waters.* International Atomic Energy Agency, Vienna. Publ. No. STI/PUB/126. [^{32}P].

Hoss, D. E., D. S. Peters, W. F. Hettler, and L. C. Clements. 1978. Excretion rate of ^{65}Zn: Is it a useful tool for estimating metabolism of fish in the field? *J. Exp. Mar. Biol. Ecol.* **31**(3):241–252.

Huckabee, J. W., F. O. Cartan, G. S. Kennington, and F. J. Camenzind. 1973. Mercury concentration in the hair of coyotes and rodents in Jackson Hole, Wyoming. *Bull. Environ. Contam. Toxicol.* **9**(1):37–43. [Neutron Activation]

Hunding, C., and B. T. Hargrave. 1973. A comparison of benthic and microalgal production measured by C^{14} and oxygen methods. *J. Fish. Res. Board Can.* **30**(2):309–312.

Hutchinson, G. E., and V. T. Bowen. 1950. Limnological studies in Connecticut. IX. A quantitative radiochemical study of the phosphorus cycle in Linsley Pond. *Ecology* **31**(2):194–203.

Ilyenko, A. I., I. A. Ryabtsev, and D. E. Fedorov. 1975. A study of territorial conservatism in open-nesting passeriformes by radioactive marking of the population. *Zool. Zh.* **54**(11):1678–1686 (in Russian with English summary). [^{90}Sr]

Inglis, J. M., L. J. Post, C. W. Lahser, and D. V. Gibson. 1968. A device for automatically detecting the presence of small animals carrying radioactive tags. *Ecology* **49**(2):361–363.

International Atomic Energy Agency. 1962. *Application of Isotope Techniques in Hydrology.* IAEA, Vienna, Tech. Rep. Ser. No. 11. Publ. No. STI/DOC/10/11. 33 pp.

International Atomic Energy Agency. 1963. *Radioactive Dating.* Proceedings of a symposium, Athens, Greece, November 19–23, 1962. IAEA, Vienna. Publ. No. STI/PUB/68. 443 pp.

International Atomic Energy Agency. 1964. *Isotope Techniques for Hydrology.* IAEA, Vienna, Tech. Rep. Ser. No. 23. Publ. No. STI/DOC/10/23. 38 pp.

International Atomic Energy Agency. 1967. *Nuclear Activation Techniques in the Life Sciences.* Proceedings of a symposium, Amsterdam, May 8–12, 1967. IAEA, Vienna. Publ. No. STI/PUB/155. 720 pp.

International Atomic Energy Agency. 1967. *Radioactive Dating and Methods of Low-Level Counting*. Proceedings of a symposium, Monaco, March 2–10, 1967. IAEA, Vienna. Publ. No. STI/PUB/152. 744 pp.

International Atomic Energy Agency. 1972. *Nuclear Activation Techniques in the Life Sciences—1972*. Proceedings of a symposium, Bled, Yugoslavia, April 10–14, 1972. IAEA, Vienna. Publ. No. STI/PUB-310. 672 pp.

International Atomic Energy Agency. 1979. *Isotopes and Radiation in Research on Soil–Plant Relationships*. Proceedings of a symposium, Colombo, Sri Lanka, December 11–15, 1978. IAEA, Vienna, Publ. No. STI/PUB/501. 660 pp.

Ivanova, M. V. 1959. Assessment of sulfur cycle processes in lakes using radioactive sulfur. pp. 160–166. In: *Transactions of the 6th Conference on the Biology of Inland Waters*, June 10–19, 1957. (*Trudy VI Soveschchaniya po Problemam Biologii Vnutrennykh Vod*, 10–19 Iyunya 1957g.) (B. S. Kuzin and S. I. Kuznetsov, eds.). Publishing House of the USSR Academy of Science, Moscow and Leningrad. [English translation: AEC-tr-6880 (1969).]

Ivie, G. W., H. W. Dorough, and H. E. Bryant. 1974. Fate of Mirex-^{14}C in Japanese quail. *Bull. Environ. Contam. Toxicol.* **11**(2):129–135.

Jennings, D., N. Cutshall, and C. Osterberg. 1965. Radioactivity: Detection of gamma-ray emission in sediments *in situ*. *Science* **148**(3672):948–950.

Kanevskiy, Yu. P., and D. G. Fleyshaman. 1971. Investigation of food chains in an ichthyocoenosis of Lake Dal'nyi (Kamchatka) according to the concentration of rhubidium and cesium in hydrobionts. *Ekologiya* **2**(3):5–8. [English translation: *Sov. J. Ecol.* **2**(3):191–193.] [Isotope dilution]

Karulin, B. E., L. A. Khlyap, N. A. Nikitina, Yu. V. Kovalevskii, E. B. Teslenko, and S. A. Al'bov. 1974. Activity and use of refuges of the common shrew (from observations of animals labelled with radioactive cobalt). *Byull. Mosk. Obshch. Ispyt. Pri. Otd. Biol.* **79**(1):65–72 (in Russian).

Karulin, B. E., V. Yu. Litvin, N. A. Nikitina, Yu. V. Okhotsky, and L. A. Khlyap. 1974. Methods of radioisotope marking of rodents in ricks, straw stacks and cocks in ecological and epizootological investigations. *Zool. Zh.* **53**(9):1401–1406 (in Russian with English summary).

Karulin, B. E., V. Yu. Litvin, N. A. Nikitina, L. A. Khlyap, N. S. Zenkovich, and S. A. Albov. 1974. A study of activity, mobility and daily range in *Microtus arvalis* by marking with ^{60}Co. *Zool. Zh.* **53**(7):1070–1078 (in Russian with English summary).

Kawabata, T. 1955. Studies on the radiological contamination of fishes. I. A consideration on the distribution and migration of contaminated fishes on the basis of the compiled data of radiological survey. *Jpn. J. Med. Sci. Biol.* **8**:337–346.

Keast, D., and L. G. Walsh. 1979. The use of ruthenium-103 for the determination of the rate of passage of food through the gut of captive wild birds. *Int. J. Appl. Radiat. Isot.* **30**(8):463–468.

Kirby, H. V. 1971. Effect of temperature on the feeding behavior of *Daphnia rosea*. *Limnol. Oceanogr.* **16**(3):580–581. [^{32}P]

Kline, J. R., J. R. Martin, C. F. Jordan, and J. J. Koranda. 1970. Measurement of transpiration in tropical trees with tritiated water. *Ecology* **51**(6):1068–1073.

Kline, J. R., C. F. Jordan, and P. Kovac. 1972. Use of tritiated water for determination of plant transpiration and biomass under field conditions. pp. 419–437. In: *Isotopes and Radiation in Soil–Plant Relationships including Forestry*. International Atomic Energy Agency, Vienna. Publ. No. STI/PUB/292.

Kline, J. R., C. F. Jordan, and R. C. Rose. 1972. Transpiration measurement in pines using tritiated water as a tracer. *Isot. Radiat. Technol.* **9**(3):348–350.

Koczy, F. F. 1965. Radioactive tracers in oceanography: Natural radionuclides in the ocean. *Int. Union Geodesy Geophys. Monogr.* **20**:1–9.

Koide, M., K. W. Bruland, and E. D. Goldberg. 1973. Th-228/Th-232 and Pb-210 geochronologies in marine and lake sediments. *Geochim. Cosmochim. Acta* **37**(5):1171–1187.

Kröll, V. 1954. On the age-determination in deep-sea sediments by radium measurements. *Deep-Sea Res.* **1**(4):211–215.

Ku, T.-L. 1965. An evaluation of the U^{234}/U^{238} method as a tool for dating pelagic sediments. *J. Geophys. Res.* **70**(14):3457–3474.

Lean, D. R. S. 1973. Movements of phosphorus between its biologically important forms in lake water. *J. Fish. Res. Board Can.* **30**(10):1525–1536. [^{32}P]

Lean, G. H., and M. J. Crickmore. 1963. Methods for measuring sand transport using radioactive tracers. pp. 111–131. In: *Radioisotopes in Hydrology*. International Atomic Energy Agency, Vienna. Publ. No. STI/PUB/71.

Lee, R. F., R. Sauerheber, and G. H. Dobbs. 1972. Uptake, metabolism and discharge of polycyclic aromatic hydrocarbons by marine fish. *Marine Biol.* **17**(3):201–208. [^{14}C,^{3}H]

Likens, G. E., and A. D. Hasler. 1960. Movement of radiosodium in a chemically stratified lake. *Science* **131**(3414):1676–1677.

Lind, O. T., and R. S. Campbell. 1969. Comments on the use of liquid scintillation for routine determination of ^{14}C activity in production studies. *Limnol. Oceanogr.* **14**(5):787–789.

Linn, I. J. 1978. Radioactive techniques for small mammal marking. pp. 177–191. In: *Animal Marking: Recognition Marking of Animals in Research* (B. Stonehouse, ed.). Macmillan Press, London.

Litvin, V. Yu., B. E. Karulin, N. A. Nikitina, E. V. Karaseva, L. A. Khlyap, S. A. Albov, Yu. V. Okhotsky, and N. D. Sushkin. 1974. Activity, mobility and daily range of *Microtus oeconomus* (observations of animals marked by ^{60}Co). *Zool. Zh.* **53**(8):1233–1240 (in Russian with English summary).

Lucas, A. C., Z. G. Burson, and R. E. Lagerquist. 1966. Design of a shielded source for the irradiation of natural animal populations. Edgerton, Germeshausen and Grier, Inc., Santa Barbara, U.S. AEC Rep. CEX-63.10. 44 pp. [Nuc. Sci. Abstr. **20**(22):40518]

Makowski, Ye., and G. Grissener. 1967. Quantitative measurement of maritime sediment movement using radioactive tracers. pp. 181–189. In: *Isotopes in Hydrology*. International Atomic Energy Agency, Vienna. Publ. No. STI/PUB/141. (in Russian with English summary.)

Marcum, L. C. 1974. An evaluation of radioactive feces-tagging as a technique for determining population densities of the black bear (*Ursus americanus*) in the Great Smoky Mountains National Park. M.S. thesis, University of Tennessee, Knoxville. 95 pp.

Marshall, S. M., and A. P. Orr. 1955. Experimental feeding of the copepod *Calanus finmarchicus* (Gunner) on phytoplankton cultured with radioactive carbon (^{14}C). *Deep Sea Res.* **3**(Suppl.):110–114.

Mavrodineanu, R. (ed.). 1977. *Procedures Used at the National Bureau of Standards to Determine Selected Trace Elements in Biological and Botanical Materials*. National Bureau of Standards, U.S. Department of Commerce, NBS-Spec. Publ.-492 x + 287 pp. [Includes neutron activation]

McErlean, A. J., and H. J. Brinkley. 1971. Temperature tolerance and thyroid activity of the white perch *Roccus* (= *Morone*) *americanus*. *J. Fish. Biol.* **3**(1):97–114. [^{125}I]

McEwan, E. H., and P. E. Whitehead. 1971. Measurement of the milk intake of reindeer and caribou calves using tritiated water. *Can. J. Zool.* **49**(4):443–447.

McNaughton, D. L., and P. Wurzel. 1972. Tritium in rain as an indicator of air mass source. *Tellus* **24**(3):255–259 (in English with Russian summary).

Mejstrik, V. 1970. Uptake of ^{32}P by different kinds of ectotrophic mycorrhiza of *Pinus*. *New Phytol.* **68**(2):295–298.

Menhinick, E. F. 1966. ^{90}Sr plaques for beta irradiation studies. *Health Phys.* **12**(7):973–979.

Merlini, M., F. Girardi, and G. Pozzi. 1967. Activation analysis in studies of an aquatic ecosystem. pp. 615–629. In: *Nuclear Activation Techniques in the Life Sciences*. International Atomic Energy Agency, Vienna. Publ. No. STI/PUB/155.

Mitchell, H. C., W. L. McGovern, W. H. Cross, and N. Mitlin. 1973. Boll weevils: Tagging for hibernation and field studies. *J. Econ. Entomol.* **66**(2):563–564. [^{65}Zn, ^{32}P]

Moore, W. S. 1972. Radium-228: Application to thermocline mixing studies. *Earth Planet. Sci. Lett.* **16**(3):421–422.

Moore, W. S., and S. Krishnaswami. 1974. Correlation of X-radiography revealed banding in corals with radiometric growth rates. *Proc. Second Int. Coral Reef Symp.* **2**:269–276.

Moore, W. S., S. Krishnaswami, and S. G. Bhat. 1973. Radiometric determinations of coral growth rates. *Bull. Mar. Sci.* **23**(2):157–176.

Münnich, K. O., and W. Roether. 1967. Transfer of bomb ^{14}C and tritium from the atmosphere to the ocean: Internal mixing of the ocean on the basis of tritium and ^{14}C profiles. pp. 93–104. In: *Radioactive Dating and Methods of Low-Level Counting.* International Atomic Energy Agency, Vienna. Publ. No. STI/PUB/152.

Myllymäki, A. 1969. Trapping experiments on the water vole, *Arvicola terrestris* (L.), with the aid of the isotope technique. pp. 39–55. In: *Energy Flow Through Small Mammal Populations* (K. Petrusewicz and L. Ryszkowski, eds.). PWN-Polish Scientific Publishers, Warsaw, Poland.

Myllymäki, A., and A. Paassikallio. 1972. The detection of seed-eating small mammals by means of P 32 treatment of spruce seed. *Aquilo Ser. Zool.* **13**:21–24.

Myllymäki, A., and A. Paasikallio. 1976. Scots pine seed depredation by small mammals, as revealed by radioactive tagging of the seeds. *Annales Agriculturae Fenniae* **15**:89–96.

Nimlos, T. J., W. P. Van Meter, and L. A. Daniels. 1968. Rooting patterns of forest understory species as determined by radioiodine absorption. *Ecology* **49**(6):1146–1151.

Nishimura, M., M. Sakuta, K. Okamoto, and N. Urakawa. 1974. Distribution and excretion of ^{115m}cadmium and its transfer to egg and bone in laying female and estrogenized male Japanese quail. *Jpn. J. Vet. Sci.* **36**(2):133–143.

Olsen, S. 1964. Phosphate equilibrium between reduced sediments and water. Laboratory experiments with radioactive phosphorus. *Verh. Int. Ver. Limnol.* **15**(1):333–341.

Olsson, I. U. (ed.). 1970. *Radiocarbon Variations and Absolute Chronology.* Proceedings of the 12th Nobel Symposium, Institute of Physics, Uppsala University. John Wiley, New York. 655 pp.

Orr, H. 1967. Excretion of orally administered zinc-65 by the cotton rat in the laboratory and field. *Health Phys.* **13**(1):15–20.

Osterberg, C., W. G. Pearcy, and H. Curl, Jr. 1964. Radioactivity and its relationship to oceanic food chains. *J. Mar. Res.* **22**(1):2–12.

Paris, O. H., and A. Sikora. 1967. Radiotracer analysis of the trophic dynamics of natural isopod populations. pp. 741–771. In: *Secondary Productivity of Terrestrial Ecosystems,* Vol. II (K. Petrusewicz, ed.). Institute of Ecology, Polish Academy of Science, Warsaw.

Parisi, V., M. G. Mezzadri, D. Bedulli, and P. Poli. 1977. Thermal pollution studied by radioecological techniques. *Rapp. Comm. Int. Mer Medit.* **24**(3):85–88.

Pelton, M. R., and L. C. Marcum. 1977. The potential use of radioisotopes for determining densities of black bears and other carnivores. pp. 221–236. In: *Proceedings of the 1975 Predator Symposium* (R. L. Phillips and C. Jonkel, eds.). Montana Forest and Conservation Experiment Station, Missoula.

Pendleton, R. C., and W. C. Hanson. 1958. Absorption of cesium-137 by components of an aquatic community. *Proc. 2nd UN Int. Conf. Peaceful Uses Atomic Energy* **18**:419–422.

Peroni, C. N. 1976. Results about the transfer of ^{32}P to copepods through contaminated bacteria. *Rapp. Comm. Int. Mer Medit.* **23**(7):143–144.

Perrier, E. R., K. R. Stockinger, and R. V. Swain. 1966. Scintillation counter for measuring thermal neutrons in a soil-water system. *Soil Sci.* **101**(2):125–129.

Peterle, T. J. 1980. Radioisotopes and their use in wildlife research. pp. 521–530. In: *Wildlife Techniques Manual,* 4th ed. (S. D. Schemnitz, ed.). The Wildlife Society. Washington, D.C.

Peterson, H. T., Jr. 1971. Stable element and radionuclide reconcentration in aquatic ecosystems. I. Stable element effects in the equilibrium situation. pp. 289–328. In: *Proceedings of the Symposium on Health Physics Aspects of Nuclear Facility Siting*. Proceedings of the Fifth Annual Health Physics Society Midyear Topical Symposium, November 3–6, 1970, Idaho Falls, Idaho. Vols. 1–3 (P. B. Voilleque and B. R. Baldwin, comps.).

Petrusewicz, K., and A. Macfadyen. 1970. Chapt. 6. The study of respiration and energy flow in relation to secondary production: Measurement of elimination rates including the biological half-life of isotopes. pp. 141–146. In: *Productivity of Terrestrial Animals: Principles and Methods*. IBP Handbook No. 13. Blackwell, Oxford, England.

Pugh, P. R. 1973. An evaluation of liquid scintillation counting techniques for use in aquatic primary production studies. *Limnol. Oceanogr.* **18**(2):310–319.

Quay, P. D., W. S. Broecker, R. H. Hesslein, and D. W. Schindler. 1980. Vertical diffusion rates determined by tritium tracer experiments in the thermocline and hypolimnion of two lakes. *Limnol. Oceanogr.* **25**(2):201–218.

Ravera, O., and G. Premazzi. 1971. A method to study the history of any persistent pollution in a lake by the concentration of ^{137}Cs from fall-out. pp. 703–718. In: *Proceedings of the International Symposium on Radioecology Applied to the Protection of Man and His Environment*. Commission of the European Communities, Rep. EUR 4800 d-f-i-e.

Reid, C. P. P., and F. W. Woods. 1969. Translocation of C^{14}-labeled compounds in mycorrhizae and its implication in interplant nutrient cycling. *Ecology* **50**(2):179–187.

Rerabek, J., and A. Bubenik. 1956. Study of the mineral metabolism of antlered animals using radioisotopes. *Int. Congr. Game Biol.* **2**:119–123 (in German with French and English summaries).

Richmond, C. R., T. T. Trujillo, and D. W. Martin. 1960. Volume and turnover of body water in *Dipodomys deserti* with tritiated water. *Proc. Soc. Exp. Biol. Med.* **104**(1):9–11.

Riekerk, H. 1978. Mineral cycling in a young Douglas fir forest stand. pp. 801–816. In: *Environmental Chemistry and Cycling Processes* (D. C. Adriano and I. L. Brisbin, Jr., eds.). U.S. DOE Symp. Ser. 45, Rep. CONF-760429.

Rigler, F. H. 1964. The phosphorus fractions and the turnover time of inorganic phosphorus in different types of lakes. *Limnol. Oceanogr.* **9**(4):511–518. [^{32}P]

Rodhe, W. 1958. The primary production in lakes: Some results and restrictions of the C^{14} method. *Rapp. P. V. Reun. Cons. Int. Explor. Mer* **144**:122–128.

Rodina, A. G. 1957. Application of the radioactive tracer method for the solution of the food selectivity problem of aquatic animals. *Zool. Zh.* **36**(3):337–343 (in Russian with English summary).

Romberg, G. P., W. Prepejchal, and S. A. Spigarelli. 1977. Temperature exposure measured by the use of thermoluminescence. *Science* **197**(4311):1364–1365.

Rosholt, J. N., C. Emiliani, J. Geiss, F. F. Koczy, and P. J. Wangersky. 1961. Absolute dating of deep-sea cores by the Pa^{231}/Th^{230} method. *J. Geol.* **69**(2):162–185.

Rowland, F. S. 1976. Cosmogenic radioisotopes as stratospheric tracers. pp. 333–334 (abstract). In: *Measurement, Detection and Control of Environmental Pollutants*. International Atomic Energy Agency. Vienna. Publ. No. STI/PUB/432.

Ryther, J. H., and D. W. Menzel. 1965. Comparison of the ^{14}C-technique with direct measurement of photosynthetic carbon fixation. *Limnol. Oceanogr.* **10**(3):490–492.

Saas, A., and A. Grauby. 1974. Study techniques of the diffusion and the migration of radionuclides in soils. pp. 341–349. In: *Tenth International Congress of Soil Science*, Vol. II, Commission II. Science Press, Moscow (in French with Russian, German, and English summaries).

Saas, A., and A. Grauby. 1975. Techniques for rapid determination of effects of synergy between radionuclides and pollutants. pp. 145–152. In: *Combined Effects of Radioactive, Chemical and*

Thermal Releases to the Environment. International Atomic Energy Agency, Vienna. Publ. No. STI/PUB/404 (in French with English abstract).

Saunders, G. W., F. B. Trama, and R. W. Bachmann. 1962. *Evaluation of a Modified C^{14} Technique for Shipboard Estimation of Photosynthesis in Large Lakes.* Great Lakes Research Division, Institute of Science and Technology, University of Michigan, Ann Arbor. Publ. No. 8. ii + 61 pp.

Schell, W. R., and R. S. Barnes. 1974. Lead and mercury in the aquatic environment of western Washington State. pp. 129–165. In: *Aqueous-Environmental Chemistry of Metals* (A. J. Rubin, ed.). Ann Arbor Science Publishers, Ann Arbor.

Schindler, D. W. 1968. Feeding, assimilation and respiration rates of *Daphnia magna* under various environmental conditions and their relation to production estimates. *J. Anim. Ecol.* **37**(2):369–385. [^{14}C]

Schindler, J. E. 1971. Food quality and zooplankton nutrition. *J. Anim. Ecol.* **40**(3):589–595. [^{14}C]

Schumacher, G. J., and L. A. Whitford. 1965. Respiration and P^{32} uptake in various species of freshwater algae as affected by a current. *J. Phycol.* **1**(2):78–80.

Scott, D. P. 1962. Radioactive cesium as a fish and lamprey mark. *J. Fish. Res. Board. Can.* **19**(1):149–157.

Shealy, M. H., Jr., and C. A. Carlson. 1973. Accumulation and retention of strontium-85 marks by young largemouth bass. pp. 307–317. In: *Radionuclides in Ecosystems* (D. J. Nelson, ed.). U.S. AEC Rep. CONF-710501-P1.

Shellabarger, C. J., A. Gorbman, F. C. Schatzlein, and D. McGill. 1956. Some quantitative and qualitative aspects of I^{131} metabolism in turtles. *Endocrinology* **59**(3):331–339.

Shura-Bura, B. L., and V. P. Kharlamov. 1961. Autoradiography as a method of identifying labelled rodents and their ectoparasites when studying migration problems. *Zool. Zh.* **40**(2):258–263 (in Russian).

Shuvalov, V. S. 1959. Experiment with radioactive calcium (^{45}Ca) in the study of inorganic fertilization of ponds. In: *Transactions of the 6th Conference on the Biology of Inland Waters* (B. S. Kuzin and S. I. Kuznetsov, eds.). Publishing House of the USSR Academy of Science, Moscow and Leningrad. [English translation: AEC-tr-6880, pp. 33–40 (1969).]

Skauen, D. M., N. Marshall, and R. J. Fragala. 1971. A liquid scintillation method for assaying ^{14}C-labelled benthic microflora. *J. Fish. Res. Board Can.* **28**(5):769–770.

Small, L. F. 1962. Use of radioisotopes in laboratory energy assimilation investigations with *Daphnia. Nature (London)* **196**(4856):787–788.

Sonenshine, D. E. 1971. Mass rearing of radioisotope-tagged larval ticks for ecological investigations. *J. Econ. Entomol.* **64**(6):1423–1429.

Sonenshine, D. E., and G. Esch. 1970. Radio-labeling *Dermacentor variabilis* with strontium-90 and strontium-90 plus carbon-14 mixtures. *J. Econ. Entomol.* **63**(5):1635–1638.

Spellerberg, I. F., and I. Prestt. 1978. Marking snakes. pp. 133–141. In: *Animal Marking: Recognition Marking of Animals in Research* (B. Stonehouse, ed.). Macmillan, London.

Stewart, N. G. 1960. Radioactive tracers in the atmosphere. *Endeavour* **19**(76):197–201.

Stuiver, M. 1970. Tree ring, varve and carbon-14 chronologies. *Nature (London)* **228**(5270):454–455.

Stuiver, M. 1973. The ^{14}C cycle and its implications for mixing rates in the ocean–atmosphere system. pp. 6–20. In: *Carbon and the Biosphere* (G. M. Woodwell and E. V. Pecan, eds.). U.S. AEC Symp. Ser. No. 30.

Swingland, I. R. 1978. Marking reptiles. pp. 119–132. In: *Animal Marking: Recognition Marking of Animals in Research* (B. Stonehouse, ed.). Macmillan, London.

Talmage, R. V., S. B. Doty, and C. W. Yates. 1962. The effect of temperature on the uptake of radioiodine by the thyroid gland of the frog, *Rana pipiens. Gen. Comp. Endocrinol.* **2**(3):266–272.

Taylor, R. E. 1978. Radiocarbon dating: An archaeological perspective. pp. 33–69. In: *Archaeological Chemistry*, Vol. II (G. F. Carter, ed.). American Chemical Society, Washington, D.C., Adv. Chem. Ser. No. 171.

Thomas, W. A. 1969. Accumulation and cycling of calcium by dogwood trees. *Ecol. Monogr.* **39**(2):101–120. [^{45}Ca]

Thurber, D. L., W. S. Broecker, R. L. Blanchard, and H. A. Potratz. 1965. Uranium-series ages of Pacific atoll corals. *Science* **149**(3679):55–58.

Timofeyev-Resovskiy, N. V. 1957. The application of irradiation and irradiators in experimental biogeocenology. *Bot. Zh.* **42**(2):161–194 (in Russian).

Triulzi, C. 1973. Analyses of U and Th in marine sediment samples by different methods. *Thalassia Jugosl.* **9**(1/2):119–125.

Van Hook, R. I., and D. A. Crossley, Jr. 1969. Assimilation and biological turnover of cesium-134, iodine-131, and chromium-51 in brown crickets, *Acheta domesticus* (L.). *Health Phys.* **16**(4):463–467.

Waisel, Y., and A. Fahn. 1965. A radiological method for the determination of cambial activity. *Physiologia* **18**(1):44–46. [^{14}C]

Watson, J. P. 1971. Comparison of chromium^{51}-versenate and tritiated water movement in a termite mound and soil. *Soil Sci.* **111**(3):188–191.

Webb, K. L., and J. W. A. Burley. 1965. Dark fixation of $C^{14}O_2$ by obligate and faculative salt marsh halophytes. *Can. J. Bot.* **43**(2):281–285.

Wegorek, W., K. Glogowski, and E. Czaplicki. 1965. Investigation of hibernation of *Perillus bioculatus* Fabr. tagged with ^{60}Co. *Ekol. Pol.* **13**(23):451–462.

Wessen, G., F. H. Ruddy, C. E. Gustafson, and H. Irwin. 1977. Characterization of archaeological bone by neutron activation analysis. *Archaeometry* **19**(2):200–205.

Willis, J. N., and N. Y. Jones. 1977. The use of uniform labeling with zinc-65 to measure stable zinc turnover in the mosquito fish, *Gambusia affinis*. I. Retention. *Health Phys.* **32**(5):381–387.

Woods, F. W. 1969. Root extension of forest trees: A method of investigation using radioactive tracers. pp. 413–417. In: *Root Growth* (W. J. Whittington, ed.). Butterworths, London.

Woods, F. W., and W. T. Lawhon. 1974. Gamma densitometry of increment cores. *For. Sci.* **20**(3):269–271.

Woods, F. W., and M. L. McCormack. 1963. Two scintillation probes for radioecological investigations. pp. 205–209. In: *Advancing Frontiers of Plant Sciences*, Vol. 2 (R. Vira, ed.). Institute for Advancement of Science and Culture, New Delhi.

Woods, F. W., W. A. Hough, D. O'Neal, and J. Barnett. 1965. Gamma ray attenuation by loblolly pine wood: An investigation of integral counting. *For. Sci.* **11**(3):341–345.

Woods, J. A., and A. R. Mead-Briggs. 1978. The daily cycle of activity in the mole (*Talpa europaea*) and its seasonal changes, as revealed by radioactive monitoring of the nest. *J. Zool. (London)* **184**(4):563–572.

Wright, C. N., and W. F. Splichal, Jr. 1973. Portable cesium counter for field use. *Health Phys.* **25**(5):516–517.

Yoshida, T., F. Takashima, and T. Watanabe. 1973. Distribution of ^{14}C PCBs in carp. *Ambio* **2**(4):111–113.

Young, S. E., J. D. Dodd, and E. R. Ibert. 1970. Tritium collection and extraction techniques for plant-water relationship studies. *Ecology* **51**(3):535–537.

Yousef, Y. A., T. J. Padden, and E. F. Gloyna. 1975. Diurnal changes in radionuclides uptake by phytoplankton in small scale ecosystems. *Water Res.* **9**(2):181–187.

Zhadin, V. I., S. I. Kuznetsov, and N. V. Timofeyev-Resovskiy. 1958. The role of radioactive isotopes in solving problems of hydrobiology. *Proc. 2nd UN Int. Conf Peaceful Uses Atomic Energy* **27**:200–207.

Index